The Silent Showman

Michael Tallis, DSc, researched mathematical problems in genetics, biology and medicine, and is affiliated with the University of Adelaide. His wife, Joan Tallis, has extensive experience in genealogical and historical research work and enjoys a challenge. With respect to this book, the pair 'started with nothing and came from nowhere' as Melbourne *Punch* might have put it. Gradually, as the story unfolded, they became fascinated by the JC Williamson Firm, its origins and size, its touring of big theatre companies, its part in the beginnings of film and radio – later to become gigantic financial hedges for Williamson's – the main players, and their interrelations and squabbles, mergers and takeovers. How did George Tallis fit into the kaleidoscope?

WAKEFIELD PRESS

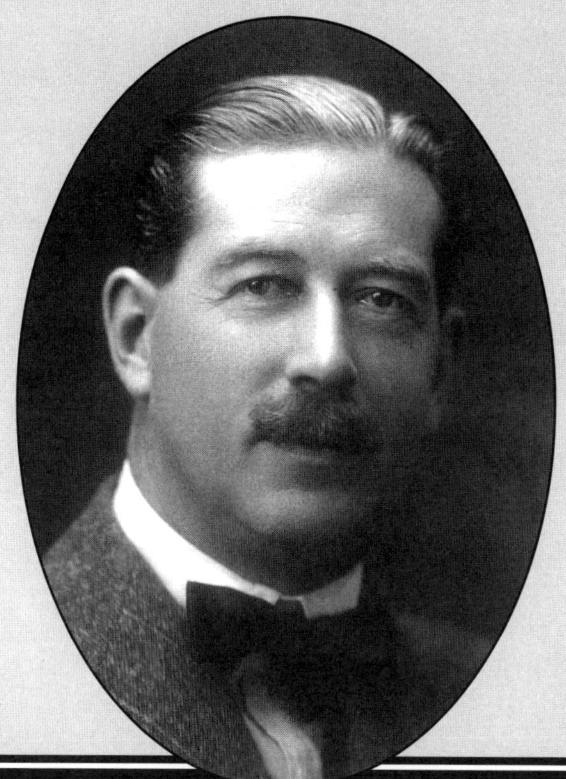

The Silent Showman

Sir George Tallis, the man behind the world's largest entertainment organisation of the 1920s

MICHAEL AND JOAN TALLIS

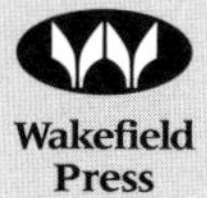

Wakefield Press

Wakefield Press
1 The Parade West
Kent Town
South Australia 5067
www.wakefieldpress.com.au

First published 1999
This revised edition published 2006

Designed by Liz Nicholson, designBITE
Typeset by Clinton Ellicott, Wakefield Press
Printed in China at Everbest Printing Co. Ltd

National Library of Australia
Cataloguing-in-publication entry

Tallis, G.M. (George Michael).
The silent showman: Sir George Tallis, the man behind the world's largest entertainment organisation of the 1920s.

ISBN-13: 978 1 86254 735 3
ISBN-11: 1 86254 735 1

1. Tallis, George, 1869–1948. 2. J.C. Williamson (Firm) – History.
3. Theatre – Australia – History. I. Tallis, Joan.
II. Title.

792.092

Contents

Foreword

Journalists, actors and private researchers have been the mainstay in the recording of Australian theatre history. Fascination with its colour, with its heroes or heroines; or the yearning to rescue from oblivion a relative or give form and meaning to one's own life and work, have been the incentives; and this work has over time produced a rich and eccentric library of memoirs and memories.

This book, however, is in another class. To bring to life the shadowy form of his grandfather may have been the motive of Michael Tallis and his wife, Joan, but this is much more than a family history. Its masterful grasp of the material, its revelations from private records, its abundance of photographs – many hitherto unpublished – and its narrative skill, make *The Silent Showman* one of the most important books on the Australian theatre yet to have been produced. It has taken the authors many years of research and reading to absorb not only the facts of George Tallis's life but the context of his achievement. The wait has been worth it.

Sir George Tallis became a junior in JC Williamson's office as a teenage Irish immigrant. As a partner and financier it was largely his drive that made the Firm into the greatest entertainment production company in the world. He was, as *Punch* called him, 'the man behind', whose character and importance has until now escaped the attention of theatre historians. This book fully reveals for the first time the extent of the company's investment not only in theatrical entertainment, which extended to South Africa, North America and Britain, but also in film-making and exhibition, and popular radio broadcasting.

With the aid of family documents, including Tallis's own unpublished memoirs, and a wealth of correspondence between him and JC Williamson and later with the Tait brothers, the book gives a unique insight into the business methods and the colourful, often discordant, personalities who made up the Firm. First-hand accounts of the share dealings and board shufflings are particularly revealing.

In their researches the Tallises found a press comment by myself at the time of JCW Ltd's centennial in 1974:

The Firm is famous for its private strife and its public unity and this has been part of its strength. Crisis is part of the JCW way of life, like every other theatrical management. That's show biz.

At the time I was thinking of its later history. But this book shows for the first time that private strife and not always public unity were at the core of the company from the start. It's a story full of drama, humour and, in those unregulated days when fortunes were won and lost, more than a little skullduggery. Through it all the retiring figure of Sir George Tallis – shrewd, unfailingly courteous and always forward-looking – emerges serenely as not only the man behind but the mind behind the great days of the Williamson legend.

The book's appearance is timely as well as welcome. Australian theatre history has recently entered the school curriculum; and students will find here a rich source of personalities, events, methods and mores written in a way that engages them. I know it captured me from the first page.

I sincerely congratulate Michael and Joan Tallis and their colleagues for the skill and diligence with which they have corrected the errors of earlier accounts, distilled public and private events from a mass of ill-assorted family records, legends and stories and brought to life a vivid, coherent and beautifully designed narrative that makes a major contribution to Australian theatre research.

I recommend it to theatre-lovers everywhere.

Katharine Brisbane, Sydney, 1998

Preface

The only direct familial link with George Tallis now is through his four grandchildren, who remember him clearly, although perhaps each in a different way. They would agree, though, that grandfather George presented as an imposing, well-built man of dignity, who carried his years well. Although he had kind words for children, for them he was hard to reach.

Time eroded George Tallis's Irish brogue, leaving only a trace of an accent to splay his speech mildly. This was enough to add to his magnetism and mystery. Who had he been? Where had he come from? Both good questions demanding answers from a generation reluctant to respond, and slow to divulge the past. We gleaned that grandfather had been a great theatre man, and that he came from the small town of Callan, in Ireland. There was no news of his early family, or wild stories of exploits. In the end, George Tallis's grandchildren grew up knowing nothing of him. They had stopped asking questions long ago, and there was the perception, tinged with truth it seems, that no one really knew him.

A string of theatre histories appeared after George died in 1948. A number overlooked him altogether; others propagated a few old stories about him, some incorrect. Since Tallis occupied such a prominent position in Australian entertainment, how had this occurred? Here was reason enough to research his life, and to look for the 'man behind'.

We had luck in uncovering George's Irish origins, and luck again in finding informative public records, old legal documents, letters, press cuttings, pictures and memorabilia that now forms the Sir George Tallis Theatre Collection. This material from six countries confirms Tallis's position at the top of world entertainment, while noting his modesty and easy manner. Collectively it provides fresh and independent insight into some fables told about Australian theatre management. It was a bonus that our research revealed a saga extending far beyond live theatre, for which Tallis is traditionally known.

We wish to thank sincerely Katharine Brisbane of Currency Press, theatre publisher and critic, for making strong, clear suggestions about the structure of this book and for her generous foreword; and Peter Downes, New Zealand theatre writer and researcher, for encouragement and a dedicated reading of a late manuscript. We also thank Bruce Horsley, grandson of JC Williamson, for many interesting conversations and for providing details on the history of JC Williamson Ltd; the Horsley family, for photographs and kind permission to publish extracts of letters written by JC Williamson; Sir Roy McKenzie, son of Sir John McKenzie, for information concerning the takeover of JC Williamson Ltd by the New Zealand investment company Rangatira; Lindsey Browne, journalist and theatre critic, for permission to publish an extract of his writings; Mark Tapping, South African researcher, for information about JC Williamson Ltd's takeover of the B&F Wheeler theatre company in 1913; Jack Tallis, youngest son of George Tallis, for his stories and his enthusiasm for this biography; Michael Bollen, Clinton Ellicott and the team at Wakefield Press for engrossing themselves in the project; designer Liz Nicholson for her brilliant work, Patsy Kirk for her support; family and friends in Australia and Ireland for photographs and anecdotal contributions; and others too numerous to mention.

Michael and Joan Tallis, Adelaide 1998

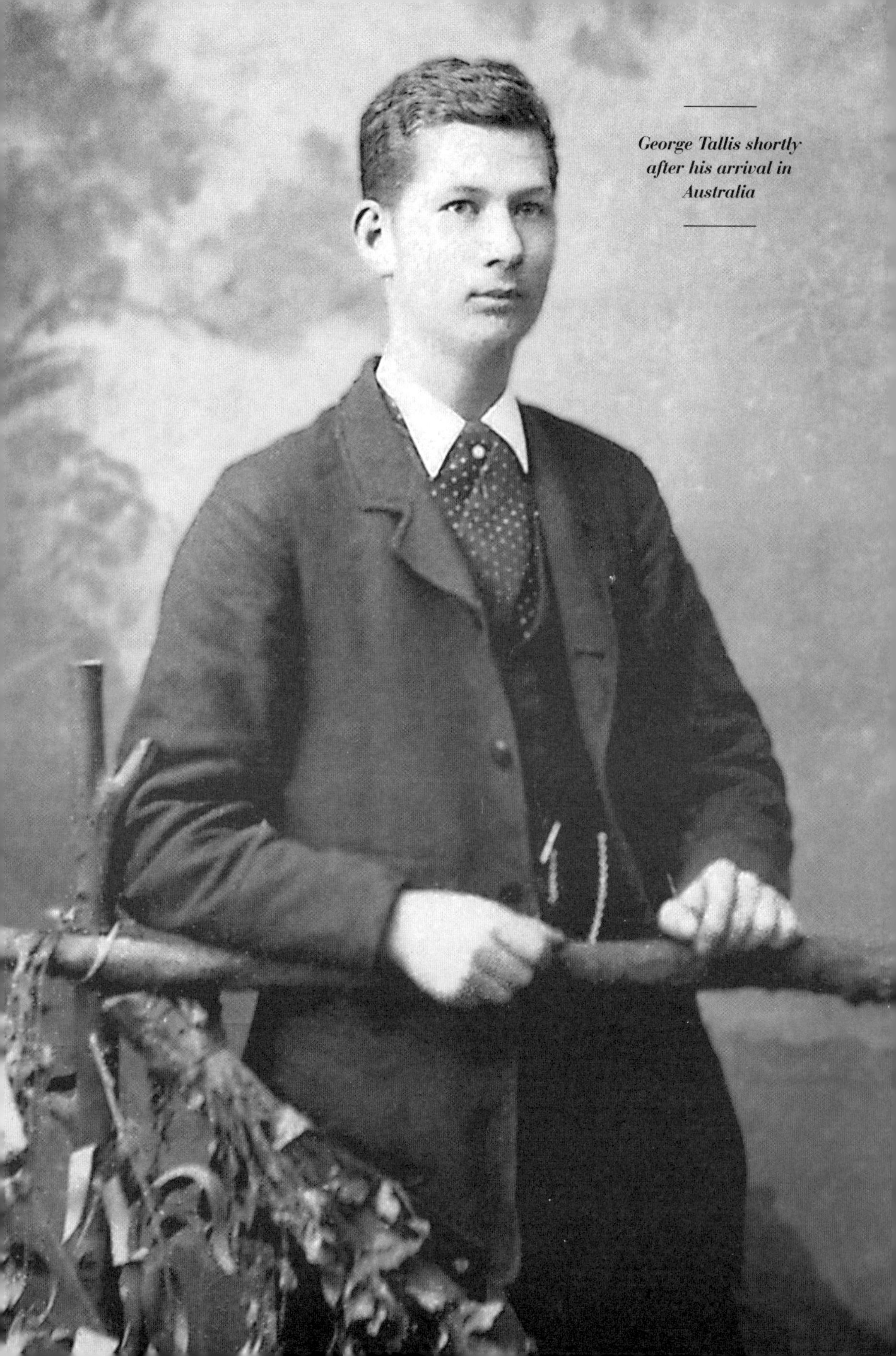

George Tallis shortly after his arrival in Australia

CHAPTER ONE

With a Little Bit of Luck

For late November, Melbourne had turned on a drab day. Dark clouds gathered to reinforce the rain already falling. Only people with pressing business were on the streets.

The young man leaving the White Hart Hotel turned left into Spring Street, and headed for the noise a block away. There he found frenzied builders and tradesmen giving their finishing touches to the Princess Theatre,[1] which was being rebuilt in grand style.

Although the entrance was crawling with men, its magnificence took the young man's breath away. From the foyer he gazed on the auditorium, with its stalls, dress and family circles, and private boxes wedged between Corinthian columns. Electric lights and gas flames threw the blue and gold decor into relief.

But the lad was obstructing traffic. A workman ordered him to move on.

'Is Mr Williamson here?'

'The American? No. Try the Theatre Royal three blocks down Bourke Street,' the man replied.

As he reached the pavement, the young man nearly fell over an advertising sign: '*The Mikado,* Opens Dec 18, Book Now.' Urgency gripped him as he turned west into Bourke Street and started to run. Wind ripped at his eyes and ballooned his coat. He swore softly. Had he come all this way expecting sunshine only to find an Irish winter in an Australian spring?

One block, two blocks, three blocks and there it was: the Theatre Royal. He tapped his pocket to make sure that the two letters he had been carrying were there. The main theatre door was open, although it was still morning.

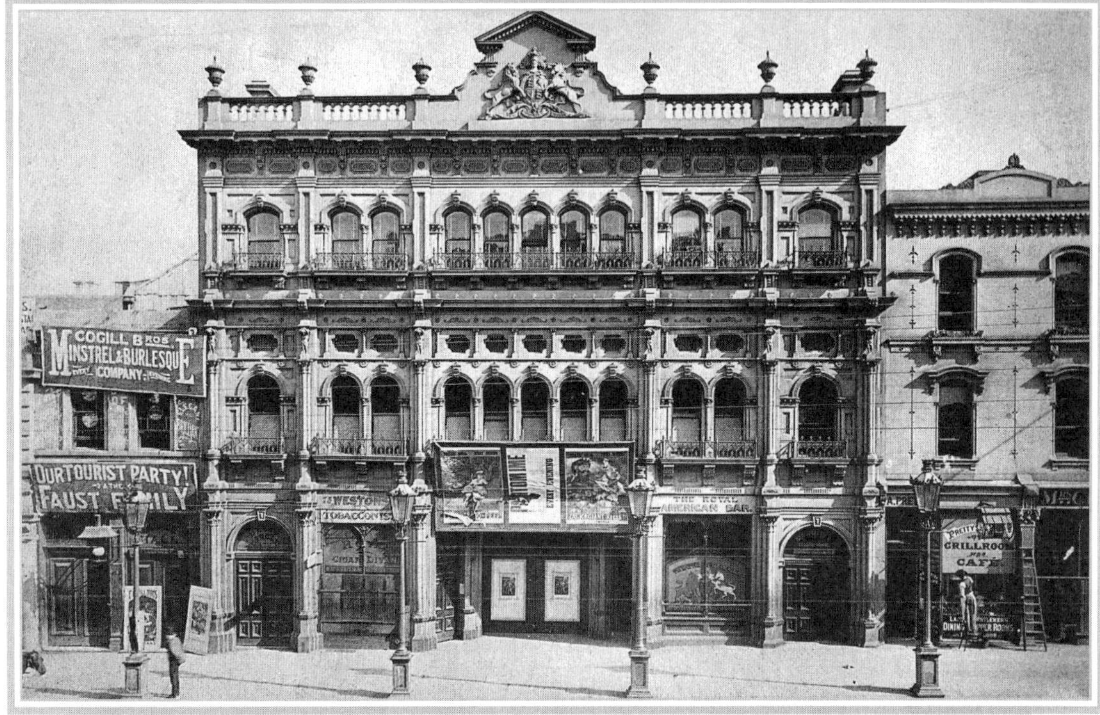

Theatre Royal, Melbourne, 1885

He wrestled with excitement as he entered the hallway that led to the main vestibule. This was not as impressive as the one he'd just left, but it would do.

A few lights burned feebly, yet he could see that the theatre was enormous. The ceiling dome stretched sixty feet high, and from it hung a glittering chandelier. The dome boasted paintings of city scenes, barely distinguishable in the half-light. An ornate proscenium surrounded the stage.

The young man looked over the rows of seats, and guessed the theatre's capacity at between three and four thousand, with every pocket catered for: soft and roomy seats, hard and skimpy chairs. Just how many patrons would turn up every night? Little did he know that star players of the day regarded the Royal as a barn. It was dusty, and the amenities for actors and audiences alike were primitive.

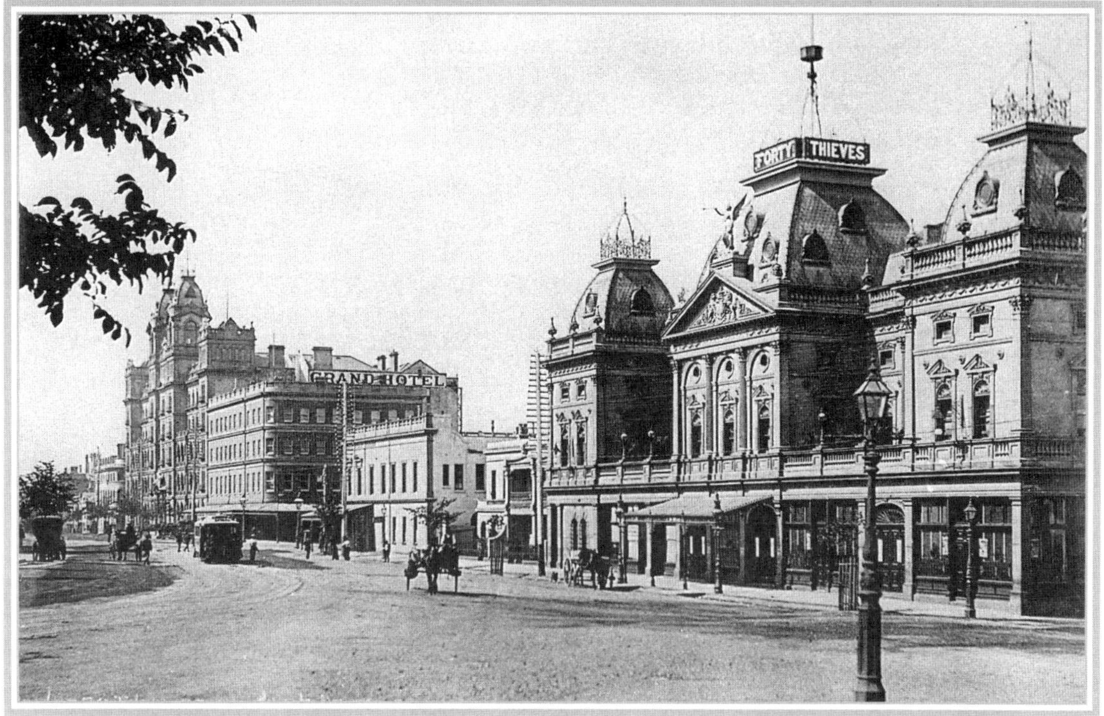

Princess Theatre, White Hart Hotel and Grand Hotel, Spring Street, Melbourne, 1892

He stood and listened to the silence of an empty theatre. The Royal cafe, billiard room and saloon were dark and deserted, and the whole place seemed asleep. A billboard near the main entrance told him that the Royal Dramatic Company was producing *Human Nature,* and that the show was in its last weeks.

Footsteps behind him interrupted his reverie. Then he heard a man's voice: 'What are you doing, young fellow?'

An American accent! The quest was over. 'Mr Williamson, I have a letter for you.' He turned to be confronted by an imposing figure.

JC Williamson was about forty, stockily built, handsome, moustached and well-dressed. His demeanour invited no liberties.

Williamson examined this boy who had identified him so readily. Just another Irish lad escaping the woes of home? Perhaps not. This one stood tall and lean; he had brown, wavy hair and steely blue eyes. His gaze was unwavering: not arrogant or disrespectful, but as if he meant business.

Williamson read the letter and put it in his pocket. 'All right, so you are George Tallis, you are seventeen and you have worked as a cadet reporter for two years on the *Kilkenny Moderator*. You are also a young man who wants to achieve. Do you have any other letters of introduction?'

'Yes, sir, I have one for the *Argus* newspaper.'

'Well, with a background like yours, why not apply there for a job first?'

'Because I don't want to be a reporter, sir. I want to work for you.'

'Do you have anything special you can offer me?'

'Yes, sir: hard work, application, loyalty and Pitman shorthand.'

Williamson was silent. Then he said quietly: 'They all offer me the first three, but none ever mentions the fourth. I doubt if they have even heard of Pitman.'

Then the showman went on with words that young George had not expected. Williamson said, speaking half to himself, that the time was coming when the management of Australian theatre would be by professional business brains. The actor–manager could no longer do it alone. The big managers of the future would leave the acting to others and concentrate on the business side – the production, management, promotion and booking of shows.

But, warned Williamson, if you start with no acting background at all, there is everything to learn. The new managers must be prepared to come in at the bottom, help clean theatres, move scenery, act as ushers, and assist with the takings and bookkeeping. They would have to learn backwards the mechanics of managing a theatre before they could take charge.

Williamson eyed the young man. 'It is a long, tortuous climb; are you sure you want to try it?'

'Yes sir,' answered George without hesitation.

'Right. You will start work here at the Theatre Royal. I will watch your progress, and maybe one day we will make use of your Pitman shorthand.'

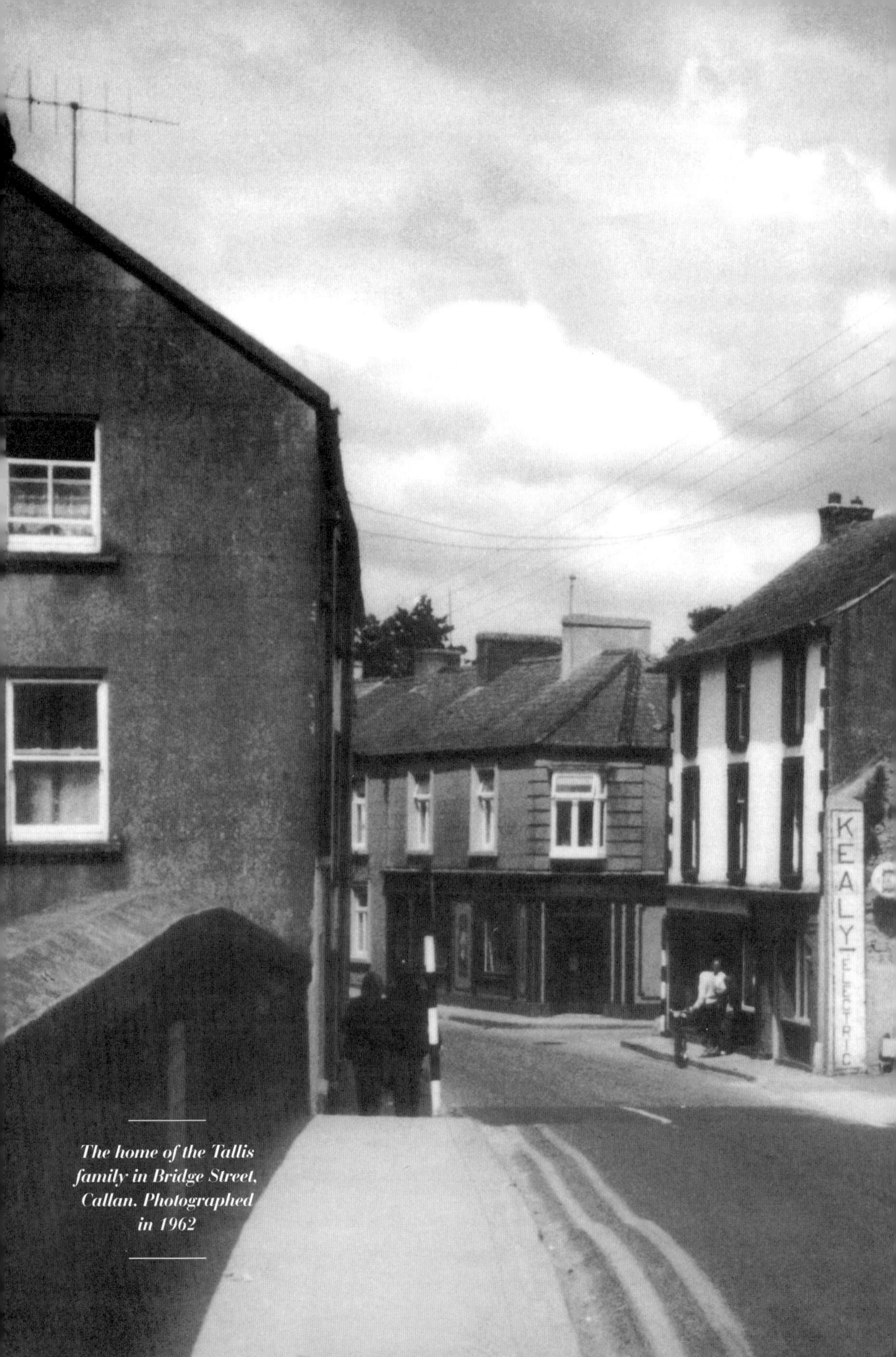

The home of the Tallis family in Bridge Street, Callan. Photographed in 1962

CHAPTER TWO

The Irish Connection

Everybody has heard of 'the man behind'; he is the unknown genius who does all the work unapplauded.

The 'man behind' the theatrical show is, paradoxical as it may seem, really the 'man in front'. For the 'man in front' is the business manager, and the business manager is the brain of the show.

On him depends in greatest measure its success or failure. He has to possess a mixture of all the qualities which go to make success in other professions. He must have the guile of a lawyer, the eloquence of a parson, the astuteness of the stock and share broker, the urbanity of the popular physician; and joined to all this he must know his theatrical world like a book. He has to deal with the most difficult, the most touchy, the most contradictory class of human beings that exists – the stage folk.

So began a piece of whimsy in Melbourne *Punch* in 1908. The writer's purpose was to extol George Tallis's success in the theatrical profession, and he went on to suggest that two qualities had been particularly important in George's rise, one of them coming naturally to an Irishman, the other rather rarer:

Somehow it seems that such an agglomeration of virtues can only be expected in the men of one race. The Irish temperament, materialised into that mysterious something which the Irish themselves call 'blarney', is peculiarly suited to the woes and worries of business management. In proof of this Irishmen have shown themselves to be pronounced successes. The difficulty is to get the Irishman with the business acumen essential for the job.[1]

A family friend would later attest to George's talent for 'blarney' when she said that 'he was the kind of man who had the knack of making everyone he met feel the most important person he had ever spoken with. He had a lovely play with words, and he could charm a bird off a tree'. In business dealings, where he was inclined to combine tactical silence with the 'friendly chat' to win his way, Tallis steered syndicates through large and delicate corporate manoeuvres without fracturing relationships. Only a few – mainly competitors within his own organisation – would remain unconvinced by his personal charm. And few would doubt that this Irishman was blessed with 'business acumen': his investments over decades helped to make both his firm and himself, as one newspaper wag put it, 'rich beyond the dreams of actors'.[2]

George Tallis was born on 28 October 1869 at 18 Bridge Street, Callan, County Kilkenny. There were ten children belonging to John and Sarah Tallis, five girls and five boys. George was the youngest.

The Tallis home is today known as Avon Ree House, and it stands near the Kings River Bridge. Bridge Street is very narrow, but it would have done nicely in the horse-and-buggy era. It formed part of the main route connecting the cities of Cork and Dublin, and for that reason alone the small town of Callan was an important centre. The coach, which ferried passengers between the two cities, rattled through Callan at the dead of night and became the subject of a disturbing folktale. One version told to George was passed on by him to his children:

Did you ever hear about the Headless Coach? Well, I saw it! It was a winter night, and the cold was upon the ground. I went out to bring in some turf for the fire, when I heard the sound of horses. I looked up, and there was a coach against the moon, racing like the bats of hell. And I swear that neither the coachman nor the passengers had a head to hang a hat on. It was the Headless Coach for sure, and I ran home and couldn't speak for the trembling. And no one believed me.

No doubt the Tallis children rehearsed this story well as they fell asleep so close to the route of the Cork–Dublin flier. With the clatter of horses' hooves on the Kings River Bridge still ringing in their ears, Sarah probably had little difficulty in convincing her children to stay in bed at night.

Good story-telling was part of the Irish social fabric, and the best tales were a mix of truth and the occult. This was the breeding ground of great authors like Oscar Wilde, WB Yeats, George Bernard Shaw, James Joyce and many others, who formalised a distinctive Irish oral tradition for comedy through their writings. George's early immersion in folklore may have guided him in selecting shows that would work in the world of theatre, where audiences had to be at once thrilled and convinced by the story unfolding before them.

As the youngest child in a clutch of ten, he had incentive to learn a way with words to help him hold his own, and reason also to develop the facility sometimes attributed to him, of being able to 'slip away' from disputes and confrontation to pursue his own goal.

George's oldest son, Mick, told some stories of his father's Irish ways:

I am six years old. I know this for a fact because my dad just told me while he shaves in his dressing room. I obediently cup my hands in preparation for Colleen's curls, which are beginning to take shape as he expertly guides a sharp knife around a large green apple.

And now with the curls safely within my grasp, I turn to go. 'What do you do with them?' he asks with interest. 'I give them to Maggie and she puts them in a bowl.'

'And what does Maggie do with them then?' But this last question is rhetorical, because father has started his day.

If this story is any reflection on George's early upbringing by his own father, John, then it is plain to whom George owed a debt for his blarney.

For his business acumen he had much to thank his mother, who was twenty years younger than John. The house at 18 Bridge Street was part of an off-licence spirit and grocery store. John, Sarah and their first four children had moved there in 1861 from the thirty-acre farm John had inherited. John died at seventy when George was just seven, but even before that Sarah had been the driving force in managing the family store. She made sure that the children helped with all the duties, and some of George's siblings later became successful manufacturers and shopkeepers.

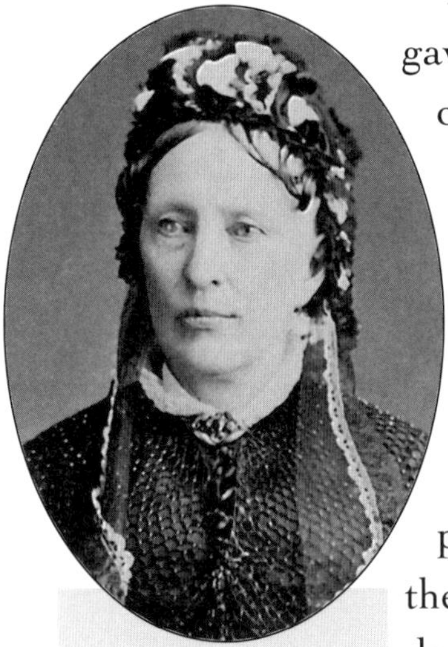

In her letters to George in Australia Sarah often gave advice about money, and related the vicissitudes of the family's small businesses. She was an extremely capable woman and a fund of business advice. George would later claim that while he couldn't read a balance sheet, he knew where to find the bottom line!

Sarah Tallis

Life in the Callan days must have been hard. Money was tight, the living crowded, peace and privacy victims of the off-licence. Few stories of these times have percolated through to the present day; certainly neither George nor his sisters spoke freely of their time in Bridge Street.

Sarah and John were Church of Ireland and St Mary's in Bridge Street was the family church of worship, all the other churches in Callan being Roman Catholic. The Protestant Church of Ireland was, and still is, the minority denomination in Southern Ireland. George Tallis the businessman was often described as aloof and single-minded in his decision-making habits. He listened to opinions when offered, especially those from his inner circle, but relied on his own counsel.

Perhaps his early years in a family of religious outsiders give some hint of a reason.

Like many an Irish youth, George became intrigued at an early age with 'grand houses'. Running errands on behalf of the family store, he would have visited nearby Desart Court[3], and perhaps experienced its crowning glory, a double staircase with carved foliage instead of a banister. He may even have met the mansion's resident ghost, of whom weird tales abounded. You can imagine the local Callan lads peering over the fences of this magnificent old estate, with its ample gardens housing a central building with flanking wings. George, however, may have seen past the thrills of taunting Lord Desart, and dreamt of a grand lifestyle far away from the crowded off-licence.

Sarah's business continued to provide work and money for the family until 1883, when the children dispersed. The most traumatic departure was that of George's brothers, John and Henry, who sailed for Australia in late June. They were in poor health and hoped that Australia's climate would offer a cure. Moreover, their destination was said to be a land of opportunity.

George and three of his sisters moved to the larger town of Kilkenny, where the sisters set up a couturier business providing employment to local seamstresses. Not to be outdone, their mother moved to Dublin with her youngest daughter, Charlotte, to open a similar operation. These twin enterprises spread the risks and straddled the markets, providing a comfortable income for Sarah and her daughters long into the future. At her home in Dublin, Sarah worked tirelessly in the workshop, shrewdly monitored business matters, and made suggestions that her family found wise to consider.

Sarah was disturbed by John and Henry's emigration. In part, she blamed her brother, Richard (Dick) Nicholson, who had emigrated to Australia years before, and who wrote glowing reports home. The Tallis children absorbed his news, and Sarah presided over the fragmentation of her family.

At that time, and since, Ireland provided one of the main streams of young migrants to America and Australia. While this drained Ireland's pool of native talent, the vigour and intelligence of its youth helped mould the future of these two rapidly developing countries.

George lived with his sisters in Kilkenny for three years, and after the first year joined the *Kilkenny Moderator* as a cadet reporter. He soon recognised the importance of being able to record speeches and events rapidly, and decided to add the recently developed shorthand of Pitman to his typing skills. Taking down the long Sunday sermons at St Canice's Cathedral gave him excellent practice and, as his speed and accuracy improved, he earned the respect of his employer by providing full accounts of what the bishop had actually said.

Brothers John and Henry, meanwhile, fared very badly in Australia. They landed in Sydney towards the end of 1883 and lived in the thriving Rocks area of the harbour, near Circular Quay. John worked as a grocer, Henry as a jeweller. But within eighteen months of his arrival John was taken seriously ill. At just twenty-two he died at Sydney Hospital and was buried in the Anglican section of the Rookwood Cemetery. Henry travelled by the special hearse-train out west of the city to accompany his brother on his last journey.

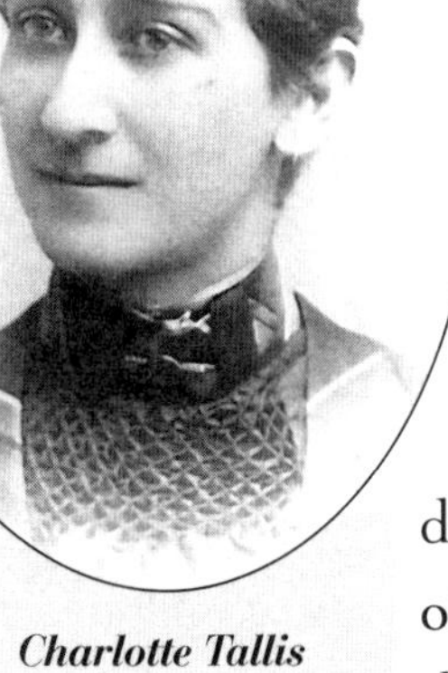

Charlotte Tallis

News of the appalling situation in Australia trickled back to Ireland. Henry had no money, and could not find regular work. He had read of a job at Silverton, near Broken Hill, and was wondering if his uncertain health could tolerate the rigours of the outback. At home in Ireland, the family saw the need for drastic action.

Charlotte, a strong-minded twenty-four, decided to take matters into her own hands. She would go to Australia and attend to Henry herself. This arrangement must have cheered George, who had been harbouring his own ambitions to try his luck in the new country. At the age of seventeen, however, his mother would hardly countenance his travelling alone. On the other hand, if he accompanied his sister Charlotte on her mission to straighten matters out in Australia . . .

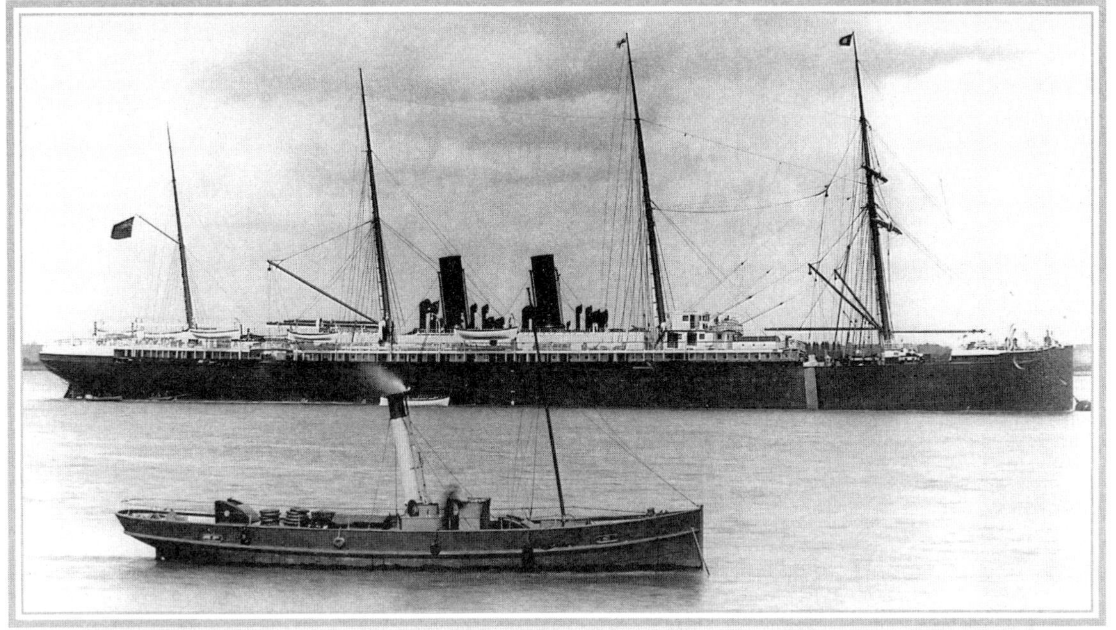

SS **Orizaba** *(maiden voyage 1886)*

Charlotte and George boarded the *Orizaba* on 30 September 1886, and arrived in Melbourne on 24 November. For the first few days they stayed at the White Hart Hotel in Spring Street, the same hotel that had attracted JC Williamson and his new wife, Maggie Moore, on their first trip to Australia twelve years before.

Henry Tallis, meanwhile, had moved to the small gold-mining town of Maldon, about sixty miles north of Melbourne. In spite of the mercy mission from Ireland, he died suddenly late in 1888, two days before his twenty-fourth birthday. Soon after the funeral Charlotte returned home alone, having failed to persuade George to go with her.

By that time George was already over a year into his long career in Australian theatre management. Unlike his poor brothers, he had fallen on his feet, and was relishing the climate, freedoms and opportunities of this new land. Anne, his oldest sister, wrote in June 1893 unwittingly reminding him of his good fortune:

When are you coming home for a holiday George? You could stay with your cousins at Pottlerath. The mud really isn't so bad this year . . . Hope you are well, and not the worse for the wetting you got when rabbit shooting. What a pity you didn't go some place on a week day instead of a Sunday. No wonder you had no luck.

Anne also counselled George to beware of 'play people', reminding her youngest brother 'that there is very little thought of such people here'. Indeed, there is no evidence that any of George's forebears had ever trodden the boards or worked in theatre. So what attracted him to the theatre world?

It is likely that George, while working as a cadet reporter for two years on the *Kilkenny Moderator*, had seen local and international press references to the Williamson activity in Melbourne. JC Williamson and Maggie Moore had taken a company to Dublin in 1877 as part of a three-year world tour from America that included a long season in Australia. The repertoire had been immensely popular in Dublin, with its Irish-American principal players and Irish dramas, as well as the Williamsons' evergreen triumph, *Struck Oil.* From time to time Tallis may have had assignments in Dublin, where intriguing stories circulated about Williamson and his emergence as the biggest theatrical operator in Australia. So when his sister Charlotte decided to go to Australia in 1886 to see what was up with brother Henry, no wonder ambitious young George's ears pricked up.

George would be joining good company. Although officially Australia was just six per cent Irish, a disproportionate number of young Irish men and women were in the theatre business and either came from Dublin, or had trained there. They included serious actors, comedians, managers, playwrights and ... the list was endless. Dublin then, as now, was a thriving theatre centre that exported its products world-wide. So while George Tallis's family background would not have led him directly to the theatre, as a young Irishman he would have been well received in Australia's theatre scene. And as it turned out, both Williamsons had ancestors from Ireland, nicely completing the Irish connection.

In any event, Tallis had obtained two letters of reference before he left for Australia, most probably from his employer at the *Kilkenny Moderator*. One letter was addressed to JC Williamson, and the second to Dr Cunningham, chief-of-staff of the *Argus* newspaper in Melbourne.[4]

Of the ten Tallis children, three emigrated to Australia. But of those three, only George had luck, opportunity and, above all, good health. That he chose the precarious world of the theatre, rather than continue a career in newspapers, speaks for his adventurous spirit and as well, perhaps, for his Irish heritage.

Bourke Street and the Theatre Royal Melbourne c 1886

— CHAPTER THREE —

The Firm

As George Tallis strolled away from his meeting with JC Williamson, he would have been impressed by the bustle of Melbourne's Bourke Street. It was a thoroughfare swarming with Cobb & Co. hansom cabs, cyclists and carts. For the tired pedestrian or frazzled businessman there were coffee palaces, tea rooms and pubs galore. For casual shoppers and tourists there were stalls, bookshops, jewellers, shoe and leather goods shops, barbers and a large emporium or two. Photographers spruiked: 'Excuse me sir, let me take a picture of you with your lovely lady.' Pop, click. Night revellers were offered a variety of billiard halls, taverns and dives. Theatres, large and small, advertised plays, concerts, musicals, opera and vaudeville. Bourke Street was the vibrant hub of Melbourne and its breathless pace was infectious. It gathered up all who had energy, ambition and imagination and propelled them into the exciting future of a rapidly growing colony.

'Melbourne,' British novelist Anthony Trollope had written in 1873, 'looks as though she were boasting to herself hourly that she is not as other cities'.[1] Yet only fifty years before Tallis's arrival in 1886, Melbourne had just thirteen buildings, eight of them turf huts. Then it bore the quaint name 'Dootigala',[2] which it might well have kept had it not been for unprecedented progress, and politicians.

By the 1850s Melbourne, stimulated by the discovery of gold at nearby Ballarat, was said to be the richest city in the world. Katharine Brisbane, theatre critic and publisher, puts to rest the old story that Australia was a forgotten backwater of entertainment when she describes a colonial society:

> *with a huge disposable income spent on grand public buildings, parks and private houses, and on food, drink and entertainment. Entrepreneurs built theatres and hippodromes the size of our present arts complexes in the major cities and on the goldfields, widening the opportunities for touring and attracting opera singers, tragedians, circus stars and low comedians from around the world.*[3]

By the time George Tallis arrived, Australia was already established as a land where theatre fortunes could be won and lost. One early great impresario was the amazing George Selth Coppin, sometimes called the father of Australian theatre. Coppin was a twenty-two-year-old English actor playing comic roles in Dublin when, in 1843, he decided, on the throw of a dice, to take his talents to Australia. With his companion, the American actress Maria Burroughs, Coppin packed Sydney's Royal Victoria Theatre for its manager, Joseph Wyatt, but soon left to follow his own star. Over the next sixty-three years he managed to cram several careers into one lifetime. He was in turn, and often at once, actor, theatre-builder and manager, hotelier,

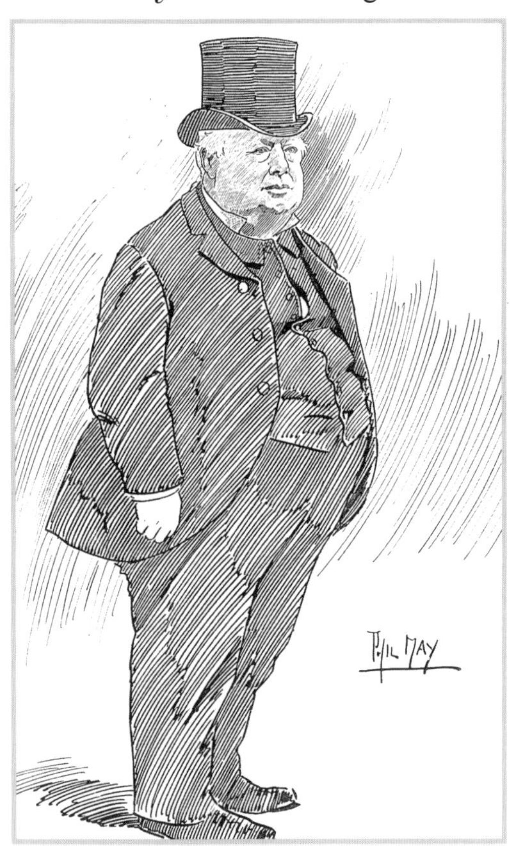

George Coppin

politician, philanthropist and entrepreneur, importing stars, spectacles and pantomimes, and mounting lavish shows. Always a visionary and gambler, he made and squandered riches with equal abandon.

No move that Coppin made in his startling life was more consequential than his decision in 1873 to bring to Australia the American husband-and-wife acting team of James Cassius Williamson and Maggie Moore. Williamson, at twenty-nine, was the leading comic character actor at San Francisco's California Theatre, having learnt his trade at New York's Wallack's, then America's leading theatre and its finest training ground. Of his journey to Australia with his bride and a new star play, *Struck Oil,* that he had acquired in its original draft from an Irish-American backwoodsman, Williamson later recalled:

After three years of San Francisco I determined to try a trip to Australia. Horace Greeley's advice, 'Go West, young man! go west!' was a popular saying in America about that time and we determined to go still further West. Well, we came to Australia and landed in Melbourne in 1874, and opened at the Theatre Royal with Struck Oil.[4]

The rather flippant tone is uncharacteristic of Williamson, who throughout his career was cautious and shrewd. He was shrewd enough to open his Melbourne season with *Struck Oil,* despite gloomy predictions that Australian audiences wouldn't understand its Dutch dialect comedy. Of the play a critic once remarked:

If our readers will take the trouble to recollect, they will see that comedian star plays have been, without exception, merely dramatic shells, owing their life and vigour to some one central character, into which the genius of the actor has infused human nature . . . [they] are all of them dramatic absurdities, and yet they have all drawn and will draw thousands to see and hear them. And so it is with Struck Oil, *and such will be Mr Williamson's luck with the piece.*[5]

Williamson and Moore made a smash hit of the play in their Melbourne and Sydney seasons. They left for a world tour in 1875, but were to return – with a vengeance. In the meantime the pair had charmed audiences across five continents, proving Williamson's uncanny ability to read the popular Victorian taste for novelty.

George Coppin was not the Australian theatre's only impresario in the 1870s. Another influential figure was Irishman William Saurin Lyster who, over two decades of management, toured international opera companies to the larger cities, and also presented drama and variety seasons. While Coppin helped introduce Williamson to Australia, Lyster was instrumental in the careers of the two men who would become JC Williamson's partners in the most potent theatrical force in Australia during the 1880s – the 'Triumvirate' of Williamson, Garner and Musgrove.

Arthur Garner was a softly spoken, elegant English actor who had worked at the Melbourne Theatre Royal and toured country Victoria with the Williamsons. He was married to the well-known actress Blanche Stammers. Under Lyster's instructions, Garner assembled a London comedy company which, with its fine repertoire of light plays and players, superb scenery, stage accessories and costumes, had Melbourne and Sydney critics in raptures in 1879 and 1880.

George Musgrove was Lyster's nephew. He had learnt opera in his uncle's office at the Opera House in Bourke Street before somehow borrowing money to travel to England and engage a company to play Offenbach's comic opera *La Fille du tambour-major*

The Triumvirate in order: J C Williamson, A Garner and G Musgrove

in Australia in 1880. Musgrove's companion, the great actress and singer Nellie Stewart, later wrote:

Nothing like [this production] had ever been attempted in Australia before, and I know of no other example of such enterprise in a young man of twenty-six. He brought out his complete company from England and every member of it had scored at least one individual success on a big scale ... Mr Musgrove carried his innovation still further, he was the first Australian manager to import and introduce showgirls. He brought out eight, all most beautiful, among them the famous Consuelo, nearly six feet of blazing loveliness.[6]

JC Williamson and Maggie Moore returned to Australia in 1879 to play again under the management of George Coppin, but Williamson was soon taking his own steps into theatrical management. He had arrived bearing the exclusive Australian and New Zealand performing rights to Gilbert & Sullivan's *HMS Pinafore*. He was unimpressed to find a number of 'pirated' versions of the operetta already playing, and expressed his dissatisfaction through the courts, serving a stiff warning that English copyright laws would apply equally in Australia. The London D'Oyly Carte company noticed Williamson's professional approach, and over the years allowed him to secure all of the new Gilbert & Sullivan works at a very good price. These comic operas continued to feed the coffers of companies bearing the Williamson name until the 1960s.

In order to stage Gilbert & Sullivan and popular French light operas, Williamson in 1880 set up the Comic Opera Company, soon renaming it the Royal Comic Opera Company. Now busy presenting both drama and comic opera, Williamson needed a base, and in September 1881 he took up the lease of the Theatre Royal in Melbourne, even though he had said that he would never go in for permanent management, 'because, you see, a manager's life is never his own. He has to be at work all the time'.[7]

Williamson was soon to learn the soundness of his intuition, later describing his activities as a one-man management:

I stage-managed the productions of these delightful comic operas, and [these have] become 'traditional' here. At that time I had not even an assistant stage-manager – just a prompter. There was work in plenty then. In addition to producing new pieces I watched the business side, and wrote all my own advertisements. The post of treasurer and business manager was one. It is very different now.[8]

Given the strains, it is not surprising that Williamson agreed when first Arthur Garner, and then George Musgrove, asked him to join them in partnership after the death of their mentor WS Lyster in 1880. The firm of Williamson, Garner and Musgrove was instituted in May 1882, and this marked the beginning of the mighty Williamson theatre organisation. For over eighty years it was to be the principal purveyor of theatrical entertainment in Australia and New Zealand. Even George Coppin was a sleeping partner for a while before he again lapsed into temporary impecuniosity.

These two mergers of rival groups became models that succeeding Williamson firms adopted. As time went on, the mergers became larger, until they assumed the form of amalgamations. The philosophy, which never wavered, was this: it is better to eat at the table in a civilised manner than to fight over the meal. By combining abilities and resources, the partners were demonstrating a method by which theatrical managements could grow and outlast their principals. No longer would all the responsibility rest on the shoulders of the particular actor–manager or entrepreneur.

Of course there were reactive cries of monopoly, and they grew louder over the decades. But in the first years at least, criticism was muted when dire predictions of lowered theatrical standards and crushed oppositions, in the interest of partnership profits, failed to materialise.

At the same time, an experienced hand like George Coppin, in a letter written to Henry Edwards in 1882, foresaw that there might be problems of conflict in this 'super-group':

The only difficulty I see is the improbability of their agreeing very long together – both Williamson and Garner are very self-opinionated with bad tempers. This draw back with wife actresses will make it rather difficult for them to work in harmony unless they separate – one taking the management in Melbourne and the other in Sydney – keeping Mr Musgrove travelling.[9]

The Williamson, Garner and Musgrove combination had youth as well as experience on its side – in 1882 the men were thirty-six, thirty-one and twenty-nine respectively – and the three were ideally placed to take advantage of the vacuum left in theatrical management by Lyster's death and Coppin's roller-coaster fortunes.

The Triumvirate set the stage for great development. Within four years it gained control of the Theatre Royal and the Princess's Theatre in Melbourne, the Sydney Theatre Royal, and set up an arrangement with the Adelaide Royal. This flourished into a large-scale business that was quickly noticed by producers and agents on the other side of the world. The early success of the Triumvirate lay in the partners' ability to import players and the latest shows from overseas, often within twelve months of their premiere. Country touring involved whole companies, which were transported from town to town for short seasons of a few days. Occasionally shows crossed the Tasman to test the New Zealand market. Here the Triumvirate was in the vanguard, as it managed companies on tour and balanced engagements. The tyranny of distance was overcome as the partners serviced the theatrical thirst of dispersed populations, and made money besides.

At the core of the partnership was Williamson. According to *Punch*:

The JC Williamson organisation in those days was a modest affair when compared with what it is today. There was no careful subdivision of duties. Everybody did a little of everything, and JC Williamson did most of all.[10]

Williamson brought to Australia a financially responsible attitude towards all theatre management. Although he was a shrewd bargainer, he was always fair in his dealings with agents and companies. The news got around that Williamson was a man of his word; he was, in fact, the man to do business with.

Williamson had noted only too well the financial mistakes of other theatre entrepreneurs, and he had experienced Coppin's boom–bust economics himself. Clearly, that was not the way to survive, and he developed a more reliable approach to management. In his last interview in Australia he outlined the model which had brought him success over three decades:

My object has always been, in working at high pressure and going in for very expensive productions in all kinds of entertainment, to offer plays that I felt the whole audience wanted ... My desire has been to amuse and interest, to elevate if possible, and at the same time to meet all demands on treasury day.[11]

Williamson always regarded theatre as a business. By keeping this creed in full view, he became, over the years, the survivor of various partnerships as they broke up. And throughout the 1880s it was the Williamson philosophy that helped the Triumvirate to head off opposition.

But no man can build an empire on his own. Williamson had an instinct for picking the right helpers, and it seems that when George Tallis appeared in November 1886 Williamson at once saw an appropriate applicant. The eyes of the partners would be upon the raw recruit; his performance carefully measured against expectations. Said *Punch* many years later:

Tallis, no doubt, had luck in the fact that he entered a business where merit is marked out and recognised so speedily. He had luck also in the fact that James Cassius Williamson was at the head of that business. [Williamson] speedily noticed the keenness and the marked ability of the new youngster in the office. He saw that Tallis meant to get on, and that was just the sort of man Williamson wanted.[12]

This, then, was the 'Firm' that young George Tallis joined in 1886. Although his older sister counselled mistrust of 'play people' in her letters to him, she would surely have been pleased by the tenor of the show run by JC Williamson. It provided family entertainment and was run on strict business principles.

The year George arrived was an *annus mirabilis* of the Australian theatre. A letter written by Williamson in February 1886 confirms just how busy the Triumvirate then was:

Frank Thornton and our Private Secretary company have just returned from New Zealand . . . and are now playing at the Bijou . . . At our Theatre Royal, Melbourne, our opera company are now finishing their ninth week in The Mikado, *which has been an enormous success. We shall run it through Easter . . . At our Bijou Theatre, Melbourne, the Majeronis begin a season, on Saturday, with* Queen Elizabeth. *At the Opera House we produce* Falka, *at the same date. In Sidney [sic] our stock dramatic company, now in the seventh week to excellent business, produce* The Magistrate *next Monday. At the Gaiety,* The Great Pink Pearl *is running well.*[13]

And the Triumvirate, of course, was not the only show around. Tallis recalled in his unpublished memoirs other great managements of the day, including one that began its long influence on the Australian stage in the year of his arrival:

A partnership was formed by two well known London actors, Robert Brough and Dion Boucicault. An organisation which had a profound effect on the future of the Australian Theatre was created in 1886. The Bijou Theatre, Melbourne, and the Criterion Theatre, Sydney, both intimate houses and eminently suited to Comedy, were secured and the new company Brough and Boucicault surrounded themselves with a brilliant company of overseas artists . . .

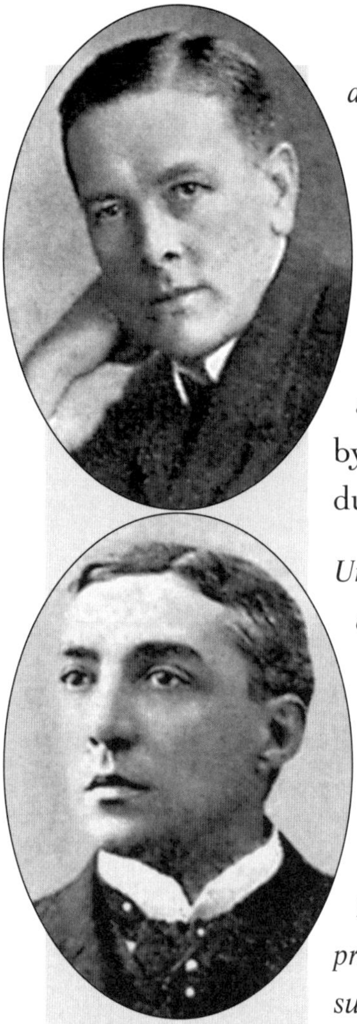

Tallis discussed this 'fruitful and prolific period in the theatre world', during which playwrights Pinero, Wilde, Chambers, Shaw, Barrie and others 'were drawn upon for their best' by Brough and Boucicault. Their works were faultlessly staged by Boucicault, regarded as one of the greatest producers in the world in his time. George continued:

Unfortunately, these high class plays and comedies were to a great extent caviar to the average theatre goer at this early stage . . . but the seed was well and truly sown and bore fruit later.

Nor was robust drama neglected during these remarkable years of profusion. The Adelphi and Drury Lane London were in their prime and Mr and Mrs Bland Holt, supported by a strong and virile dramatic company, presented all the great London Adelphi and Drury Lane successes at the Theatre Royal Melbourne. So, in this very interesting period starting in 1886 playgoers were provided with a very varied and excellent fare with elaborate pantomimes, of course, at Christmas.

Thus from the nineties to a time before the introduction of the Radio or the Talkies may well have been the Golden period of Australian theatre.

Robert Brough and Dion Boucicault

The Brough–Boucicault and Holt companies, among others, were competition for Williamson and partners, although the friendly associations that existed between these entrepreneurial groups led to more cooperation than opposition. They were all part of the 1880s surge of theatre of all kinds. This energy was felt in local halls, on the streets and in the outback. Groups of painted buskers and players roamed the cities, and travelled by train and Cobb & Co. to remote settlements. Formalised into bush stock companies these barnstormers left hardly a trace; that is unless the ring master was Dan Barry, who was described by JC Williamson as the 'worst actor and the best showman in Australia'.

There were no frills in the tough business of bringing fun and enlightenment to the frontiers of the colonies. Barry plagiarised good scripts, and with faithful bulldog Paddy at his heels roamed the hinterlands of Australia – where he was better known than Williamson himself. Dan and Paddy often appeared in the same show, when it was difficult to decide which of the two had put on the worse performance.

With Australian theatre so very alive, no wonder the Triumvirate was looking for young men with management potential. And those young men would need to look sharp because the 1880s were rich in plays, players and managements competing for audiences. George Tallis had joined the biggest and most professional outfit in town, and the one that would outlast all its rivals.

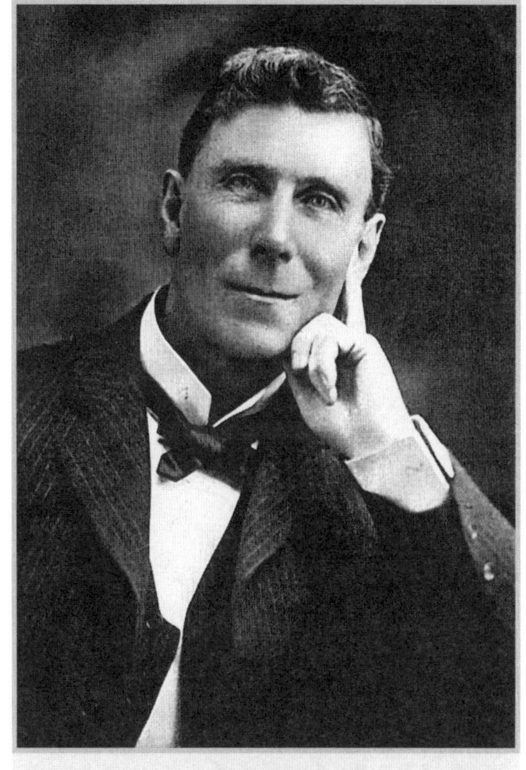

Bland Holt

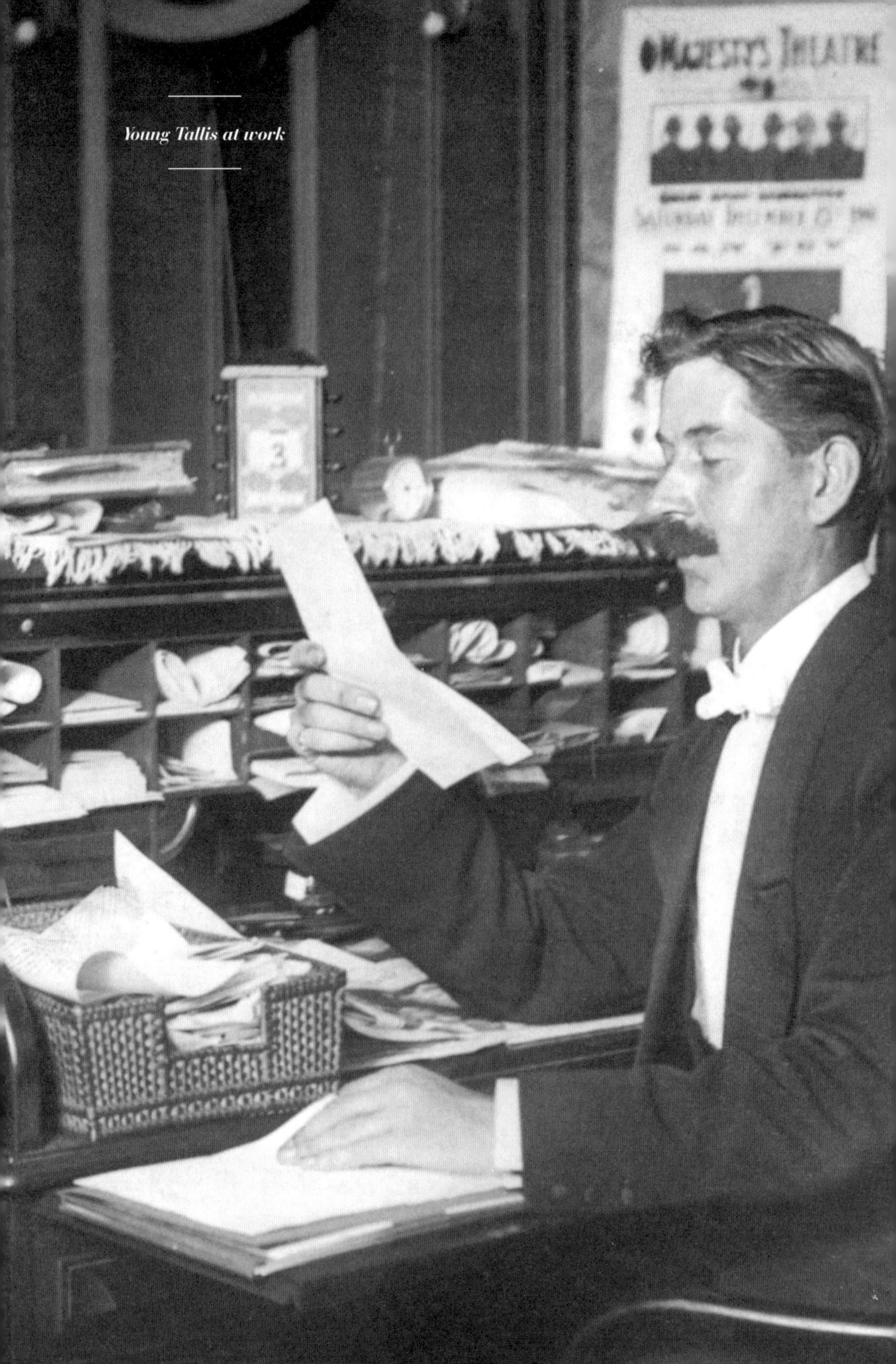

Young Tallis at work

CHAPTER FOUR

Preparation of an Irish Immigrant

When George Tallis arrived in Melbourne as a seventeen-year-old he was 'the freshest of fresh Irish importations, [with] a soft brogue that would have served to identify his race anywhere, and a pair of Irish blue eyes'. In this respect, George was no different from hundreds of other young Irish men working in humble jobs in the city. However, according to the writer of those words, underneath his soft Irish manner Tallis had 'a keen brain, with an enormous capacity for taking pains with his work – a desire to learn, and apply all that he learnt'.[1]

Bert Levy, who became a world-renowned theatre journalist, worked as a young man alongside Tallis for the Triumvirate and came to know him well. He wrote affectionately in 1920:

[He] is a silent man, undemonstrative and strictly business. I have a mental picture of an immaculately tidy young Tallis at the Theatre Royal, Melbourne, thirty years ago – when he, as treasurer, paid me my first salary, an immaculately clean, one pound note. He paid me as seriously as if the amount was one hundred pounds, and he demanded a properly signed receipt, and he would not permit any jokes or familiarities.[2]

Jokes and familiarity? There must have been plenty in those early days, as young actors and actresses, artists, stage hands and managers mingled. But George resisted the bohemian lifestyle although, as he wrote in his memoirs:

It was an amazingly colourful world into which I entered in 1886, under the aegis of the original firm of Williamson, Garner & Musgrove. A world in which melodrama, with good honest retribution in the third act, ruled on the Melbourne stage! Typical of this was Human Nature, *the play then running at the Theatre Royal. That show had its big scene in the British campaign in the Sudan, and was full of lofty and patriotic sentiment.*

George's family background in middle-class Irish shopkeeping would have promoted a business-like ethic, and perhaps his sister's words of warning about 'play people' rang in his ears as he kept actors at what Levy called a 'respectful though not unfriendly distance'. From Ireland he also received well-intentioned advice from a family medical friend, 'not to keep late hours at the theatre', 'to keep out of the crowds and the strong lights' and 'to try to go for a walk during the performance'. All somewhat impractical for a rising young man of the entertainment world.

George may also have inherited a certain aloofness at work from his boss JC Williamson, who was known not to play favourites. 'It is this characteristic which has earned him the respect of everyone in theatrical Australia' wrote Bert Levy of Tallis in 1920. 'His words – like the words of the Guv'nor [Williamson] – mean something. He never wastes them.'[3]

George grew to love the theatre, but unlike his mentor Williamson, or Williamson's great predecessor George Coppin, he had no aspirations as an actor. In this respect, at least, he stands closer to George Musgrove who, like his uncle William Lyster, was from the start an entrepreneur, rather than an actor–manager. Musgrove, of course, had background and training in theatre through his family. Tallis had none. Yet he rose rapidly in theatre management. *Punch* explained the apparent anomaly like this:

Every immigrant who comes to Australia has only to get a list of this country's leading men in every profession and investigate something of their history to find that four out of every six began with nothing and started from nowhere. But brains and ability and, most of all, hard work have carried them to the top of the tree . . .

[An immigrant] is held down by no clogs of habit and custom. He can look round, pick his height, choose his pinnacle, and shape his course for it.

Tallis came from outside. He had no stage history, no tradition of the footlights to hamper his judgement. All theatrical problems he could face with an unbiased mind, could consider them in their proper business perspective – a feat which JC Williamson as an old actor could never perform. Though there were two other partners in the firm – Garner and Musgrove – it was to Tallis that JC Williamson turned most often.[4]

Even allowing for the hyperbole of hindsight, the *Punch* assessments make sense in that George was forever interested in innovation and modern practices and technology, as evidenced early on by his decision as a junior reporter to learn the new shorthand of Pitman. Much later he would show the same innovative streak in his embracing of the new media of cinema and radio. And for an ambitious young man interested in novelty and business, there was no better place to be than Williamson's growing theatre enterprise in the Australia of the 1880s.

From these sketches of the young Tallis at work, a picture emerges of a rather enigmatic character. In an 'amazingly colourful world' he was hard-working, immaculately tidy, somewhat aloof, forward-looking and keen to advance. But he was not an aggressive figure; his soft brogue and personal charm made him well-liked and trusted. He might have been without any theatrical background but he had inherited a goodly portion of what Williamson's firm needed most in order to grow: business sense. With all this, he was blessed with the faculty of being in the right place, at the right time.

These themes – hard work, ability, innovation, speculation, personal charm and luck – recur in their positive and negative guises as we tell Tallis's story.

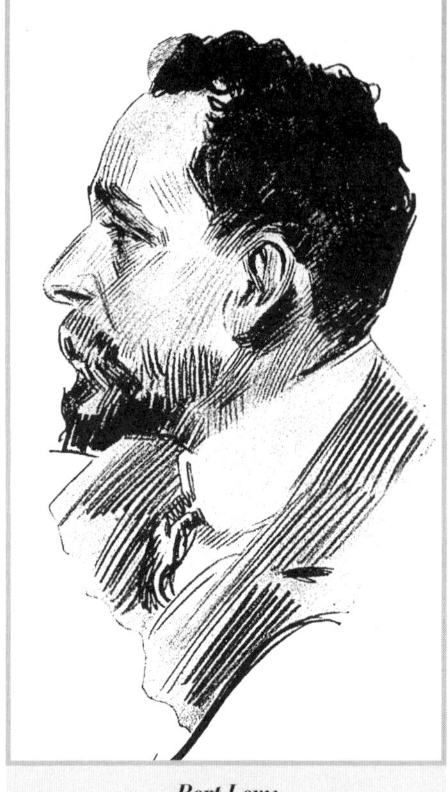
Bert Levy

Beginning as an assistant at the Melbourne Theatre Royal, George acted as clerk, messenger, usher and general factotum. Unlike his friend Bert Levy, whose introduction to theatre life was as an understudy to the Firm's house scenic artist George Gordon, Tallis was at the nerve centre, and in the thick of it from the start. He had opportunities to meet all the right people, and to learn from them and the partners of the Triumvirate.

A month into his job, George would have helped in the preparations when the partners opened the lavishly refurbished Princess Theatre in December 1886. Gilbert & Sullivan's comic opera *The Mikado* was presented by the Royal Comic Opera Company with the people's idol, Nellie Stewart, as Yum-Yum. What an initiation! 'Overnight the Princess became the outstanding theatre in Australia,' wrote George later in his memoirs.

Over the Christmas and New Year period of 1886, the Williamson Pantomime Company staged *Robinson Crusoe* at the Royal. Pantomimes were standard holiday fare for Williamson partnerships; in time they became a tradition. There followed more serious work presented by actor–manager George Rignold, supported by Kate Bishop and Bland Holt. Mid-year there was a Maggie Moore–JC Williamson season, featuring the tenth revival of *Struck Oil.* Further plays and pantomimes rounded out 1887 for the Royal.

Mid-year at the Princess, the musical *Dorothy* was another great success. Alfred Cellier, the composer, came out from England to conduct. George Gordon was putting the finishing touches to the set even as Cellier was bowing to the first-night applause. The musical left lingering memories, and Melburnians went home humming:

From daylight a hint we might borrow,
And prudence may come with the light,
But why should we wait til tomorrow,
You're queen of my heart for tonight.

Whether anyone was queen of young George Tallis's heart in these days we have no idea. Maybe so. Old photographs suggest that he had a cheerful personality and, after all, there was a bevy of actresses and showgirls in his ambit.

George was short of relatives in Australia, but his cousin Fred Nicholson, son of Uncle Dick, had a bank job in Melbourne, and it is likely the pair roomed together for a time to share expenses. This was one way of spinning out a salary of about one pound a week. Even so, there would not have been much left over to invest in the property market, which later became one of George's passions.

There was an early illustration for Tallis of the virtues of caution in property investment. In 1886 his brother Henry was duped in a land scam that involved the ghost settlement of Rugby, north of Sydney. Mother Sarah berated Henry for this entrepreneurial splurge, encouraging him to save for the future and use the banks. Stung, Henry wrote to sister Anne in Ireland: 'I sunk money in it, but it may be of great value yet, or worth next to nothing. Still I got a lesson from it.'

Henry, of course, did not live long enough to benefit from the lesson, and George took over the responsibility for the blocks. He enquired of a Sydney land agent early in 1889, and then again some eighteen months later, about the health of the investment. Bad news indeed: the price did not appear to be lifting as expected. That remained the case until 17 July 1971, when the Gosford Council finally terminated the non-existent township of Rugby and put the site under water. The outstanding rates were $15,883.86, owed by a legion of investors who had vanished into the history of this country.

But there was ample food for thought here. Touts, scams and wasted money; they added up to the requirement of 'due diligence' for all investment in Australia's future. Moreover, there was trouble aplenty from the family in Ireland if news of any speculation trickled through. Silence and due diligence then; they would be George's golden rules, and he stuck to them.

Back at work, George was confronted by an early illustration of how fragile theatre life can also be. The venue was the Princess, the date 3 March 1888, the production Gounod's *Faust* – starring Nellie Stewart as Marguerite, the English tenor Clarence Leumane as Faust, and the English bass Frederick Baker – Federici – as Mephistopheles. Young George Tallis and Bert Levy were looking forward to experiencing some grand opera. They got more than they bargained for, as Tallis later explained:

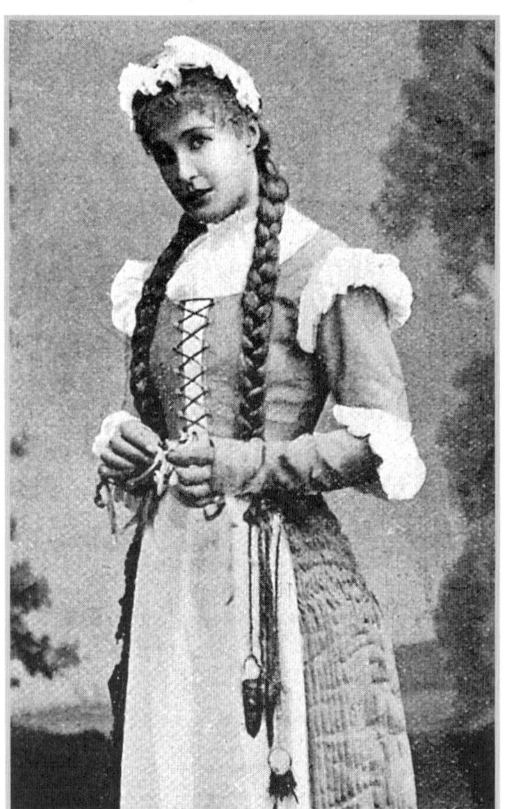

Nellie Stewart as Marguerite in Faust, 1888

At the end of the first performance Alfred Cellier, the conductor, noticed a tremor in Federici as he descended to hell with Faust in the last scene. The singer suffered from heart disease. From the cellar they carried him up to the greenroom,[5] *where he died a minute later, surrounded by the principals in costume. By a marvellous effort of self will he had kept himself going until the last note.*[6]

There are still sightings of Federici's ghost at the Princess!

Perhaps Federici's demise was an omen. The following year Melbourne's boom went bust, ushering in years of economic uncertainty. Banks and credit unions collapsed as land prices tumbled, and borrowing became a dirty word. For a year or so the messages were mixed. In 1891 James McMahon, a Melbourne theatre manager, was in America telling all who would listen how well theatre was doing in his city: 'There is no such thing as absolute poverty in Australia, and where all enjoy prosperity to a certain extent the theatres are sure to prosper.'[7]

One year later the financial crisis in Victoria worsened. Credit restrictions skittled more banks, and undid companies and institutions. McMahon's bravado was looking ill-timed.

In 1893 George was still able to send his mother and sister a present of 'two beautiful rugs'. In July of that year, however, his mother sent him money and wrote:

I hope you will be able to put it with your savings in a safe bank. I was sorry to see such a dismal picture of the state Melbourne is in at present – the papers say things are beginning to mend, which I hope for your sake is the case. I did not expect to hear your salary would be curtailed, which I hope will be no inconvenience to you.

Many years later, when the Great Depression of the 1930s was taking its toll, George was to say that 'theatres were, if anything, more severely hit in the boom smash of the nineties than at present'. Furthermore, the economic malaise lingered. As if orchestrated by the financial woes, a disastrous drought started in 1896, delaying full recovery until the next century. Williamson's company was reeling. The cost of importations had risen but, more importantly, there had been a dearth of suitable overseas shows, especially pantomimes. One of these, and a good one at that, was needed urgently for the 1896 season.

In desperation Williamson decided to write one himself and called in his staffer Bert Royle as collaborator. Together they created the unusual plot of *Djin Djin*, which tells how an Australian prince, Eucalyptus, rescued a Japanese princess from evil. There was ample scope for spectacular ballet sequences and the novel effects that audiences had come to expect from end-of-year shows. The music was by the Firm's conductor, Leon Caron, and everything was geared for a grand Christmas special. But there was a major problem. There was no money.

How this crisis was overcome has been the subject of several stories over the years, but we cling to George Tallis's version. He told it to a newspaper in 1931:

An interesting scene during the crash in the nineties had some point for us today. The crash came practically overnight. An opera season was on at the Princess Theatre. Williamson called the company together on the stage after the performance. Standing on a chair he gave them the bad news. A catch came into his throat, there was a tear in his eye. But, before he had finished, Florence Young and other principals caught his hand and reassured him, and the whole company, from stage hand up, made a voluntary reduction of a third of their salaries.[8]

Djin Djin played, and it filled the seats. It was exactly what the people wanted, and it was what the Firm needed. The pantomime toured for months across Australia and New Zealand, saving the company from ruin.

Despite the problems of depression, the 1890s were years of professional advancement for Tallis. In 1889 the Triumvirate rewarded his diligence by appointing him treasurer at the Theatre Royal and then treasurer of the up-market Princess Theatre in 1892. Around the same

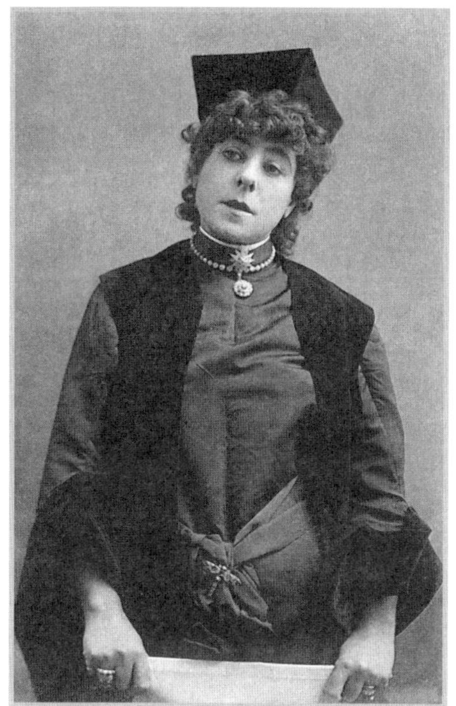
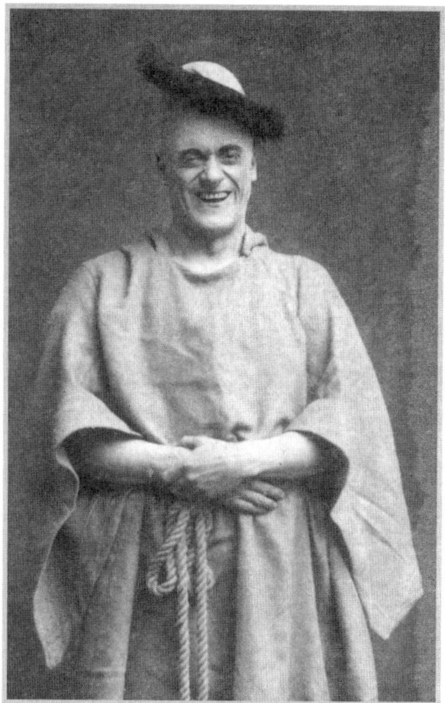

***The famous London Gaiety company, with Nellie Farren (left), Fred Leslie (right) and brilliant comedians, singers and dancers, opened at the Princess in 1888 with* Monte Cristo.**

time, JC Williamson asked him to become his private secretary at the Theatre Royal, 'where the name of Williamson was a spell to draw the public'.[9] *Punch* later suggested that it was George's shorthand skills that ensured him the job:

Even a small business man today dictates his letters to a stenographer. Thirty years ago he wrote them himself, or dictated notes which were taken in long hand. Williamson decided to instal a private secretary who was a stenographer. Tallis had learnt shorthand.[10]

George's new position would have involved long hours with his employer, as Williamson revealed:

Often I come home from my office and bring my work with me, and my secretary to deal with a heap of correspondence that can't be crammed into the day; and then, maybe, it's necessary to sit up till two or three in the morning reading plays, or looking over the English and American dramatic papers, so as to miss nothing that will be of service.

It's not [only] keeping the companies going – though that is no light task in itself – but sometimes I have to take part in stage management . . . Then there is the continual labour of keeping in touch in order to be up-to-date. Weekly letters come from our agents in London and New York telling us what is going on there, and these have to be carefully considered. You have to keep an eye open for new men – for rising talent both in the field of authors and in the acting field. You have to see not only that the whole machine works, but that every part of it works so well that there is the least possible friction.[11]

What a crash course for a budding theatrical entrepreneur.

Unfortunately, even if the internal workings of the 'machine' were smooth enough, there was friction at the top. Initially this was to Tallis's advantage as the Williamson partnerships went through various permutations.

In 1890 George Musgrove withdrew following a dispute involving Nellie Stewart. Due to financial difficulties, Arthur Garner left the following year. In 1892, Musgrove rejoined Williamson in a partnership that lasted until the end of the decade. From 1895, however, Musgrove was mainly in London, and Tallis became Williamson's closest business ally. By the turn of the century Williamson and Musgrove had split permanently and George had become pretty much a *de facto* partner. With all these changes, George had an early glimpse of how brittle partnerships could be, particularly in the theatrical world where egos ruled supreme.

Actors, of course, are also fractious people, as twenty-one-year-old George learnt in 1891 when he supervised some of the arrangements for touring the great Sarah Bernhardt. Born in Paris in 1845, a magnetic personality and a '*voix d'or*' helped to establish her as the most significant actress of her time. It was a triumph for the partnership of Williamson and Garner that they had induced her to visit Australia.

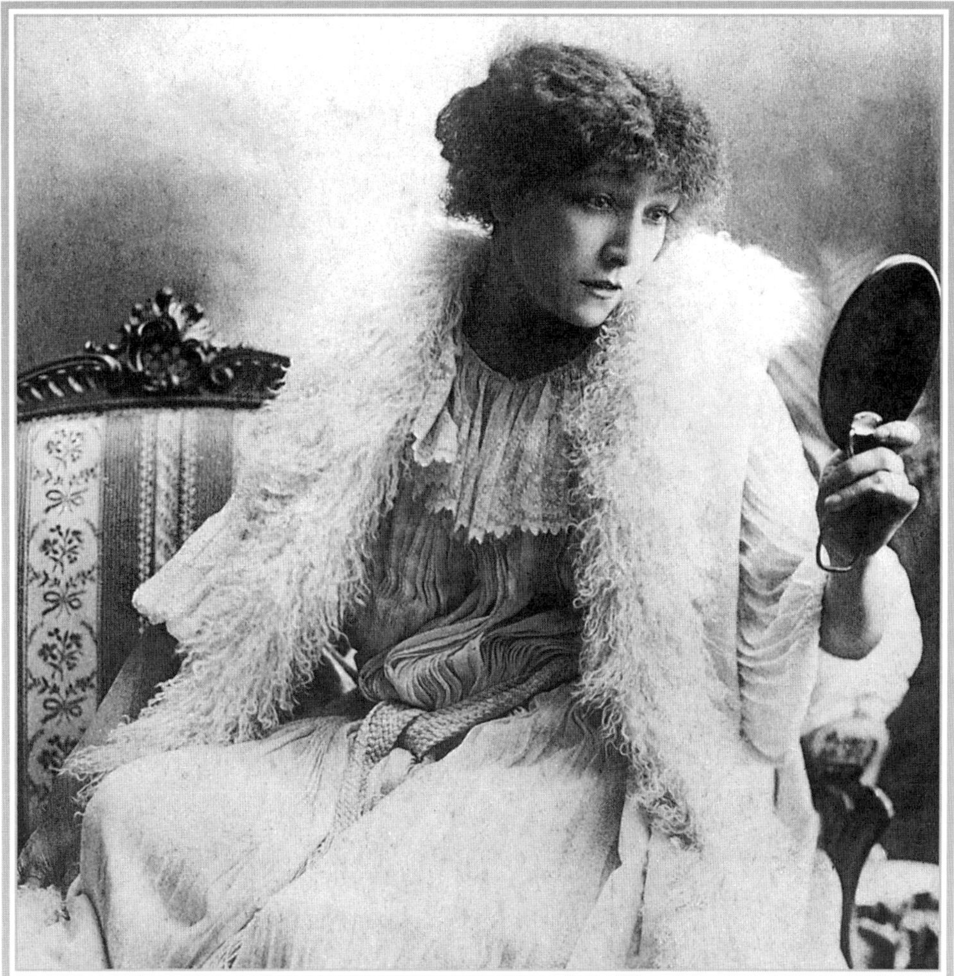

Sarah Bernhardt in La Dame aux camelias, *1891*

In May, Bernhardt disembarked in Sydney with hundreds of tonnes of luggage that was to see her through a ten-week tour hailed as the social and theatrical event of the decade. Her company performed *La Dame aux camelias,* known locally as *Camille,* and nine other serious plays. Under auditorium lighting, the audience tried to keep up with the French text by reading English translations during the performances. The rustling of the pages distracted Bernhardt who, in turn, kept audiences waiting with excessively long intervals. There was, therefore, some disenchantment both sides of the curtain, and at least once Bernhardt kept a management and a full theatre on edge by … but this is George's story:

Stars were appearing in the theatrical firmament of Melbourne. One had to learn to use a great deal of tact in handling celebrities. Tact, they say, comes easily to an Irishman. However that may be, all the tact in the world was sometimes needed. I found that out in meeting Bernhardt, one of the earliest and most interesting celebrity engagements of the Firm.[12]

One incident is as real in my mind as though it happened yesterday. One Saturday, after two performances – a matinee of Fedora *in the afternoon and* Tosca *at night – Bernhardt and her whole company left the city, in an open drag, for the Dandenongs and a weekend shoot. What they were to shoot, I had not the faintest idea, but it was mid-winter and bitterly cold for midnight driving in open drags.*

On the Monday evening 7 o'clock came with no Bernhardt. The theatre was a sell out. Half-past seven; a quarter to eight. Still no Bernhardt. At ten to eight, bugles were heard blowing in the street and Bernhardt arrived in her drag and descended with an air of unconcern. Her performance was a memorable one, which fully compensated for the anxiety she had caused.[13]

Tallis also recalled that Bernhardt's season in Adelaide led to drama for the organisers when she objected to the terrible train trip from Melbourne, and insisted that she return by ship. There was not a great choice at Port Adelaide, so they got to work on the *Adelaide,* an intercolonial passenger ship on the Adelaide–Melbourne run. Two cabins became one, and a lightning refurbishment delayed the ship's departure until one in the morning, when Bernhardt arrived after her last performance. The captain, crew, wharfies and a host of eager passengers met her – and her doctor, manager and maids with hatboxes.

Bernhardt climbed aboard the small vessel and inspected the promised luxury. Spontaneously, it seemed, her disdain of the 'inferior' interstate train service softened. All was forgiven; without a word she fled Port Adelaide to see if that 'lovely train' was still available.

The Sarah Bernhardt tour was a prime example to George of enormous effort and financial risk in the face of dubious rewards. The

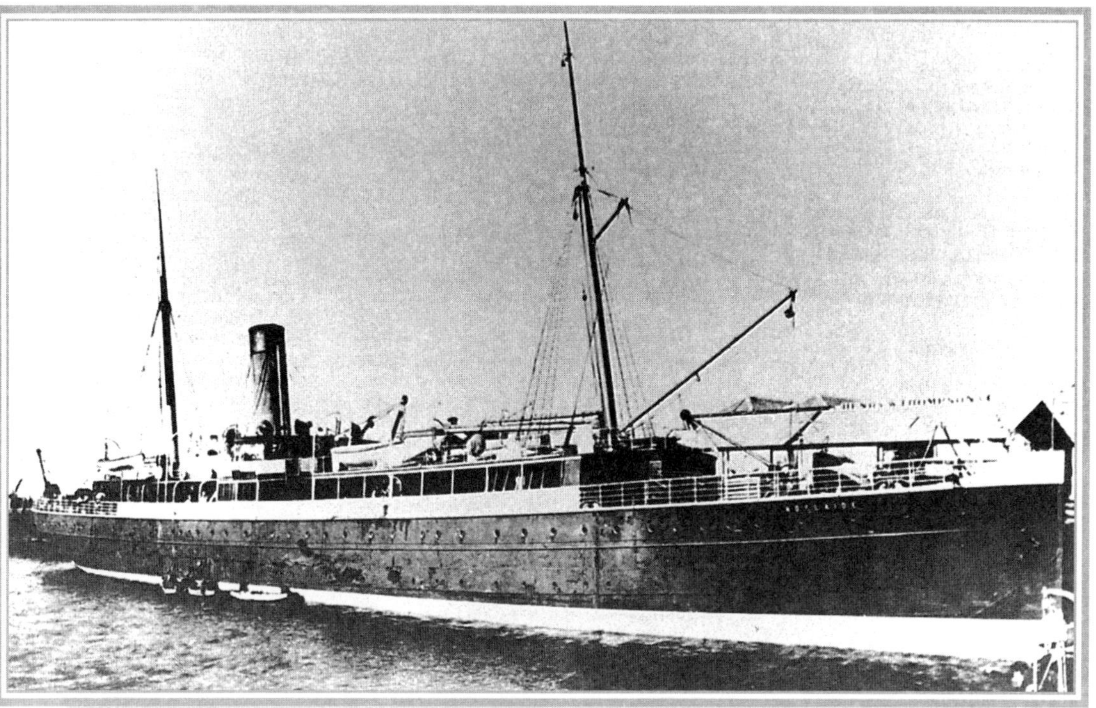

The Adelaide – *10 yards wide, 100 yards long, weighing in at less than 2000 tons*

season was an artistic success during which fulfilment outran expectations; it was generally appreciated by Melbourne, Sydney and Adelaide audiences. As a bonus, the presence of the world celebrity elevated theatrical morale and the prestige of sponsors, Williamson and Garner. But the story goes that money was lost when expenses swamped receipts, and at the close of counting Garner was forced to retire from the partnership.

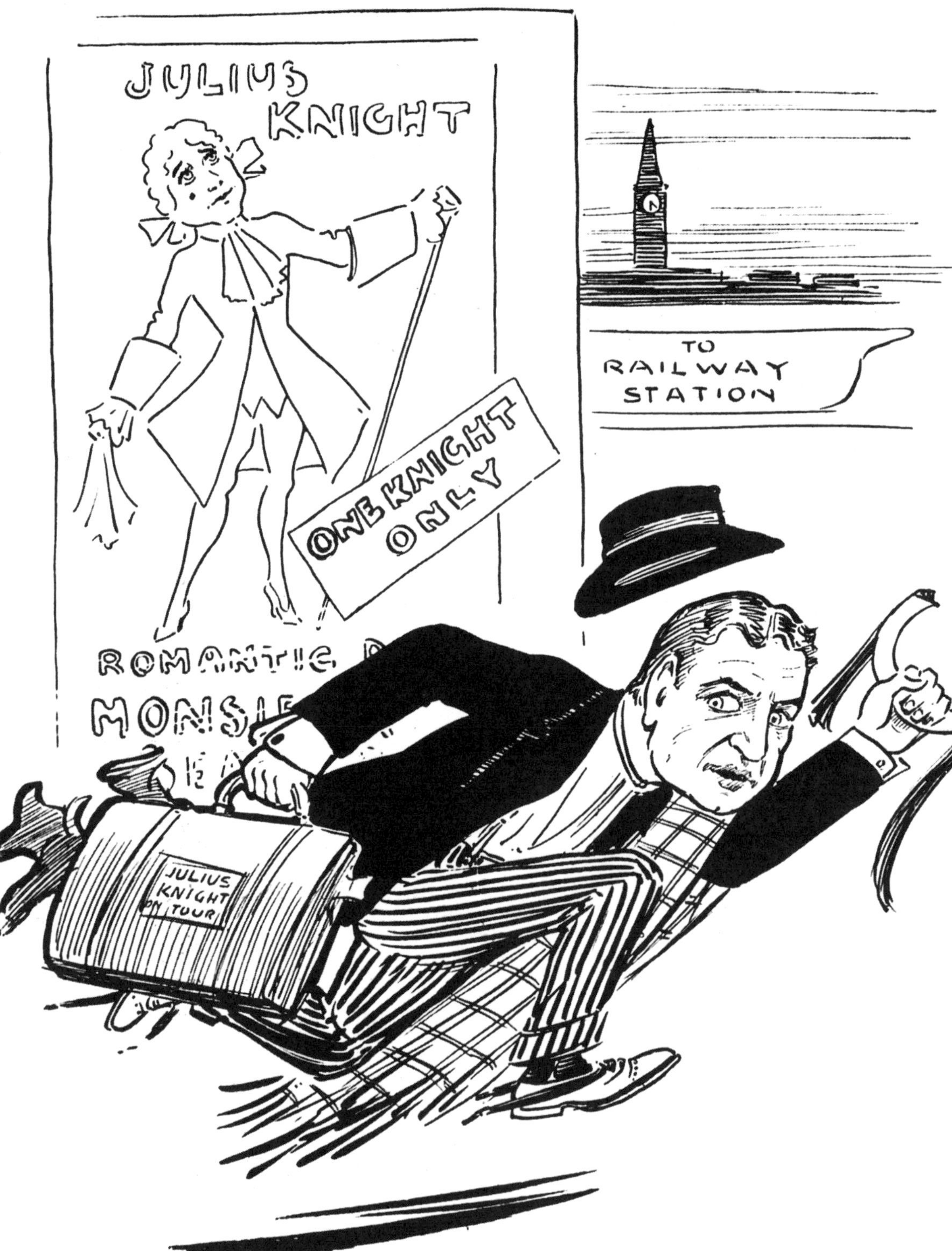

THE EARLY MORNING STAR.

Julius Knight on tour

CHAPTER FIVE

Tour Manager

In a throwaway line in his history of the Sydney Theatre Royal, Ian Bevan suggests that George Tallis learnt all about the theatre business from the cloisters of JC Williamson's office.[1] Perhaps this statement reflects a prejudice against professional theatre business managers in favour of high-profile actor–managers. George may have been 'the man behind', but he saw a lot more of Australia than simply his boss's desk.

As early as 1891, Tallis was involved with the Bernhardt tour, and he frequently led the 'roving life' managing touring companies. By the mid-1890s, the circuit included the main cities of Australia and New Zealand, and up to eighty country centres in between. Irish family letters between 1892 and 1897 tell George how it is 'grand for you to have seen so much of Australia' and how they are 'glad to see you are enjoying yourself travelling about', while at the same time hoping that he is 'again settled down in Melbourne' where he 'will not feel the same amount of responsibility as when going from place to place'. But George Tallis revelled in the touring.

One with whom Tallis shared the circuit was Johnny Farrell, who joined Williamson around 1880 as an office boy, and graduated to an acting career specialising in Gilbert & Sullivan. In time he was given managerial roles, and at the end of his seventy years with the

Firm he was its most experienced and best-loved employee. Farrell grew into the organisation with George, and in 1931 he wrote to his friend:

With all due respect and deference to the outstanding ability and judgement of our great 'Chief', it was your genius that resulted in the extension of JCW Ltd and made it one of the biggest theatrical companies in the world.

In any emergency case that has happened during a tour when I have been in charge of a company I always tried to imagine what you would do in a like case, and I always found that this inspiration helped me to do the correct thing.

The Williamson tour managers formed a fraternity that George joined. It was life on the edge and by no means suited to all temperaments. George's quiet and unflustered disposition was particularly well-geared for crises, and decisions on the run. Good personal relations with the touring cast and stagehands minimised conflict, hurt feelings and industrial unrest.

For a period Tallis specialised in the Firm's country touring. After the bright lights of Sydney and Melbourne, it was with these tours that the real work started. George had good tutors. Initially there was Nellie Stewart's father, Richard Stewart, from the Princess Theatre days. The group also included Bert Royle, Johnny Farrell and Harold Ashton, all great characters and close friends of George. He toured Victoria and New South Wales, and often took companies to Adelaide and Brisbane. This exposure to the Australian countryside never dampened his zest for it. In later years he enjoyed driving the lonely roads that connected the main cities, analysing the farming methods he saw on the way, and relating them to how things were done in Ireland.

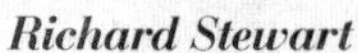

Richard Stewart

From the beginning of his days at the Firm, George saw shows loaded onto the Inter-Colonial Express bound for a season of three or four weeks in Adelaide, on the tip of the driest state on the driest continent. Maybe they then headed north to Brisbane for some hundred degree heat and hundred per cent humidity. In Adelaide they played the Royal and in Brisbane they played Her Majesty's. Some tired tour manager once said that if all the Theatre Royals and Her Majesty's Theatres across Australia suddenly vanished, country touring would cease.

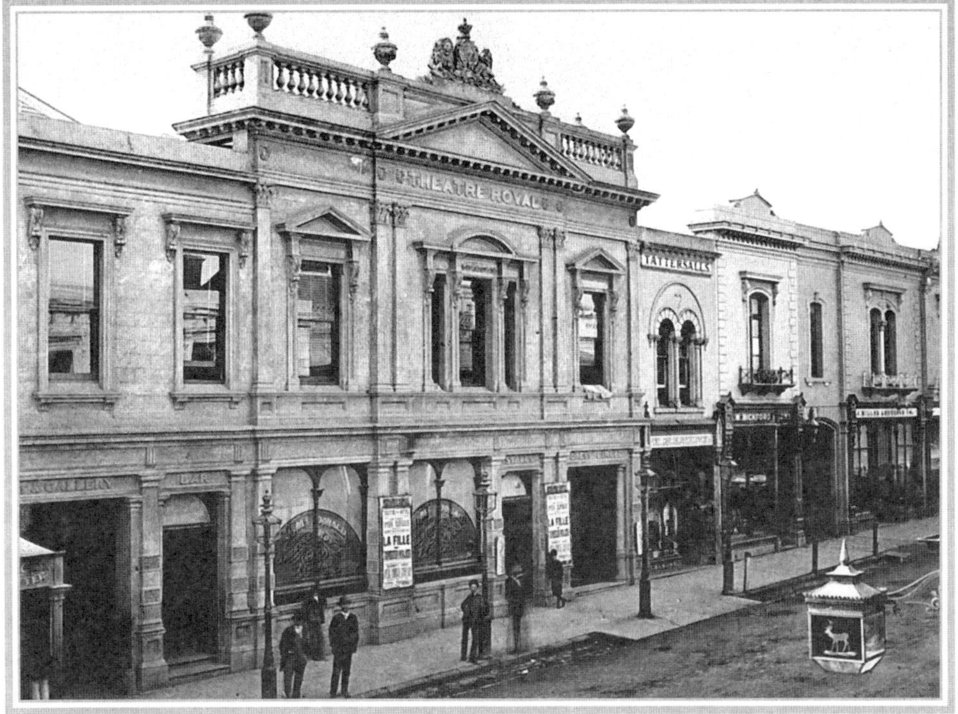

Theatre Royal, Adelaide, c 1890

A natural extension of the Adelaide season included the boat trip to Perth across the Great Australian Bight. There the season opened at the Theatre Royal, or at His Majesty's Theatre after 1904. From Perth, the tour would drop in at Kalgoorlie to brighten the nights of the miners by making the four-hundred-mile train trip east to the goldfields. The Williamson companies were always well received, but the miners had their own ideas about entertainment and the town became a touring manager's nightmare.

Because of his commitment to the touring circuit, George would have made this long trek west. He would have enjoyed the sea trip, and the challenge of steering companies of artists, with wardrobe and scenery, all the way to one of the theatrical outposts of the continent. It could be a rough voyage, but a few waves never seemed to bother him. Had he ducked the Kalgoorlie run, though, he would have missed a slice of genuine outback, and a lot of rustic fun.

There were two theatres in Kalgoorlie: the Tivoli and the Cremorne. The music-hall artists played at the Cremorne, while the dramatic and comic opera companies played the Tivoli. Thus it was that Nellie Stewart played at the Tivoli in the December of 1909 or 1910 under the banner of JC Williamson, and the miners and their partners turned up for some top 'highbrow' at 1/-, 2/- or 3/- a seat.

The temperature soared, and the hotel hosting Nellie became an inferno. Fans and blocks of ice were rigged as rudimentary air conditioning to help Nellie with her sleep and theatre performances. The system appears to have failed, for 'Sweet Nell' was made comfortable in the giant refrigerator of a meat works, where she relaxed among the frozen chickens, fish, beef and mutton. Ten minutes in the sun for defrosting, and Nell was ready to go. The heat wave took the usual course, finishing with a blow, and Nellie found herself dancing through the red dust at the Tivoli Theatre in front of an appreciative audience she couldn't even see.[2]

Touring was a military-style exercise that required precise planning and execution. Although the Firm booked everything in advance – theatres, accommodation, ship and rail transport – it was a lucky tour manager who ran unscathed the gauntlet of illness, flu epidemics, strikes and Tasman storms.

Frequently matters went wrong, and the star performers complained about their roles, or their accommodation; or the scenery

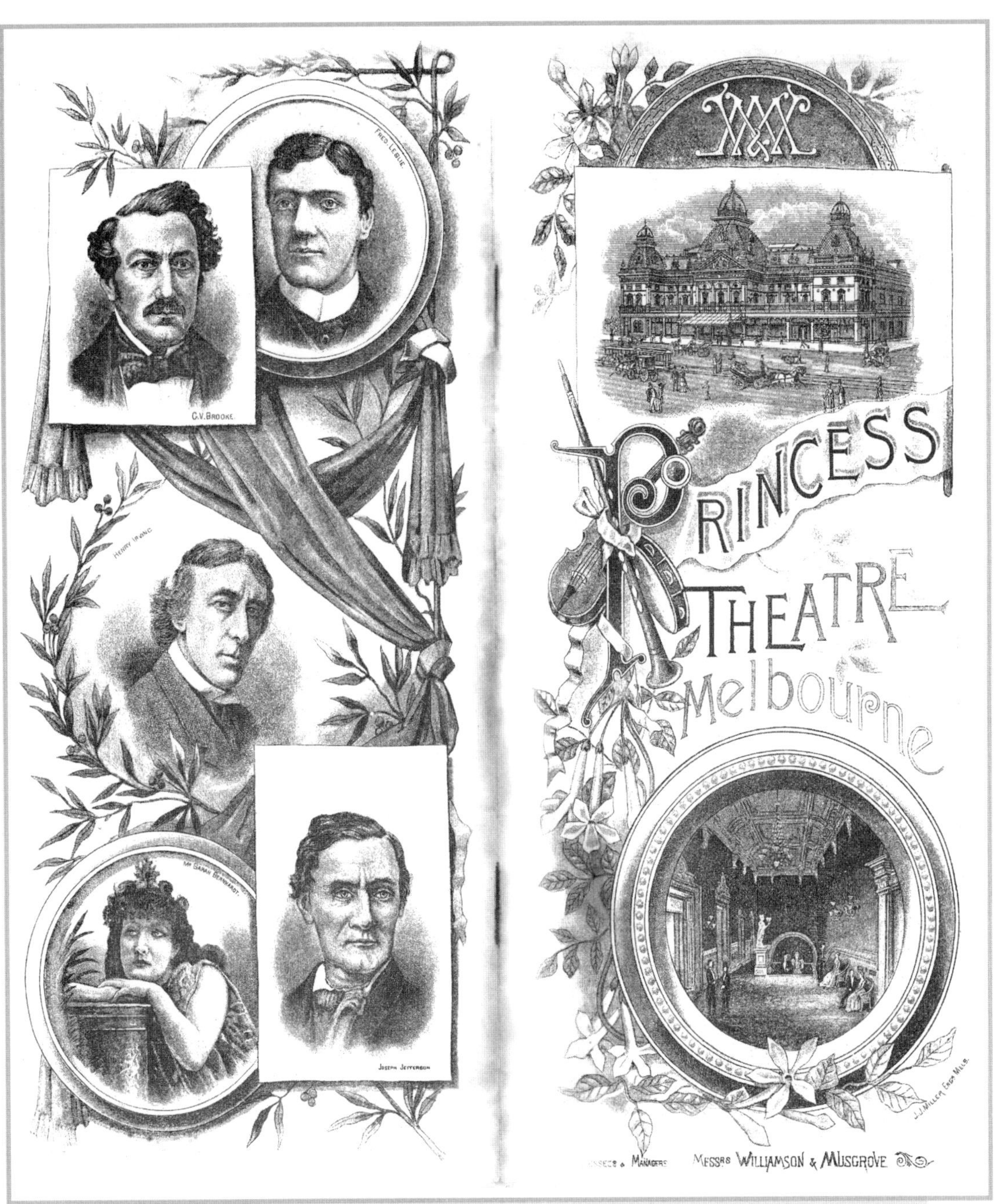

Cover for Comic Opera Programs, 1890s

PRINCESS THEATRE.

Sole Lessees and Managers:

Messrs. WILLIAMSON & MUSGROVE.

Treasurer .. .. Mr. GEO. TALLIS

1893—ANNUAL COMIC OPERA SEASON—1893.

WILLIAMSON and MUSGROVE'S

ROYAL COMIC OPERA COMPANY.

THIS EVENING.

The Mikado,

OR THE

TOWN OF TITIPU.

CAST OF CHARACTERS.

The Mikado of Japan (First time here) Mr. WM. ROSEVEAR

Nanki-Poo (First time here) ... ... Mr. HENRY BRACY

Ko-Ko (Lord High Executioner of Titipu) Mr. HOWARD VERNON
(His original Character).

Pooh-Bah (Lord High Everything-else) Mr. CHARLES RYLEY

Pish Tush (a Noble Lord) ... ... Mr. THOMAS GRUNDY

Yum Yum, Pitti Sing, Peep-Bo — Three Sisters. Wards of Ko-Ko.

- Yum Yum — Miss FLORENCE YOUNG (First time here)
- Pitti Sing — Miss VIOLET VARLEY
- Peep-Bo — Miss NINA OSBORNE (First time here)

Katisha (First time here) ... ... Miss CLARA THOMPSON
(An Elderly Lady in love with Nanki-Poo).

Chorus of School Girls, Nobles, Guards and Coolies.

didn't arrive; or the public complained of tired performances; or senior management complained of poor takings. It was then that the true metal of the tour manager was tested. By sheer diplomacy, and the ability to improvise, he would get his tour through these crises without violence or litigation. A week may well be a long time in politics, but a touring manager's crisis week was significantly longer.

All the headaches and frustration of touring erupted once in front of Taylor Darbyshire (Darby), who was one of Tallis's fellow tour managers. He reminisced to *Theatre Magazine* in 1914:

The Ben Hur Co. played Invercargill (New Zealand) one Saturday, and Melbourne (Victoria) the next Saturday. Yes; and with the same scenery. We paid the shipping company extra to speed up the steamer, and they got into Melbourne on Friday night instead of Saturday mid-day.

I remember the manager of the Ben Hur tour coming into my office the Saturday afternoon in Melbourne. His face was streaming with perspiration, and he was covered in dust. He had stood by the show in and out of the New Zealand towns, seeing that the scenery, horses and impedimenta – impedimenta was the word all right – got to the theatre from the trains, and back again to the trucks. He reported that everything was ready for the Melbourne opening.

He looked at me hard – I might say almost fiercely. Then he mopped his brow, and looked at me some more. 'That's a nice —— job you set us,' he exploded. 'It's all very well for you fellows to sit in your offices like —— prime ministers, and give orders. But you ought to go on the —— road and —— well do it!' [3]

Much of Tallis's early touring was with the Firm's famous Royal Comic Opera Company and in his memoirs he recalled those days with great affection:

In no country of the world was there an organisation in any way comparable to the Royal Comic Opera Company, with its continuity record of more than twenty years. In the early days of the 'Firm', as Williamson, Garner and

Musgrove were then designated, the Royal Comic Opera was organised to present the Gilbert & Sullivan series as they came along and the light French opera in vogue at that period. The chorus of young, well-trained voices was unsurpassed, while the principals were continually being reinforced with the finest voices and the very best talent obtainable in England or America. The productions were impeccable. The scenery was supplied by those eminent artists George Gordon and Phil Goatcher and W Coleman and most of the costumes were imported from London or Paris or manufactured in the Firm's own wardrobes under the direction of Miss Emily Nathan.

It was the custom for this organisation to play four or five months every year in Melbourne, the same in Sydney and three weeks each in Brisbane, Adelaide and Perth, with a New Zealand tour of ten or twelve weeks worked in every second or third year.

It is difficult to estimate in these prosaic days the emotional interest attached to the visit of the Royal Comic Opera to the smaller capitals. It was the outstanding event of the year. In Brisbane, hotels would be packed with opera lovers from all over the state for the entire season. Likewise in Adelaide and Perth, while in New Zealand it was not an uncommon thing to witness at least a thousand people gathered on the wharves at Auckland and Wellington to welcome the arrival, or bid farewell to the favourites when leaving.

By 1895 George Tallis was the man in the Firm who knew most about the Australasian touring circuit, and in recognition of this Williamson and Musgrove promoted him to manager in charge of touring, an appointment close to the top of the tree. At the same time he was also listed in the Firm's advertising as business manager at the Princess in Melbourne. Clearly his star was in the ascent.

The family in Ireland was naturally pleased to learn of his progress, but their pleasure was tempered with Irish caution. His sister Charlotte wrote in 1894:

I am delighted you are getting on. I saw by your ticket you are Business Manager as well as Treasurer: you are great to be able to do all, but mind your

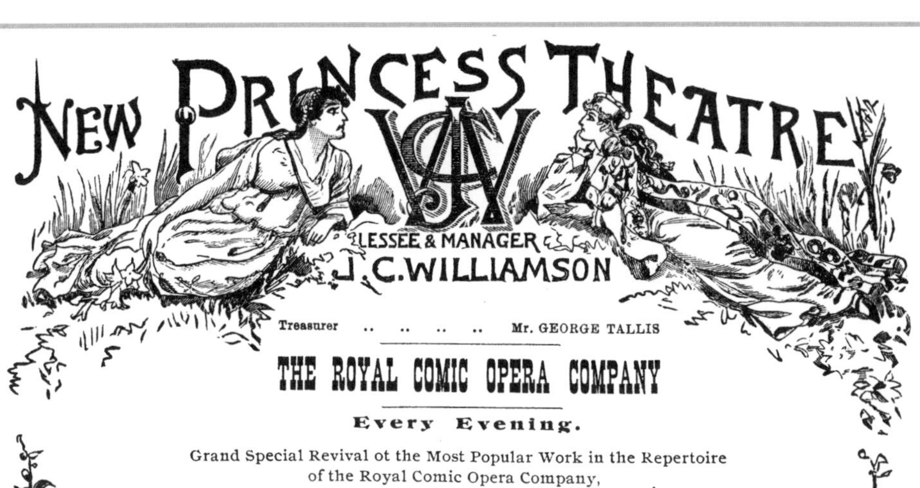

Treasurer .. .. Mr. GEORGE TALLIS

THE ROYAL COMIC OPERA COMPANY

Every Evening.

Grand Special Revival ot the Most Popular Work in the Repertoire of the Royal Comic Opera Company,

DOROTHY

By B. C. STEPHENSON.
Music by the late ALFRED CELLIER.

CAST OF CHARACTERS:

Dorothy Bantam ... ... **Miss MARIE HALTON**
(For the First Time in Australia.)
Lydia Hawthorn ... ... **Miss FLORENCE YOUNG**
(First Time.)
Phyllis Tuppett ... ... **Miss VIOLET VARLEY**
(First Time.)
Mrs. Privett ... ... **Miss ELSIE CAMERON**
(First Time Here.)
Geoffrey Wilder ... ... **Mr. HENRY BRACY**
(First Time.)
Harry Sherwood ... ... **Mr. CHARLES RYLEY**
Squire Bantam ... ... **Mr. HOWARD VERNON**
John Tuppet ... ... **Mr. T. GRUNDY**
Tom Strutt ... ... **Mr. A. LISSANT**
Lurcher ... ... **Mr. WILLIAM ELTON**
(His Original Character, and for the Last Time in Australia.)

Hop-pickers, Guests, Bridesmaids, Peasants, &c., by the
ROYAL COMIC OPERA CHORUS

THE ROYAL BALLERINAS

In New and Attractive Ballets, instructed by
Miss MARIE REDDALL.

Musical Director ... ... M. LEON CARON.
Stage Director ... ... Mr. HENRY BRACY.
Assistant Stage Manager ... ... Mr. F. GRESHAM.

Doors open at 7 o'clock. Early Door (Amphitheatre), 6.45.

In preparation—

CARMEN.

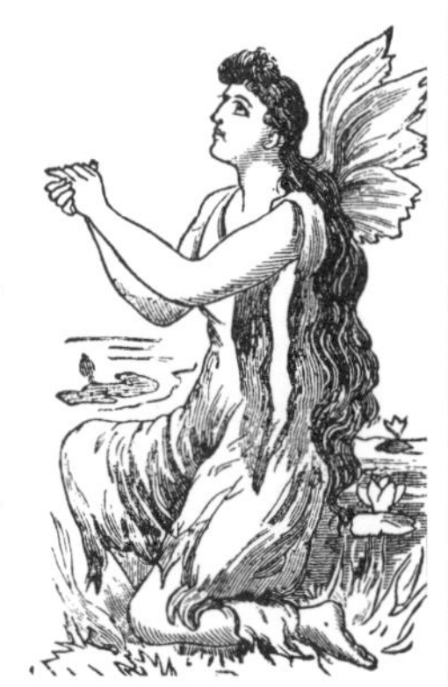

The Dress Circle Programmes are perfumed by
R. W. BEDDOME & CO.,
with ENGLISH LAVENDER Sachet Powder.

health what ever you do . . . Mind George boy, if you will want any tin just let me know and I will gladly send it. I would now if I thought you were in want of it . . . I hope you don't work too hard. I wish you would come home for a holiday. Think about it.

With George Musgrove away in London for much of the time between 1896 and 1900, and Williamson spending more time in Sydney, Tallis found he had to focus largely on Melbourne between 1896 and 1902. As manager in charge of touring his brief was to streamline the itineraries to make tours more profitable and efficient.

Just how demanding this job must have been was also discussed by Taylor Darbyshire in his illuminating 1914 *Theatre Magazine* interview. He discussed days more recent than Tallis's early ones as touring manager, but conditions by then would, if anything, have been easier:

Take the annual pantomime as a typical example. Every year it has to be moved a long journey of from 13,000 to 15,000 miles. One or two of the girls who began as children in Mother Goose, *and have been with us ever since, have travelled over a hundred thousand miles (four times around the world) with the pantomimes.*

From the regular route of this attraction there is no deviation. It starts in Melbourne at Christmas, arrives in Sydney for Easter, then goes to Brisbane, Toowoomba, Newcastle, and across to New Zealand. Then Adelaide is on the list and the 'panto' invariably makes Perth for the Show dates.

The Williamson pantomime engagement means ten months' solid work. It is the longest engagement of its kind in the world.

Darbyshire gave more examples:

The Royal Comic Opera Co. played Invercargill [in New Zealand] one Saturday, and on the following Saturday showed at Adelaide. Again the steamer was speeded up. A special train met it at Hobart, and ran express to Launceston to connect with the Loongana, *which was met by a special train on the wharf at Melbourne. I kept out of the way of the manager of that company.*

We have sent companies from Perth to Brisbane in one jump, and only this month we sent the New Comic Opera Co. from Invercargill to Perth without stopping any longer than it was necessary to make the connections with boat and rail and rail and boat.[4]

The problem of manipulating dates was another concern. It was not a matter of the manager in charge of touring balancing one company, but eight to ten at once. The sequence of attractions had to be varied, especially away from the big centres, Sydney and Melbourne. It would have been disastrous, for instance, to send simultaneously to Brisbane a pantomime, a revue, and a musical comedy.

The booking of tours was immensely complex and often emergency improvisations were made on the run. Sometimes the scenery or wardrobe would over-shoot or under-shoot the destination by thousands of miles. Opening dates had to be switched without notice. Flops caused a similar problem, as fresh shows had to be whipped up to fill the gap. All this was costly, since artists were engaged for fixed periods, and they had to be paid despite delays and foul-ups.

The weather also played a part. Like farmers, it turned theatre entrepreneurs into gamblers. New Zealand, the hot weather outlet for Australia, absorbed about three touring companies every Christmas. But a summer heatwave in Auckland could destroy the strategy, for then New Zealand theatre attendances would fall, and the companies might just as well have stayed at home.

And, according to Darbyshire, there was also a fourth dimension:

Another thing about dates is that while one acts in the living present, one is always working six or twelve months ahead of it. As an instance of this we have just arranged dates for an English company for South Africa for June. Six months after that it will be in Australia. The Australian dates have already been booked, and, of course, the route has had to be arranged with a consideration of all the exigencies already enumerated.

Many decades later operations research analysts would employ high-speed computers to handle these difficulties. In the early days, however, there was ample scope for innovation, and *Punch* noted in 1913:

Tallis' wonderful gift for organisation bore fruit in every direction. He was the date maker. He arranged the rotation of shows, and decided where productions should be put on, and in what circumstances. In this capacity he stands alone in Australia today. While he is in the country there are never overlapping productions, never audacious revivals. All goes smoothly and regularly.[5]

It is surprising that Australian theatre histories have so little to say about the New Zealand theatre industry. This is in spite of the fact that trans-Tasman theatrical tours not only became more frequent after 1880, but eventually developed into a big and lucrative business.[6] Early in 1903, Tallis raised with Williamson new initiatives for expansion.

'Did you have a good trip George?' Williamson asked when Tallis entered his office.

'Yes, thank you Mr Williamson. I rather enjoy the train trip to Sydney, it gives me time to think.' A silence followed. George looked at his boss, who appeared to have developed an interest in some papers on his desk. The ball was now clearly in the younger man's court, and he continued: 'We have often discussed building up the New Zealand touring circuit. Bert Royle is there, and Farrell will probably settle in Auckland. Couldn't we now venture more frequently, and with bigger companies, beyond our old stamping grounds? There are people hungry for entertainment outside Auckland, Wellington, Christchurch and Dunedin.'

Williamson took up the challenge. He named the theatres in the four major cities, in order Her Majesty's, the Opera House, the Royal and the Princess. 'These are all good for a two-to-four-week season, but I'm a little out of touch. Are these satisfactory houses?' he asked.

'Yes they are, and facilities at the smaller centres are improving. There are two or three towns within easy reach of Auckland, ten close to Wellington and three or four in the South Island in addition to Christchurch and Dunedin. It makes for quite a lusty tour, and the distances are nowhere near as daunting as in Australia.'

Williamson was thinking now. 'Yes, and if one town improves its theatre or hall to help attract our companies, most of the others will follow suit. It's a matter of pride.' He turned to his 1903 calendar. 'You've been a busy fellow. You are just back from an overseas trip, so what do you have in mind? Incidentally, I feel Royle is making a good fist of things in New Zealand.'

'So do I, but I think that someone else should cross the Tasman and show the flag. Bert might feel isolated, and I'd like to see him again and help with decisions he may not wish to make off his own bat. The Royal Comic Opera Company tours later in the year and I could go with them.'

Williamson looked at his recently married lieutenant. George enjoyed touring, especially with the favourite company, and the plans for expanding the New Zealand circuit needed pushing along. Tallis would be doing a lot more than chatting with Royle. Could he be spared to go? 'What will Mrs Tallis say to more long absences?'

Tallis smiled. 'We are all away too much from home and that must include you. Let's hope our wives have reconciled themselves to it. Incidentally, the last time I was in New Zealand people were asking about you, wondering if you might visit them again. It would make an attractive holiday.'

Williamson's pen was in his hand as he turned back to his business. 'All right George, have a go. It's a good idea, and if it all works out well I may take that holiday.'

Tallis toured New Zealand for part of the 1903 season. Wilson Barrett offered a considerable repertoire that included *The Sign of the Cross,* in

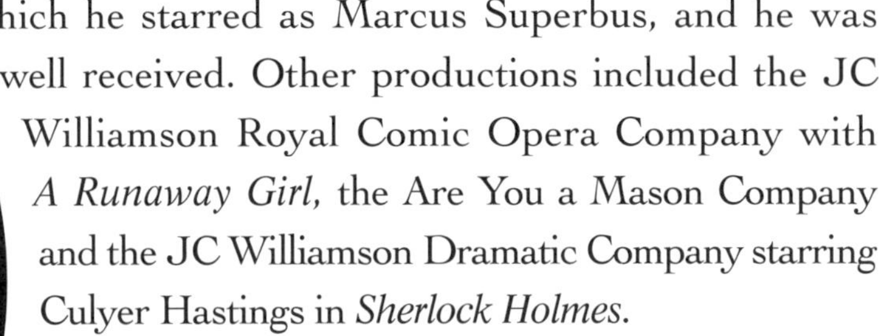

Wilson Barrett

which he starred as Marcus Superbus, and he was well received. Other productions included the JC Williamson Royal Comic Opera Company with *A Runaway Girl,* the Are You a Mason Company and the JC Williamson Dramatic Company starring Culyer Hastings in *Sherlock Holmes.*

George, working with resident Williamson representatives Bert Royle and Johnny Farrell, studied the various towns, keeping in mind the number of eager theatre-goers, ease of access and the quality of theatres. As a consequence, many country centres came on stream. From Auckland, tours began to visit Hamilton and Rotorua. From Wellington, an enlarged North Island tour circuit encompassed Masterton, Palmerston North, Wanganui, Hawera, New Plymouth, Dannevirke, Waipukurau, Hastings, Napier and Gisborne. In the South Island, Timaru, Oamaru and Invercargill now formed part of the circuit although these were not popular with Williamson companies during the winter. Wind, rain, snow, sleet and ice were common.

Only a few miles from Invercargill is the Bluff, a tiny port on the southern extremity of New Zealand. The houses nestle into the hills for protection against rogue Antarctic storms. From here the Firm occasionally loaded its touring companies onto tiny vessels for the crossing to Australia. With the prospect of mountainous seas smashing over the decks, and zealous managers urging the skippers to make better way, this was a cruel reward for tired casts after a long, hard season.

Nor were conditions in the more northern parts of New Zealand necessarily any better. Once a company was flooded at Wanganui. The men wandered the streets knee-deep in water, while the ladies floated from the hotel to the theatre in a gondola. Another time, the Are You a Mason Company encountered a land slide in the Manawatu Gorge while travelling by train. The cast had to walk up to their knees in slush through a tunnel, carrying with them all the scenery and effects.

But despite these and countless other similar experiences the vast and expanded operation in New Zealand thrived to such an extent that in 1907 JC Williamson decided to go and see for himself. This was the second of only two visits that he made across the Tasman – the first, as an actor–manager, had been in 1882 when he and Maggie Moore toured with *Struck Oil*. In 1907 he found a country vastly more developed and his own company as the premier theatrical organisation. It delighted him. At last a reliable structure for frequent and more intense touring existed, and success would be reflected in profits.

Obviously neither then nor later was the touring without problems, but in time the Williamson organisation came to favour New Zealand country tours over their Australian counterparts. It was an unusual situation, but one that was not at all difficult to explain. Said *Theatre Magazine* in 1914:

It is well known among managers that many a poor show-town has been transformed into a good one by the provision of a decent theatre. The small towns of New Zealand are, almost without exception, worth playing, because the majority of them are now provided with theatres above the average in size and comfort, both before and behind the stage. The Australian small town is generally unplayable. The average Australian is a great theatregoer, no matter where he is; but he is not going to pay to sit in a filthy, bare-walled, hard-seated, badly-ventilated hall. Small blame to him![7]

For years Williamson theatrical tours provided enhancement to the lives of New Zealanders, who were at least as isolated from world affairs as Australians. If the Firm is to be remembered as one of the great theatre companies of the world, then equally it should be remembered for its courage in setting up a giant and profitable touring program that allowed an agenda of variety and excellence to be shared across the Tasman.

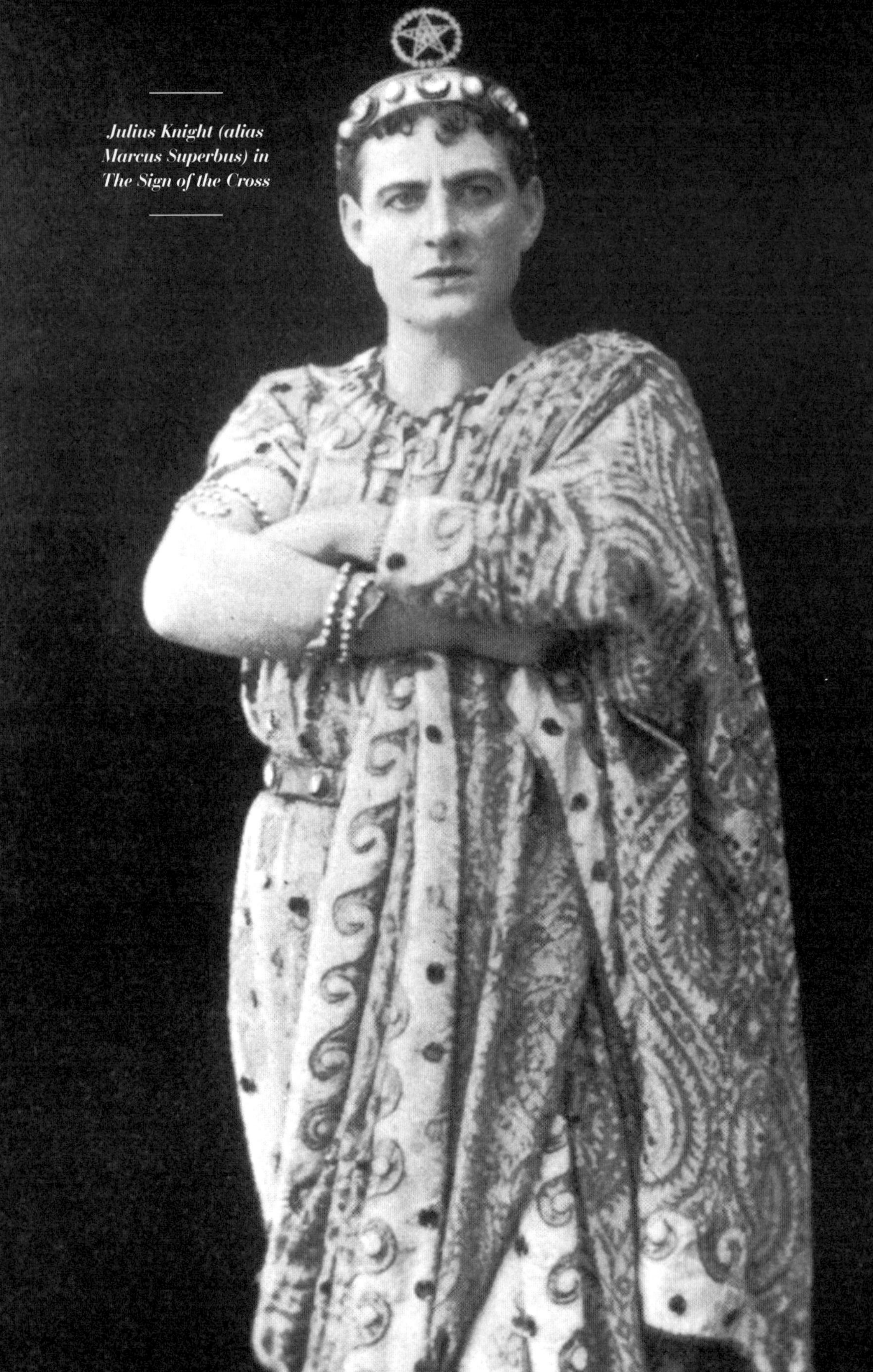

Julius Knight (alias Marcus Superbus) in The Sign of the Cross

CHAPTER SIX

Partnerships

As part of an old tradition, early theatre managers and leading performers used to stage a 'benefit' at the end of a successful season. The managers provided a theatre for an evening or a matinee session, and the stars dug deep into their repertoires for novelties to rustle up an audience just one more time. Actors and charities were the main beneficiaries of these affairs. George Tallis soon became involved in the organisation of benefits, and he must have felt the strain of making them successful, because many of the artists were his friends.

One of these was the English actor Julius Knight, who had been playing as Marcus Superbus in *The Sign of the Cross* company since 1897. *The Sign of the Cross* was a hugely successful melodrama for the Firm, playing to 250 audiences. Julius Knight was magnificent, and he began a long reign as Australia's matinee idol. He deserved a big benefit, and he got one.

But *The Sign of the Cross* was important in other ways for George Tallis and his employer JC Williamson. In the cast were their new brides, Amelia (Millie) Young and Mary Weir. This play was a high note on which the women would phase out their stage careers.

George Tallis and Amelia Young married on 8 September 1898, at St Peters Church, Melbourne. It was a small wedding. Witnesses were Millie's friend Maude Gordon and George's cousin Fred Nicholson. Millie was an actress who specialised in musical comedy and comic opera. She was from a large Melbourne family that had been badly affected by the 1893 land crash. Some of her brothers and sisters were also in the theatre, by far the most famous of them being Florence Young, known to legions of theatre-lovers as 'Flo'. She became one of Australia's most popular comic opera stars of the early twentieth century.

George Tallis

Millie, in spite of her theatrical gifts, was content to step away from an acting career in 1898 to play the role of a business manager's wife, supporting her husband at social functions, charity benefits and theatre nights.

PRINCESS THEATRE

Under the Direction of
Messrs. WILLIAMSON and MUSGROVE.

Bus. Mgr., Mr. Geo. Tallis. Treas., Mr. R. Stewart

TO-NIGHT (SATURDAY), JULY 3.
Messrs. WILLIAMSON and MUSGROVE have the honour to announce the
FIRST REPRESENTATION in MELBOURNE
of
THE SIGN OF THE CROSS,

A Remarkable Drama in Four Acts, by
WILSON BARRETT, Esq.

THE SIGN OF THE CROSS
Will be Interpreted by the following Great Cast:-
PAGANS.

Marcus Superbus .... Mr. Julius Knight
(Prefect of Rome)
Nero (Emperor of Rome) .... Mr. Caleb Porter
Tigeellinus (Counsellor to Nero). Mr. Gaston Mervale
Licinius (Aedile) .... Mr. H.J. Carvill
Glabrio { Patricians } .... Mr. W.F. Hawtrey
Philodemus { } .... Mr. Harry Hill
Metullus (a General) .... Mr. A. Lissant
Signinus .... Mr. Newton Griffiths
Servillius {(Spies and } .... Mr. J.B. Atholwood
Strabo { Informers) } .... Mr. Geo. Herron
Viturius (Captain of the Guard to Marcus) ....
.... Mr. R. Stewart
Sergius Africanus .... Mr. Grant
Berenis { (Wealthy } .... Miss Elliott Page
Dacia { Patricians) } .... Miss Linda Raymond
Poppoea (Empress of Rome) ...... Miss Nellie Mortyne
Ancaria .... Miss Florence Terriss
Cydonia (a dancer) .... Miss Mary Weir
Lesbia (a singer) .... Miss Millie Young
Daones .... Miss Alma Vaughan
Julia .... Miss Edith Russell
Cyrene .... Miss Madge Herrick
Ilione .... Miss Lucy Cobb
Zona } (Slaves) } .... Mrs. Maesmore Morris
Catin } } .... Miss Edith Sutton
Mytelene .... Miss Florence Hope
Thea .... Miss Dora D'Amele

CHRISTIANS

Mercia .... Miss Ada Ferrar
Favius .... Mr. David Glassfore
Titus .... Mr. Mario Majeroni
Melos .... Mr. Geo. Majeroni
Stephanus (a boy) .... Miss Marie Neilson
Guards, Lictors, Nobles, Slaves, Christians, &c.........
by specially-trained auxiliaries.

COMPLETE OPERA CHORUS and ORCHESTRA
Under the direction of Mr. LEON CARON

JC Williamson's wedding to *première danseuse* Mary Weir around the same time marked the end of a period of private turmoil for him. Back in 1891, celebrations at the Firm marking the conclusion of the Sarah Bernhardt season had been cut short when Maggie Moore left her husband for the actor Harry Roberts. This break-up caused Williamson at least as much professional as personal grief, because he not only lost his wife, but also control of *Struck Oil,* the show on which he had ridden to world-wide success.

After bitter and confused legal manoeuvring, Williamson failed in an attempt to gain an injunction preventing Maggie from producing the play. Over the following thirty years she starred in it until she and the play wore out. Williamson never acted in his favourite role of John Stofel again, although 'Stofel' remained the Firm's telegraphic address.

JC Williamson's second marriage was domestically more successful. Mary Williamson retired from the theatre and the couple moved to Sydney, where they settled at *Tudor,* the family home in Elizabeth Bay. This left George Tallis in charge of the Melbourne operations of the Firm, with the additional responsibility of planning for the future of his own family.

The decisions of George and Millie Tallis, and James and Mary Williamson, to pursue more (for the times) 'conventional' marriages perhaps reflects the solidifying of Australian theatre around the 1890s into a business with infrastructure beyond its principal personalities. In earlier days George Coppin and JC Williamson depended heavily for their first fortunes on their female companions' acting abilities, and Nellie Stewart – whose love and respect for her man she poignantly reveals in her autobiography *My Life's Story* – remained one of George Musgrove's prime 'assets' in his various times of sole management.

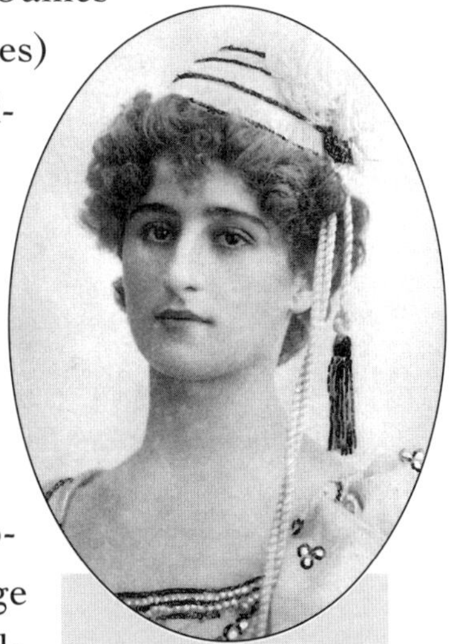

Millie Tallis

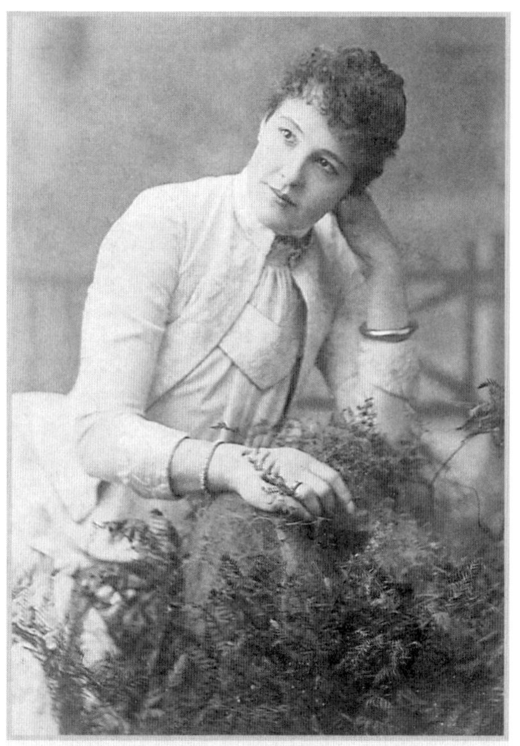

Nellie Stewart

The last decade of the century had also seen the fracturing of the Triumvirate's partnerships, and again romantic intrigues were involved. When George Musgrove left the partnership in 1890, he sailed to London with Nellie Stewart following a dispute with Williamson about her pay. Apparently Musgrove had quietly encouraged Nellie to quit the Triumvirate's employment and go into management on her own. Nellie's immediate success with her production of the operetta *Paul Jones,* and the defection of chorus members, annoyed Williamson intensely.

In 1892 Musgrove left London and again joined with Williamson, who in the meantime had bought out his other triumvir, Arthur Garner. From 1896 Musgrove spent most of his time in London and New York searching for shows to engage for Australia. In letters to Williamson he complained of difficulties that would be echoed later by the Firm's directors stationed overseas:

> *The anxiety to get material to keep theatres open is a fearful strain on the nervous system and I am heartily sick of it but I can't give up. I will not send out people I think will be failures just to keep our theatres open. You cannot from your letters have the slightest idea of the worry, work and anxiety I have getting some companies together. I'm afraid you're getting very colonial and like all people out there want impossibilities.*[1]

This was heading into the final split between Williamson and Musgrove, and it probably would not have happened had Musgrove been able to keep in more rapid communication with his partner, explaining his ideas and reasons. As it was, a major row between them was precipitated when, without consulting Williamson, Musgrove agreed to join a syndicate, to be known as Williamson and Musgrove Ltd, and leased the Shaftesbury Theatre in London.

It is easy to see the pen leaping into Williamson's hand as he wrote his reply: 'I have never been mixed up with syndicates and dealing with strangers is a very different thing to dealing with one's own partner with whose business methods one is thoroughly acquainted.'[2]

Thirty years later George Tallis would try a similar venture in London against the protests and financial fears of his partners, although Tallis, unlike Musgrove, did gain their agreement first. It is interesting to ponder how much George's London ambitions were influenced by what transpired for Musgrove at the Shaftesbury.

After initial success with a new musical comedy, *The Scarlet Feather,* Musgrove suffered losses, leaving Williamson lamenting and complaining that Musgrove should return his energies to the Firm's Australian needs. But in April 1898 Musgrove imported a show from New York that packed the Shaftesbury for two years. George Tallis tells an entertaining story in his memoirs about *The Belle of New York.* Once again, apparently, it was Nellie Stewart who unwittingly planted the seeds that hastened the dissolution of a partnership:

The story of The Belle of New York *in Australia is interesting as showing what a gamble the theatrical business can be. At that period Williamson and Musgrove were partners and George Musgrove and Nellie Stewart were in America on a three-month trip in search of suitable material for this country.* The Belle of New York *was just finalising a long and successful run at the Casino Theatre, New York. Knowing that all characters in the piece had been modelled on, or were caricatures of, famous American personalities and therefore assuming that it might be too local for Australian audiences, Musgrove postponed seeing it until his last evening in New York. At supper that night in*

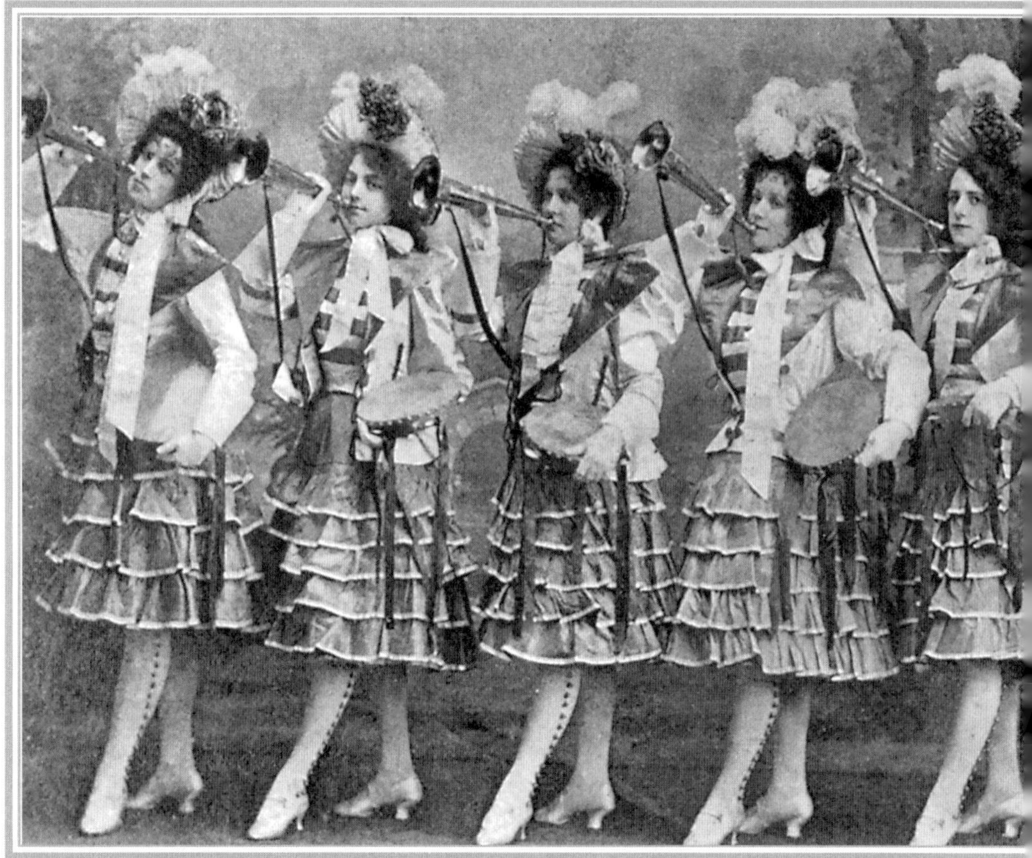

Belle of New York *chorus line*

his hotel, Nellie Stewart casually remarked, 'You know, George, I think the Belle *would have a good chance in London.' The remark said at about 1.00 am, Musgrove strolled over to the Lambs Club, where they never go to bed.*

He had to contact the Directors of the Casino, the owner of the copyright, Gustave Kerker, who wrote the music, and also the librettist. By 3.00 am terms had been debated and agreed upon. A lawyer and a couple of typists were secured and at 5.00 am Musgrove returned to his hotel with contracts in his pocket for the visit of the complete company, including Edna May, to London in a few weeks' time. Simultaneously, arrangements were also completed for the dispatch of a second Belle of New York *company to Australia.*

The success of the Belle *at the Shaftesbury Theatre London was phenomenal and overnight Edna May became the talk of the town. Unfortunately, com-*

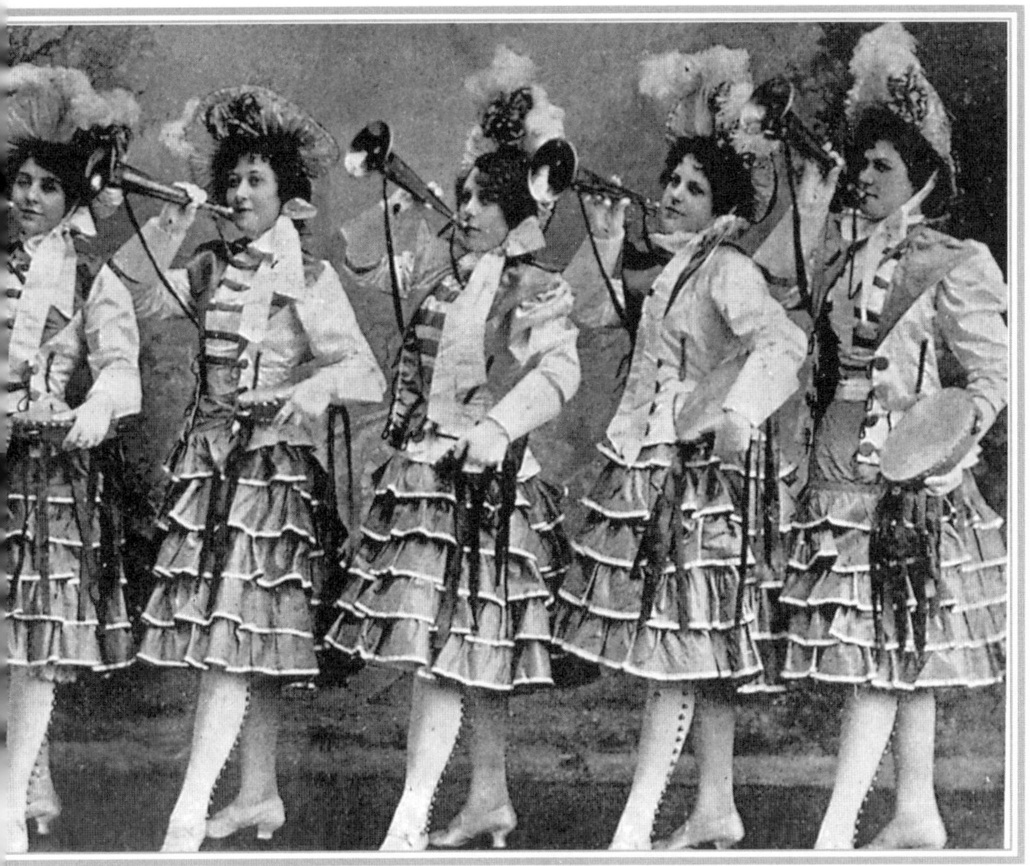

plications in connection with this engagement ensued between the two partners Williamson and Musgrove, and these led to the dissolution of the partnership.

Meantime, all the principals for the Australian company of The Belle of New York *had duly arrived in Melbourne together with a producer, Gerard Coventry, and half a dozen hefty, typical American showgirls of the period. News of its triumphant success in London had reached Melbourne and on its opening night the Princess was packed with a pleasurably excited audience. Everybody anticipated a delightful evening. Yet within a quarter of an hour after the rise of the curtain one could sense a feeling of irritation and disappointment in the behaviour of the packed gallery. Cat calls and ironic applause and laughter, a thing unheard of at the Princess, greeted the dialogue entrances and numbers and when the lady representing the Queen of Comic Opera, on making her very dramatic entrance, tripped and fell flat out on the stage, there was a roar of laughter and jeers from the gallery lasting a couple of minutes.*

This continued more or less throughout the evening until Lawton's wonderful whistling number in the second act. Here at last was something they could understand. When the curtain finally fell on a miserably despondent company everybody was convinced that the Belle *had been a colossal failure.*

And then a miracle happened. Monday's audience, though small, was appreciative, Tuesday's better still, and by Saturday evening the house was once more packed, but this time with an audience that roared with genuine laughter at the quaint humour and encored again and again the wonderful musical numbers. A brilliant success was assured and once more the Belle *had conquered a continent.*

Interestingly, George's version of the *Belle*'s success in Australia is at odds with the account given by Viola Tait in her book, *A Family of Brothers,*[3] and reiterated in Ian Dicker's biography of JC Williamson.[4] Evidently relying on a tetchy letter from Williamson to Musgrove complaining about the quality of the cast sent to Australia ('the showgirls must have been a job lot'), Dicker writes of the 'failure of the company engaged by Musgrove to play *The Belle of New York* in Australia in 1899'.

George Tallis, however, was the Firm's manager in charge of touring during the *Belle* company's Australian season. His assessment, while perhaps a little euphoric, is supported by information in the 'running order' at the end of this book. This establishes that the *Belle* opened in Melbourne on 1 April 1899 and ran for five weeks. It may not have been the blockbuster of the London version, but it certainly did not fail, and it went on to further enjoy a five-week season in Sydney. A reviewer of the first night at Her Majesty's in Sydney wrote of the *Belle*'s good reception and added 'that whatever first night misadventures the musical farce met with in Melbourne, in Sydney it is likely to "catch on" more or less in the way that it did in the city of its birth and in London'.[5] Over the next forty years the *Belle* was one of the most revived shows in the Williamson portfolio.

The Williamson–Musgrove partnership dissolved in December 1899, but wrangling ensued about the distribution of assets, and not until February 1901 were matters finally sorted out. Williamson appointed George Tallis to resolve the mess with Musgrove's old acquaintance, lawyer Theodore Fink.

As he watched old friends feuding, George may have been aware of George Coppin's comment back in 1882, the year of the Triumvirate's formation, when he predicted that friction between the partners, and the wives of the partners, could destroy their cosy agreements. As it turned out, irascibility intervened between Williamson and Musgrove, not Williamson and Garner as Coppin had thought. Coppin had also believed that Musgrove should be kept on the move, which he was, but this brought as many problems as it did solutions.

When the cashed-up Musgrove returned from England in 1900, he at first presented as a formidable rival to JC Williamson and George Tallis. He led off with a fine season of grand opera based on the English Carl Rosa company. Williamson's, stung, retaliated with popular musicals and, the following year, with its own grand opera company imported from Italy. So by Federation year, 1901, Australians had experienced an unprecedented choice of grand opera, even if it seems that the entrepreneurs lost money in their efforts to outdo each other.

In his memoirs George Tallis, an acknowledged expert in Australian opera, discussed its early days at some length:

It is difficult to accurately trace the early efforts to adequately present Italian Opera in Victoria. The names of Lyster, Madame Ristori and A Beaumont are associated with operatic ventures at the Opera House in the seventies. Likewise Martin Simonsen.

In 1887 Simonsen leased the Theatre Royal Melbourne for a venturesome season of Italian Opera with imported artists, with Simonsen himself conducting. Productions were praiseworthy but the public showed little interest and the season was disastrous financially.

A few years later in 1893, Pagliacci *and* Cavalleria Rusticana, *in conjunction with the* Blue Ballet, *were presented in an elaborate manner at the Princess Theatre, and proved a great artistic success only. Again, in 1901, another season of Italian Grand Opera was to have the same experience. In 1899, a company was carefully selected from Italy for JC Williamson by the late Signor Hazon and George Allan of Allan and Co. music publishers, Melbourne. All the principals and a number of chorus men and women together with all the costumes were imported from Milan. No expense was spared.*

One of the tenors engaged was the great Caruso, then in his teens but already with a great voice. Unfortunately at the last moment his family intervened and induced him to cancel the contract. The repertoire included La Bohème *for the first time in Australia, together with* Aida, Faust, Il Trovatore, Traviata, *and so on, yet the season resulted in a loss of 8000 pounds.*

However, audiences gradually matured, and when George Musgrove brought out an entire German company of principals for a Wagnerian season of Grand Opera in 1907, the venture was at last successful.

As his Melbourne base, Musgrove took over the Princess Theatre, in which he had a financial interest. Williamson, by now ensconced in Sydney, was left without a Melbourne headquarters. According to the Melbourne *Midnight Sun,* it was largely under George Tallis's initiative that Williamson's set about the leasing and renovation (by the architect William Pitt) of Melbourne's old Alexandra Theatre, renaming it Her Majesty's.[6] In his memoirs George Tallis plays down his own role:

Williamson took over the Alexandra, renovated and reseated it, and called it Her Majesty's; while Musgrove took a short lease of the Opera House and then settled down at the Princess.

Musgrove's first venture at The Opera House was the comic opera Paul Jones *with a great cast including Nellie Stewart and Marion Burton, and it*

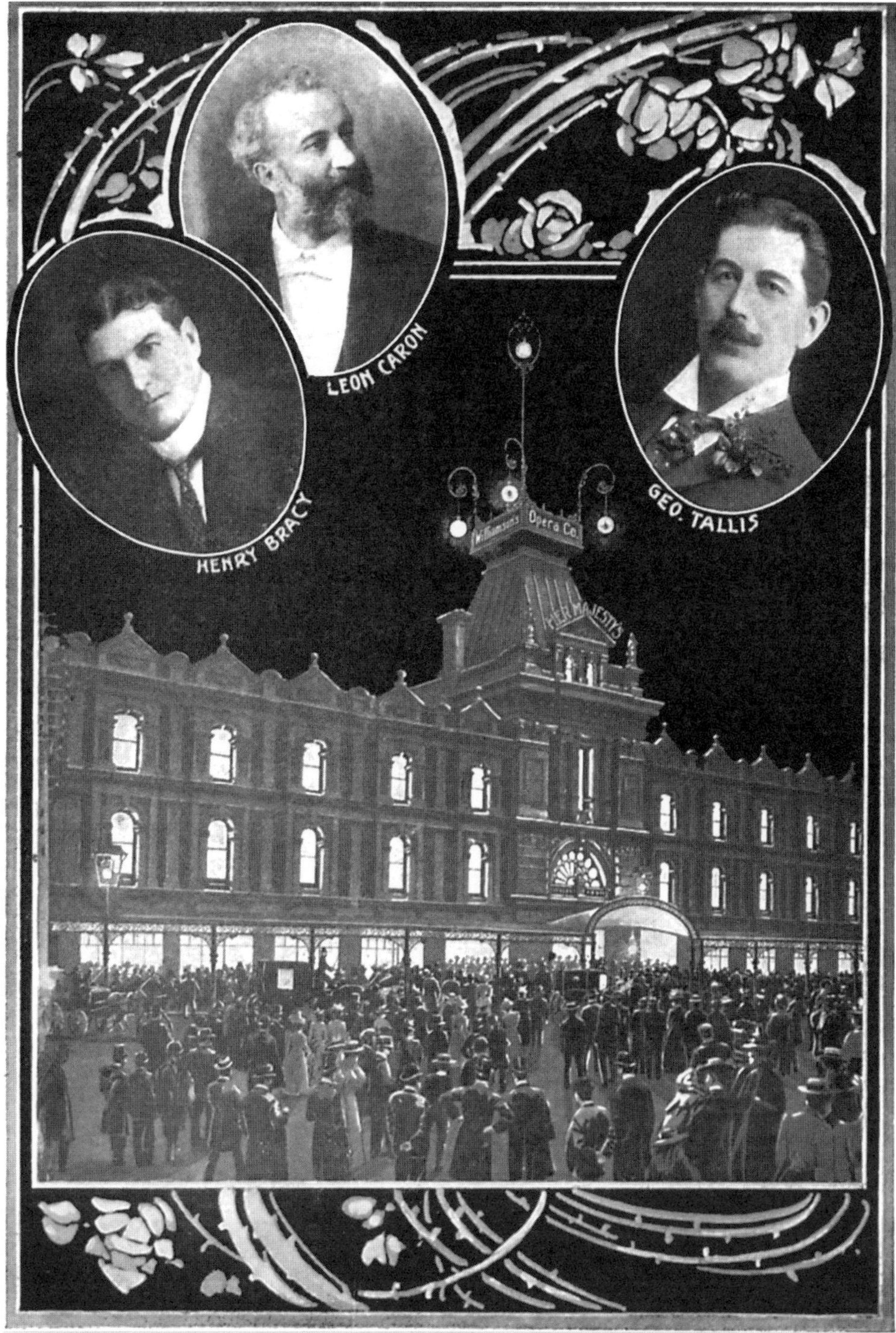

Her Majesty's Theatre, Melbourne, from the program for the 100th performance of Florodora, *28 March 1901*

achieved a record run of over 100 nights. Before very long, however, Her Majesty's became recognised as the leading theatre in Australia and it has maintained its premier position to the present day. One of its early productions was the famous Florodora, *which is supposed to have beaten all previous records. But Her Majesty's seating, 2600, was an ideal 'House for Grand Opera', and the Melba Opera Seasons (1911, 1924, 1928) at this house will long be remembered for their high standard.*

On 21 May 1900 the Melbourne *Age* praised the alterations that had transformed the old Alexandra to the new Her Majesty's Theatre:

The Alexandra in its new guise is handsomely transformed. A magician's wand had passed over the building and changed dinginess and drab into cheerfulness and harmonious colour. The gloomy exterior has been made a blaze of light, and the illumination inside gives the proportions of the house their proper effect. The cardinal architectural fault of the theatre, however, is the diminutive foyer, and the fact that access to three of the most important parts of the auditorium are all in the one vestibule, causing crowds a most uncomfortable squeeze before reaching the street.

This 'uncomfortable squeeze' must have been unacceptable, because in October the magician was called on again:

By the wave of a wand, as it were, the meanest and most cramped approaches to any theatre in Melbourne had been converted into . . . one of the roomiest and most elaborately appointed that Australian theatres can boast of.[7]

In a letter to actor–manager Bland Holt in 1899, Gustav Ramaciotti, an eventual partner of JC Williamson and George Tallis, described the effect on the Firm of the Musgrove–Williamson split. He had heard that everything was to be relocated from Melbourne to Sydney, the future headquarters of the company, and now JC Williamson's home city. Ramaciotti mentioned that, in spite of the partnership break-up, the Sydney Theatre Royal and Her Majesty's were doing brisk business for Williamson's. It was Ramaciotti's opinion that:

Of course there will be great rivalry between the two houses. Tallis will be in front at the Royal. I have my doubts as to the wisdom of running two houses – but JCW ought to know.

For the next four years George was business manager of the Sydney Royal; at the same time he remained in charge of operations in Melbourne. Overseas trips – one to Europe, and two as tour manager to New Zealand – were also somehow shoehorned into his schedule. Surely the man was overloaded!

Later *Punch* suggested that George had been offered a position by Musgrove at the time of the break, and perhaps he was tempted:

At the time Musgrove seemed to be on the top of the heap. He had made a world-wide reputation. He had scored heavily in London. It seemed as though he would be the gainer by the dissolution of partnership. Tallis was equally well appreciated by both men. He could have gone with Musgrove had he chosen; but Tallis is an acute judge of men. He had been given abundant opportunities of studying both entrepreneurs, and he knew the flaws in the Musgrove character. He decided to stay with Williamson, and, of course, he decided right, though it might be interesting to speculate how the career of George Musgrove might have been altered had he taken Tallis with him when he separated from the 'Firm'. There is no doubt that much of the success of JC Williamson has been due to . . . Tallis.[8]

With Tallis's hand firmly on the tiller, Williamson's continued to grow and prosper before the First World War. Musgrove, on the other hand, after initial successes on his own in management in Australia, died a poor man in 1916.

One of Musgrove's 'flaws' is supposed to have been his rather spendthrift ways, but another story suggests that Tallis may have been feeling that his own employer was becoming rather too conservative. He told a newspaper in 1931:

In my early days here a rising young singer, known merely as Mrs Armstrong, was touring Victoria. I have seen the playbills announcing her appearance at Ballarat – prices, 3/-, 2/-, and 1/-. It is not generally known that before she left for Europe, on the first of those trips that were to bring her fame and fortune, she promised to come back to us when she had made good. Years later [her brother-in-law] Tom Patterson brought me a cable from her. She had remembered that promise. The great Melba was ready to return. Great news, for an enthusiastic young man! That night I caught the train for Sydney, and hurried to bring the tidings to Williamson.

I found Williamson taking a leisurely midday meal at his home. He was always a great reader of newspapers, and before him on the table, when I entered, he had an early edition of the Evening News *propped against the cruet. As I poured out my story he continued to read, going on with his meal in the most deliberate way. My enthusiasm was dwindling. Then he looked up, folded his paper over, and passed it to me. His finger indicated one word, printed in large black type in an advertisement.* 'CAUTION'. *That was his verdict on the Australian tour that Melba was offering.*

Missing that engagement cost us 40,000 pounds. Melba came out, and opened her season in Sydney. She created a record by singing to a 2000 pound house on her first night. Of course, her tour was an enormous success.[9]

The pill was without doubt the more bitter for Williamson and Tallis since it was George Musgrove who secured Melba for the tour of 1902.

Yet George's decision to stay with Williamson must have been at short odds. The contact between him and his immediate boss had been on a day-to-day basis, and Musgrove had been absent overseas for nearly five years. Doubtless, in respect to taking business risks and the desire for innovation, Tallis was closer to Musgrove than he was to Williamson. When it came to business dealings, hard work and an eye for detail, however, the opposite was true.

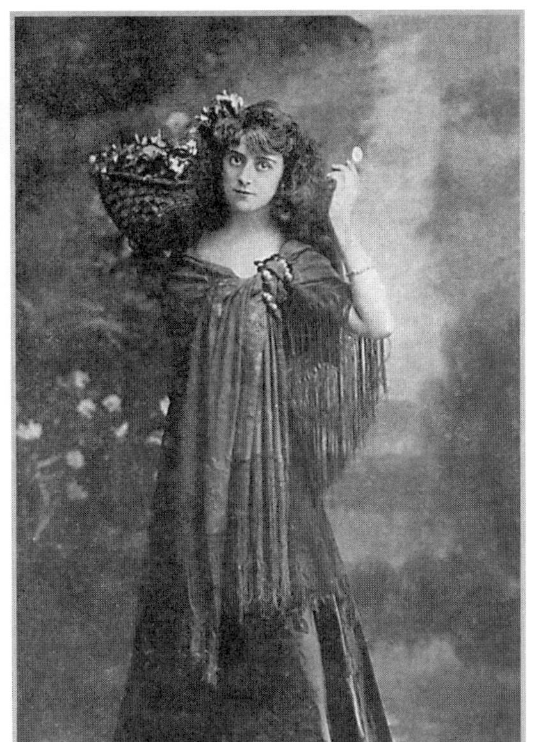

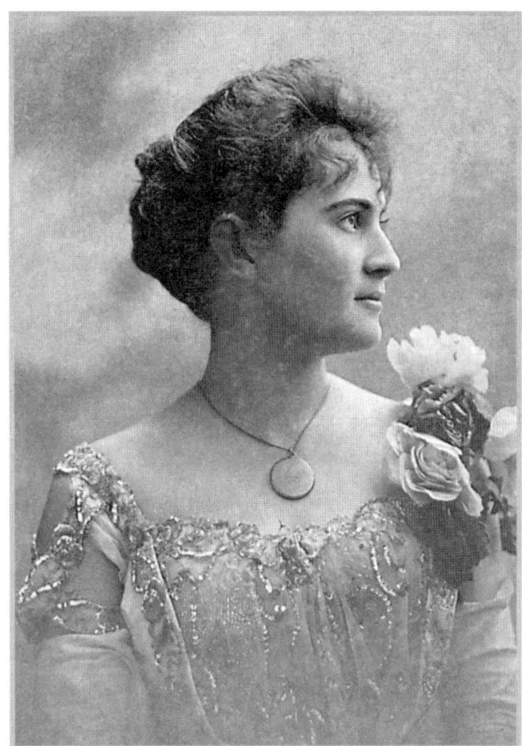

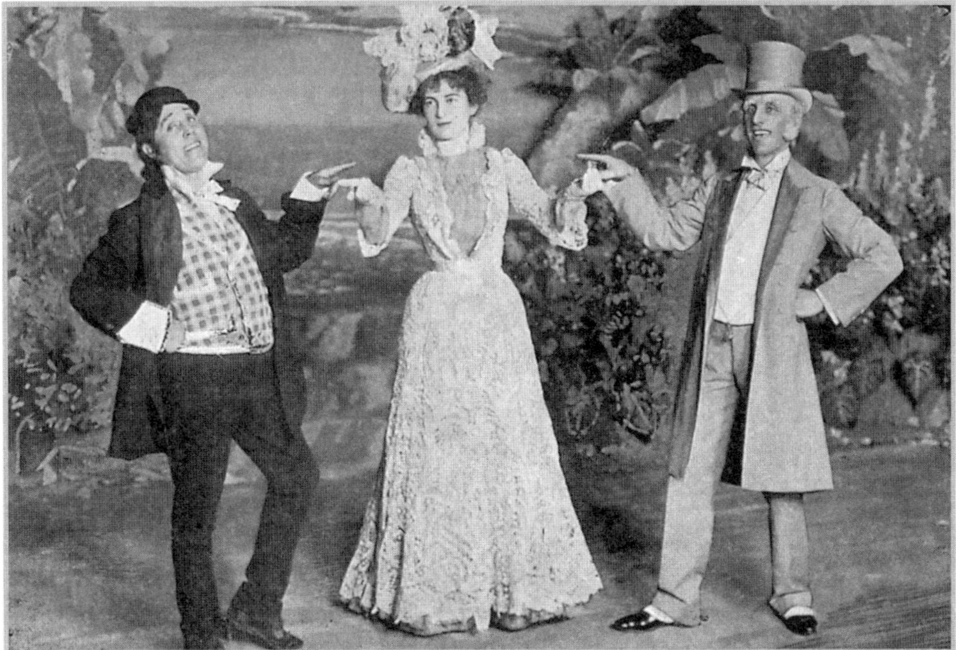

Top Left: Grace Palotta Top Right: Carrie Moore Above: George Lauri, Grace Palotta and Hugh Ward as they appeared in the 100th performance of Florodora *28 March 1901*

With Musgrove now out of the partnership, George's importance in the Williamson enterprise continued to grow. The year 1902 saw him make his first trip outside Australia or New Zealand on behalf of the Firm. He travelled part of the way with Fred Nicholson, his cousin, and his itinerary included the United States, England, Ireland and France. His brief: to buy new shows, engage actors, and investigate the new 'creature comforts' that were wooing theatre patrons in the Northern Hemisphere. Back in 1891 Sarah Bernhardt had complained about cold and drafts in Australian theatres, and she had refused a return bout on this account. In 1931 Tallis told the Melbourne *Herald*:

She found much to complain of in the discomforts of travelling between Australian cities and – whisper it! – in the Australian climate. Later we sought to engage her for a return season. Negotiations were conducted between Melbourne and France, and at last a contract arrived here for signature. Then we found that she stipulated that all theatres in which she was to perform should be heated to a temperature of 70 degrees! At that time there was no provision for heating theatres and such an installation would have meant enormous expense. We argued and protested but the temperamental Sarah stood firm. There was nothing for it but to cancel arrangements.[10]

A decade later it was time to make amends.

Landing in San Francisco, Tallis moved on to Chicago and New York. He saw two or more plays a day, and found out about theatre heating in a country where it was essential, not a luxury. New ways of selling tickets in advance intrigued him, and he inspected the modern orchestra pits. The most important innovation he found was the asbestos safety curtain that was painted as a theatrical drop. However, it was the ability to call cabs by 'electricity' that really caught his fancy.

Tallis's approach to assessing theatrical performances is revealed in his diary. At the beginning of the show he armed himself with a program, and then evaluated each actor's performance in the margin. After the performance he made notes on the content and appeal of the plot or the lyrics and music, and then he critically examined the costumes and stage settings. Finally he analysed the theatre itself – seating, comfort and the system of seat bookings. His extraordinary memory stood him in good stead when he compared New York and London productions of the same show.

Such a systematic approach to screening potential attractions for Australia was imperative. Literally dozens of shows could be viewed before a single candidate presented itself. With experience, bad ones were detected early in the performance and discarded, the selector then moving on to the next theatre. When a production showed real potential, it was marked for reassessment.

Some excerpts from Tallis's diary at this time make interesting reading:

Chicago: *Met Mr McCaull, business manager for Brady, and saw* Way Down East – *at the McVicker's Theatre, a lovely theatre (according to the letterhead the safest theatre in the world – 30 exits). Like arrangement of seats. Performance excellent, especially Collins as David and Haney as Hi Holler; not struck on Robert Gaillard as Sanderson or Archie Boyd as Squire – doing great biz.*

Saw Charles Frohman's David Harum *at Powers' Theatre – rotten.* Beauty and the Beast – *Disappointing, shabby production, comedians good especially Joe Cawthorne who was excellent. Find he has been with Alice Neilson opera co.*

New York: *Visited The Empire Theatre – Charles Frohman Manager – and saw Mr John Drew in* The Mummy and the Humming Bird – *Delightful – Splendid performance all round especially Drew as Lumley and Barrymore as Giuseppe and Margaret Dale as Lady Lumley. Marie Derickson weak.*

In New York George met Walter Jordan and America's top theatre manager, Charles Frohman, who controlled several theatres and the contracts of thirty of the leading performers of the day. Tallis was to have a long association with these two men, Jordan in the role as the Firm's American representative.

But it was time to move on:

December 6, leave for England. Sailed from New York at 10am, very cold. Ice and snow on deck. Rough passage. Arrived Queenstown Friday afternoon [12 December] and took special mail for Dublin at 6, arriving at 9 oc. Called on the Mater at 10pm, remained until 1 am.

It was the first meeting between George and his mother, Sarah, since September 1886. How might it have gone? Perhaps like this:

Good evening, Mother, you look great. No, I am not being Irish. Yes, I have grown a bit since you saw me last; no, I am not thin. Yes, I am well, and so are Millie and baby George Cassius. Why Cassius? Well, you see Mr Williamson is a Cassius. Not a good enough reason? No, I really don't miss the old home town Callan. How are Anne, Susan, Sarah, Frances, Charlotte and William? I do like my moustache – they're the going thing. Yes, Australia is far away, but I think of you all the time. I must go now, Mother. You know I will be back!

George spent a few weeks in London, and arrived in Paris on Christmas Day. He walked the boulevards, and learnt the loneliness of the itinerant theatre entrepreneur. On the train to Marseilles he felt a twinge in his good eye again. He was concerned about that eye; he had lost the sight of the other one at St Canice's Cathedral, in Kilkenny, eighteen years earlier. Some lout had pushed him on the stairs, and he had fallen on a barb. The doctor in Marseilles told him there was congestion of the nerve, and that he should take a rest. George wondered how that might be achieved.

While Millie Tallis would accompany her husband on many of his later overseas trips, she was happy to remain at home attending to their young family. George was seldom around the house and Millie bore the brunt of parenthood. In this she was no different from other wives of busy theatre men. It went with the business.

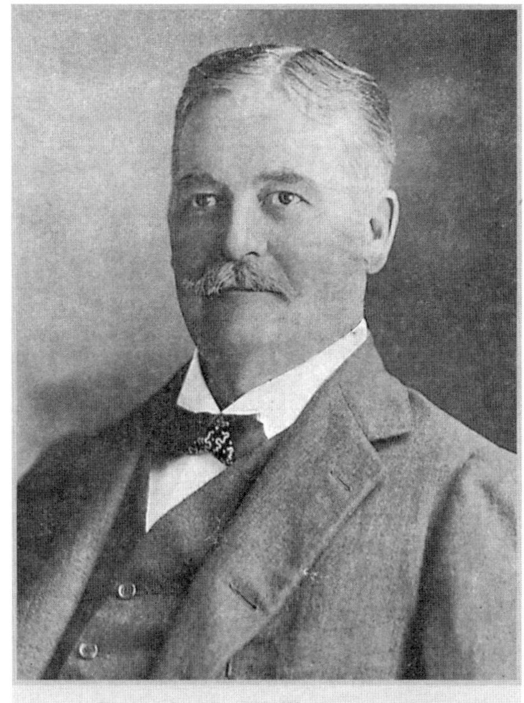
James Cassius Williamson c 1901

At first the Tallises lived in a small apartment in Melbourne, at 2 Collins Street. This was convenient while both worked in the theatre, but it was no place for more than two and they soon moved to the suburb of Camberwell. Here their first son, George Cassius (Mick), was born in 1901. Their second son, Jeffery Andrew (Pat), was born in 1904, just in time to move into the Tallises' grand new Camberwell home, *Santoi*. Two more children followed: Sunday Millicent (Bid) in 1907 and Jack Morton (Jack) in 1911. Local residents still remember the children, but their father not at all. He was rarely at home.

Perhaps this was linked with the fact that, by 1904, Williamson was tiring of managerial responsibility and, when in Australia, was enjoying home life at Elizabeth Bay in Sydney. More work therefore came the way of Tallis, who was no doubt keen to see all his effort and innovation on the Firm's behalf rewarded. He did not have long to wait.

For years Williamson had insisted that the division of his managerial interests between two widely separated cities imposed more administrative problems than he was willing to undertake. He needed two senior managers to take on the growing load in Sydney and Melbourne. On 2 July 1904, it became public that he had invited Tallis into partnership, along with Gustave Ramaciotti, popularly known as 'Colonel' Ramaciotti, whom he described as his 'legal adviser'. George he described as his 'Melbourne manager' and the two of them as 'both friends long associated with my affairs'.[11] Each bought a quarter share in the Firm, at a cost of £6250,[12] while Williamson retained fifty per cent.

Tallis's selection as one of his partners was not unexpected in theatre circles. George had come up through the ranks and had long demonstrated his suitability for a top position in the Firm. He was Williamson's second-in-command, and he was business manager in Sydney and Melbourne. Since 1895 he and Williamson had managed the Firm in Australia together. By early 1904 George had already invested in the Firm, especially the long-running Julius Knight tour in 1900 and some of the musicals presented by the Royal Comic Opera Company. A partnership would simply formalise the business relationship.

Ramaciotti's association with Williamson at this time seems largely to have been concerned with the entrepreneur's personal affairs. As managing clerk of the conveyancing department of a large Sydney legal firm, Ramaciotti advised Williamson on his private investments in Sydney. But the new partner was not without theatre experience. An inspection of his letters to Bland Holt in the late 1890s indicates that before joining the law firm Minter Simpson, he was running an agency that provided electric light plants, storage facilities and legal services to visiting theatrical companies and artists. Using the letterhead 'Electric Light Station, Theatre Royal, Sydney', he wrote to Holt that his electric light ventures were flourishing – even JC Williamson wanted particulars. At the same time he complained that he had so many irons in the fire as to make a holiday impossible. Ramaciotti had a substantial interest in the Theatre Royal from the late 1890s onward, enough to renovate it for Bland Holt and to write to him about hidden exits: 'I am making arrangements for you to escape people you don't want to see. I hope I will not be the first you will give the slip to.'

To his advantage Ramaciotti also knew many of the touring companies and individual artists, and spoke fluent Italian. Any mysteries that might have existed about his candidacy for a partnership were finally swept away by the *Sydney Morning Herald* on 2 July 1904:

Mr Williamson has refused many syndicates during past years, but on receiving a proposal of great financial advantage from two gentlemen he had esteemed for so long he thought it wiser to take the opportunity of partly releasing himself from the strenuous life.

Tallis and 'Rami' had come up with the right money!

For Tallis, the promotion was overdue, and he must have been relieved when the deal was struck. As far as Ramaciotti was concerned, he knew a sound investment when he saw one, and he turned his skills to mastering the Williamson theatre business. He and George established a lasting business and personal relationship.

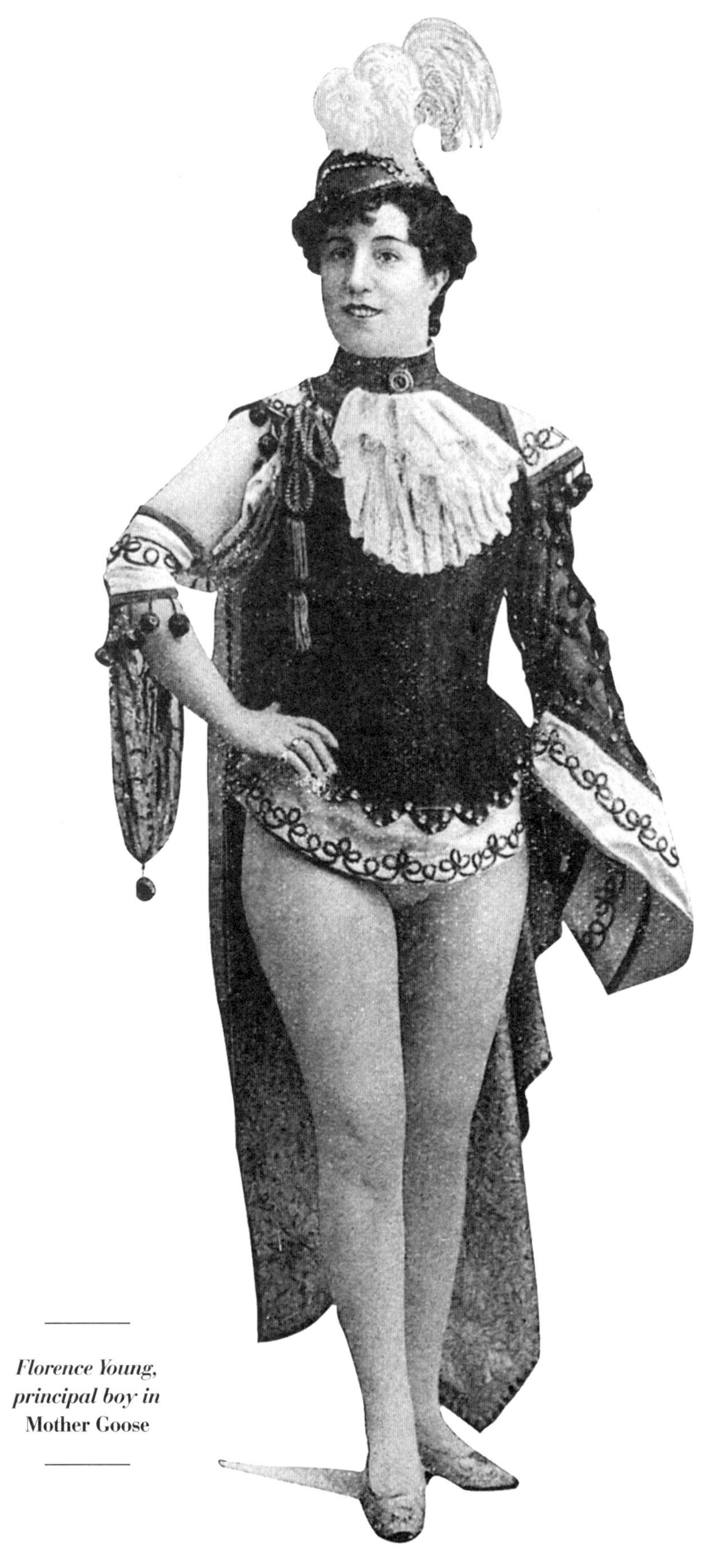

Florence Young, principal boy in Mother Goose

CHAPTER SEVEN

Very Firm

The years following the establishment of the 1904 partnership – known as Williamson, Tallis and Ramaciotti – were immensely profitable and exciting. Immediately the partners took over the management of another theatre in Melbourne – the Princess – giving the Firm full control of two theatres in that city for the first time since the Triumvirate days.

Because of Williamson's desire to retreat from day-to-day management, and Ramaciotti's lack of experience with the Firm's affairs, Tallis continued to be the administrative linchpin of the organisation. Williamson spent a large part of his time overseas during the next nine years – 'he has practically lived on steamers and trains in his many visits to America, England, and the Continent' said the *Otago Witness* in 1913[1] – leaving George and others to look after the Australian operations. Tallis did not travel internationally again until 1912.

During the era of the new partnership, it was common for the Firm to have ten to fifteen companies on tour simultaneously, and as the Melbourne *Argus* noted in 1906, George's skills and experience would have been truly put to the test in keeping all the shows on the road:

Companies now travel in a manner never dreamed of ten years ago, the most striking instance of all being provided by the record of one week in 1905.

Within seven days the Repertoire Co. started from Perth to Sydney, the Royal Comic Opera Co. travelled by special train from Sydney to Port Adelaide to catch the steamer for Perth, the Nance O'Neill Co. arrived in Sydney from San Francisco and took the train immediately for Melbourne, the Andrew Mack Co. travelled from Melbourne to Sydney, the Gilbert and Sullivan Co. from Wellington to Sydney, the Tittell Brune Co. from Melbourne to Wellington via Sydney, and the Knight–Jeffries Co. from Sydney to Brisbane. During last year the various companies covered 76,674 miles [three times around the world].[2]

The Firm managed about ten tours a year over the period 1905–1925, each of them spending around ten weeks in each of Sydney and Melbourne, and fifteen weeks in touring Brisbane, Adelaide, country centres and New Zealand. Thus, companies were out and about for thirty-five weeks, and the ten tours required some 350 weeks of management per year. Of course, these figures are averages, and they do not reflect the large, capricious, year-to-year variations. In some years the Firm handled fifteen touring companies, and in others only five or six. In any case, since one theatre requires fifty weeks of management per year, this managerial load is about the same as managing seven theatres – a convenient way of viewing the effort.

What happened to the jaded piles of old gear from the myriad of performances staged by all these touring companies? The same *Argus* article revealed that a former skating rink in Sydney was being used to store surplus wardrobe built up over twenty-five years. 'These costumes would be worth a fortune for anyone who could find a use for them,' lamented Williamson. 'In America and England managers are able to dispose of their surplus stocks for the provincial tours. Here there are no such means of recovering a portion of the initial expense.' Instead, day after day hundreds of baskets were emptied, and the contents resorted, aired and repacked with moth repellent, all in anticipation of the day when the right show would come along and justify their reuse.

A year later, a New Zealand newspaper, the *Lyttelton Times*,[3] placed a different spin on the Firm's plight. The journalist said that Williamson was ready to retire from the responsibilities of management, but that there were 'lions in the way'–the same storehouses stacked with tonnes upon tonnes of ageing scenery, wardrobes and dramatic effects. Apparently it was easier to get into successful theatrical management than it was to get out of it.

The writer in the *Argus* went on to give a fascinating insight into the employment base of the partnership. The staff at that time amounted to a large pool of temporary hired help, and 650 permanent employees of whom two hundred were actors and about one hundred musicians. Ian Bevan writes in his *History of the Theatre Royal* that the senior departmental staff included five touring managers, five orchestral conductors, four theatrical directors, two ballet mistresses, four scenic artists and four property masters. There was also a permanent wardrobe staff of eight that included four tailors, while the librarian kept track of the growing number of scripts, libretti and musical scores going back to the days of *Struck Oil*. There were in addition office staff in each of the states, and in New Zealand.

Money was mentioned in the *Argus* article. It seems that the annual running costs of the Firm were then about £200,000, and the annual profit was about £60,000. Unfortunately, we have been unable to place this partnership in the pecking order of companies of the day, and attempts to interpret the figures in modern equivalents remain unconvincing.

The partnership was responsible for consuming acres of new canvas, and miles of fresh timber for the construction of sets. Placed end to end the advertising columns in the newspapers would have also spanned miles, and the bills and posters covered acres of skyline. No matter how rubbery the figures, this was a big business, and it stimulated the general economy by its activities:

The relation of the stage to literature, to public morals, to the church are subjects of frequent discussion and controversy, its relation to the industrial life of the community is never considered ... [but] even in a population relatively small, like that of Australia, the magnitude and extent of its operations are unguessed by most of those who are excellently acquainted with it from the front of the house.

In fact, it is only necessary to consider the immense figures supplied yesterday by Mr JC Williamson to realise how much of the shilling which the playgoer pays for his amphitheatre seat is distributed again in wages to a multitude of trades. When the money has reached the treasury of the theatre the cue has come for 'Enter Omnes'.[4]

The painting of scenery and backdrops for the various productions was an art form also subject to evolution, and it was a business in its own right. Scene-painting had gone through three recent phases but the last and truly modern school of 'impressionist' scenic art allowed the artist, by means of clever lighting and paintings, to merely suggest the setting of the piece, thereby 'calling the audiences away from that world which lies just outside the theatre doors, to the one of storyland and make-belief'.[5]

No theatrical production called on storyland and make-belief more than the pantomime. In 1907, George Tallis described the economics and technicalities of staging the spectacular annual shows, while the *New Idea* journalist described how wonderful they were for audiences:

Only a child can enjoy the pantomime!

But, you object, if you look in at Her Majesty's any night after Christmas week you will see that the circle is filled with grown-ups in evening dress; rows of bald heads and wonderfully fashioned coiffures extend from the orchestra rail way back to the pit wall; up among the gods it is the same.

True, yet they're children, all children. Watch them jump when the motor party goes up in a cloud of smoke and comes down in a shower of limbs and goggles. Hear them roar when the donkey uprears himself and bites five square inches out of the policeman's trousers. That is simply the children in the men and women waking up!

Yes, the pantomime appeals to the child, whether he is four and wears velvet knickers, or forty, and sports a silk dinner jacket. That explains why we ask so much from it – and forgive so much in it. That is why we insist on a mile-long programme run off at a mile-record pace; also why we excuse the quality of the music and brevity of the skirts, provided that what there is of them both is bright and striking.

The principal boy swaggers on, and the little child says Oh-oh-oh! While the big child says 'Isn't she stunning! ... and she makes 60 or 70 pounds a week, I'm told.' In a word, the little-child sees just what is on the stage; the big-child realises that this living toy that is running for his amusement is a great and intricate machine, and that for every performer he sees in costume, there are two in shirtsleeves whom he doesn't see.

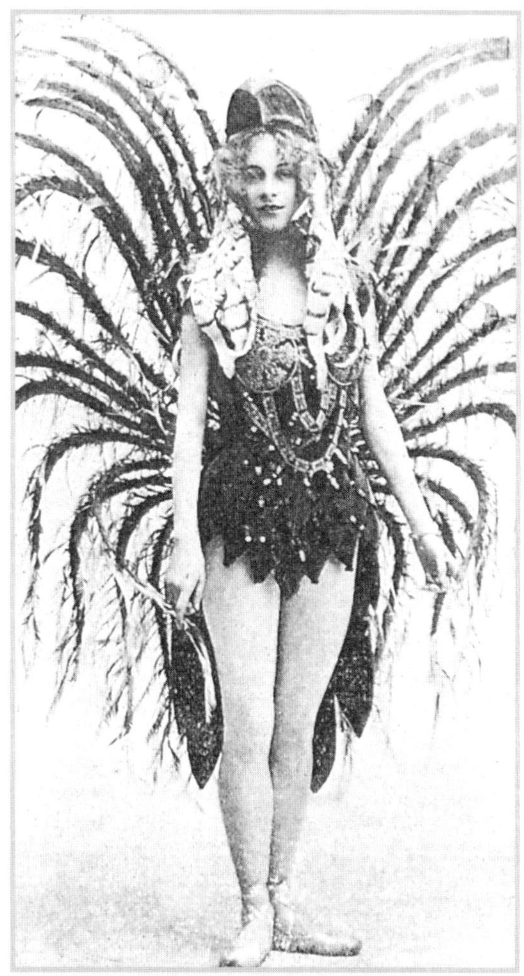

From Aladdin – *A dainty member of the Bird Ballet*

And it is a costly toy, this pantomime. 'Four thousand pounds to stage it,' says Mr Geo. Tallis.

'Four thousand pounds, without a penny of salaries or current expenses. Add to this the pay-list of property men, mechanists etc. (Something like 200 pounds a week). Weekly salaries running into four figures for the principals (two at least of whom receive bigger salaries than the Prime Minister of the Commonwealth). Add the salaries of the ballet,

the show girls, the children and the animals (ranging from 30 shillings to 5 pounds a week) and the heavy cost of lighting, advertising and so on and you will see that the booking needs to be pretty generous to make the managerial mind easy.'

How many people are employed in the pantomime? About 350 all told, including the regular working staff. The bulk of the performers are locally engaged; the stars – with several notable exceptions – are imported. Again Mr Tallis is speaking:

'Let us suppose that the subject is chosen. This by the way is not the simplest matter in the world. Dozens of books were waded through before Mother Goose *was adopted for this year. The essentials of a pantomime are fun, brilliance and startling novelty. It does not require an elaborate plot, but merely a firm line of story on which any number of specialities may be hung.*

' Mother Goose *was written by Mr J Hickory Wood, and ran at Drury Lane and at Manchester. As soon as the script arrived here it was localised, all the foreign jokes being lifted out and replaced by local ones ... The script ready, Mr Williamson at once calls the heads of departments together and scene after scene is thoroughly discussed and mapped out.*

'Then the whole thing is prepared in miniature. The scenic artists draw to scale tiny models of the scenes from which the property master, the mechanists, carpenters and painters will make the fairy palaces, the marvellous forests and the thundering waterfalls. The costume artist makes sketches, and passes them to the costumier, who fashions sample dresses. The property master also draws to scale the animals, the birds, the fairy paraphernalia, the hundred and one accessories.

'So much for the setting. Next comes the cast. Mr Williamson's agents secure the necessary talent from abroad, England and America being scoured for specialists, many of whom have to be engaged a long time ahead.

'Quite six months before the curtain went up on the first performance of Mother Goose *the work of selection of the local talent had begun in all parts of Australia. In the principal theatres of Melbourne and Sydney an hour on*

each Tuesday (between one and two) is set apart for the trying of voices, and in giving audience to any specialities that may come along. The difficulties encountered in obtaining just the right class of material may be gauged from the fact that for every ten finally selected a thousand have been tried.

'The children belong entirely to the department of the ballet mistress, Miss Jennie Brenan, and are selected mainly from her classes . . . The ballet also is

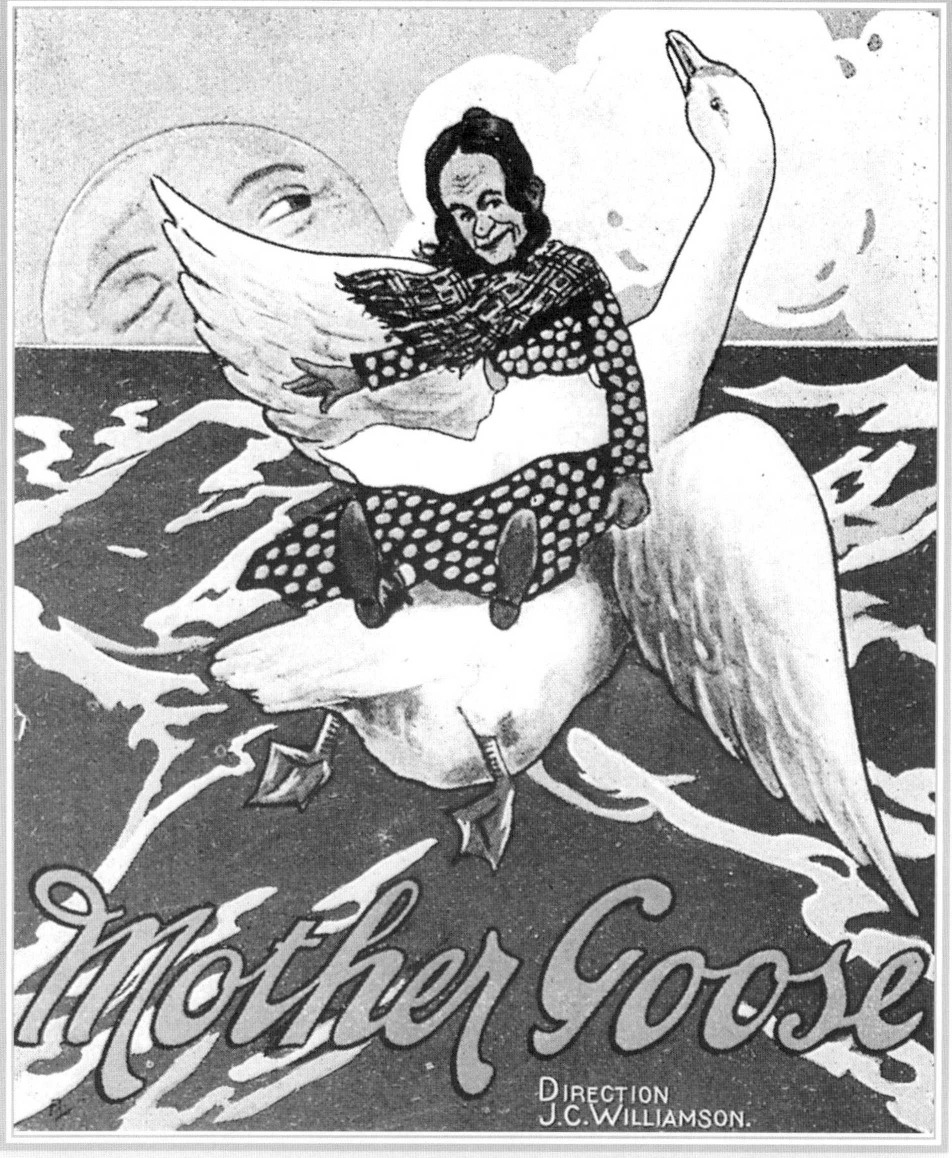

Up, up and away with Mother Goose

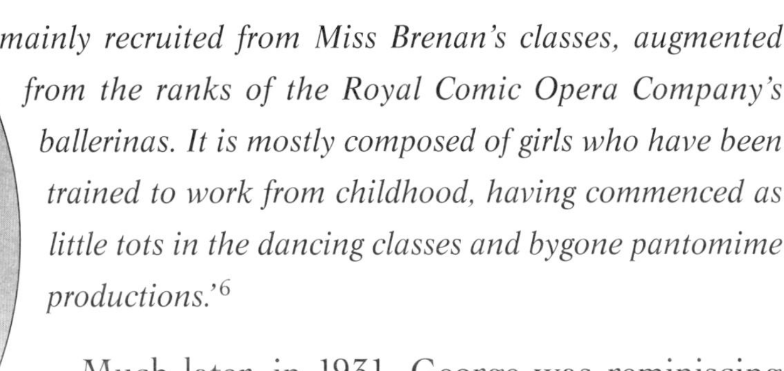

Jennie Brenan

mainly recruited from Miss Brenan's classes, augmented from the ranks of the Royal Comic Opera Company's ballerinas. It is mostly composed of girls who have been trained to work from childhood, having commenced as little tots in the dancing classes and bygone pantomime productions.'[6]

Much later, in 1931, George was reminiscing about pantomimes. One stood head and shoulders above the rest. It was *Mother Goose*. Not only had this pantomime delighted the older children and thrilled the younger ones, it had also made the 'managerial mind' very 'easy' indeed – by returning vast profits.

Dancing was a vital component of the Royal Comic Opera Company productions, as so vividly described by Edward Pask in his book *Enter the Colonies Dancing*. Starting in 1888, Marie Reddall, followed a few years later by Madame Rosalie Phillipini, developed ballet within the company to a strength of one hundred dancers known as the 'Royal Ballerinas'. An advertisement in the Melbourne newspapers read:

To young ladies desirous of acquiring a knowledge of the art of dancing according to the latest European methods, an opportunity will be afforded for free tuition in classes under the direction of Madame Rosalie Phillipini ... Apply Princess Theatre, Spring Street.

When the Firm brought the Grand Italian Opera Company to Australia in 1893, each night's performance was followed by the classical ballet *Turquoisette* (*Blue Ballet*) performed as a collaboration between the Royal Ballerinas and internationally acclaimed stars. Madame Phillipini was responsible for many wonderful and very successful ballets while working for Williamson's. She was especially

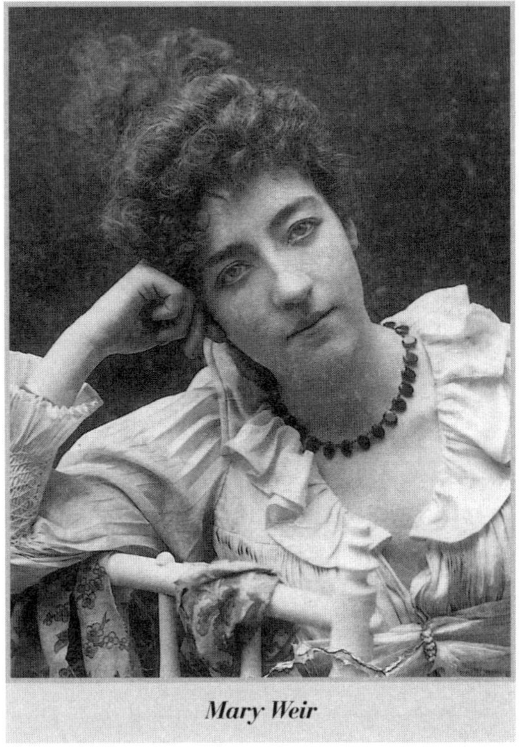
Mary Weir

remembered for the choreography in *Djin Djin* in 1895 in which Mary Weir, later to become the second Mrs Williamson, was the *première danseuse.*

At the turn of the century, other dancers were rising through the ranks to carry on the tradition set by their talented predecessors. Over a period of thirty years, Minnie Everett was for the Firm in turn *première danseuse,* choreographer and stage producer. Around the same time, Jennie Brenan was given the opportunity to further her training overseas with Alexandre Genée. She returned to a career as ballet choreographer to both JC Williamson and George Musgrove, and in this role created for Williamson's the ballets for the *Mother Goose* pantomime in 1906.

It is sobering to remember how this mighty firm was financed. Of course it hinged on the shows themselves, and their attraction to the public. There was a fine line between fortune and bankruptcy. As the *Otago Witness* put it:

Every play that has a prospect of pleasing audiences is purchased. The operations involve big finance and big risks. Probably in Australia there is no business, save horse racing, that is so speculative or more nerve-wracking. These are matters the playgoer never dwells upon, but it is just as well that he should know once in a while what elaborate machinery is employed in his service.[7]

The success of the Williamson–Tallis formula of giving the people what they wanted was demonstrated by the survival of the Firm.

Other entrepreneurs had come and gone trying to educate a seemingly unreceptive public in the ways of serious theatre. Planning for the long term was the only way forward for the partnership, allowing it from time to time to dabble in productions of enlightenment. JC Williamson, in his last Australian interview in 1913, pointed out that although he was not against the modern plays which used theatre as a forum for 'frank discussions of unpleasant subjects':

That would call for special ability and special audiences. The special ability is hard to find, and the special audiences are harder ... there is nothing I would like better than to satisfy, with discretion in selection of material, the so-called demand of the public in this. The season would probably last just as long as I cared to spend my money.[8]

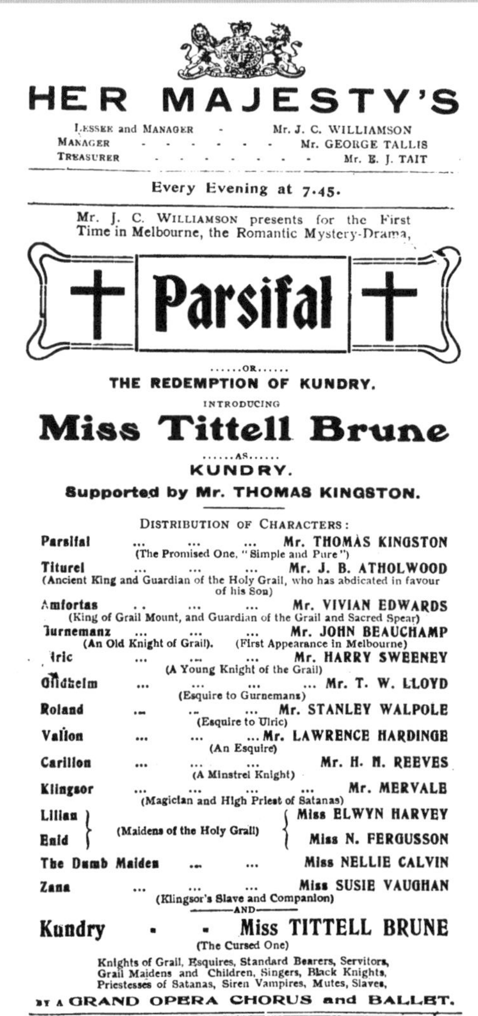
HER MAJESTY'S

LESSEE and MANAGER - Mr. J. C. WILLIAMSON
MANAGER - - - - - - - Mr. GEORGE TALLIS
TREASURER - - - - - - - - Mr. E. J. TAIT

Every Evening at 7.45.

Mr. J. C. WILLIAMSON presents for the First Time in Melbourne, the Romantic Mystery-Drama,

Parsifal

......OR......

THE REDEMPTION OF KUNDRY.

INTRODUCING

Miss Tittell Brune

......AS......

KUNDRY.

Supported by Mr. THOMAS KINGSTON.

DISTRIBUTION OF CHARACTERS:

Parsifal ... ... Mr. THOMAS KINGSTON
(The Promised One, "Simple and Pure")
Titurel ... ... Mr. J. B. ATHOLWOOD
(Ancient King and Guardian of the Holy Grail, who has abdicated in favour of his Son)
Amfortas .. .. Mr. VIVIAN EDWARDS
(King of Grail Mount, and Guardian of the Grail and Sacred Spear)
Gurnemanz ... ... Mr. JOHN BEAUCHAMP
(An Old Knight of Grail). (First Appearance in Melbourne)
Ulric ... ... Mr. HARRY SWEENEY
(A Young Knight of the Grail)
[illegible]dhelm ... ... Mr. T. W. LLOYD
(Esquire to Gurnemanz)
Roland ... ... Mr. STANLEY WALPOLE
(Esquire to Ulric)
Vallon ... ... Mr. LAWRENCE HARDINGE
(An Esquire)
Carillon ... ... Mr. H. H. REEVES
(A Minstrel Knight)
Klingsor ... ... Mr. MERVALE
(Magician and High Priest of Satanas)
Lilian } (Maidens of the Holy Grail) { Miss ELWYN HARVEY
Enid } { Miss N. FERGUSSON
The Dumb Maiden ... ... Miss NELLIE CALVIN
Zana ... ... Miss SUSIE VAUGHAN
(Klingsor's Slave and Companion)

AND

Kundry - - Miss TITTELL BRUNE
(The Cursed One)

Knights of Grail, Esquires, Standard Bearers, Servitors, Grail Maidens and Children, Singers, Black Knights, Priestesses of Satanas, Siren Vampires, Mutes, Slaves,

BY A GRAND OPERA CHORUS and BALLET.

In voicing these views, Williamson was stating the policy of his firm long into the future. Succeeding managements tended to shun avant-garde plays, for the same financial reasons.

But the new partnership was not averse to taking risks, especially when it came to producing the most spectacular and novel shows. On 22 December 1906 Williamson, Tallis and Ramaciotti took a bold step. An entirely Australian drama, *Parsifal* – written by Reverend Hillhouse Taylor and following the Wagnerian story in spirit – was produced at the recently rebuilt

Her Majesty's Theatre in Sydney. Williamson's reached deep into their special-effects bag, and came up with one of the most dramatic productions the Australian stage had seen. It surpassed even the visual impact of the lifesaving pantomime *Djin Djin* a decade earlier. In the final act, amid the flashing of lightning, the roaring of thunder, the heavens caved in and the world imploded, leaving only shattered columns, broken arches, Kundry and Parsifal.

Kundry, the leading role, was taken by the American actress Minnie Tittell Brune, and the Williamson partnership was praised for its courage in producing an untried local play. Yet the critics were divided. The *Age* described it as a most notable play full of 'mysticism and symbolism'. The *Argus* judged it as tangled and confused, but full of 'elaborate mechanical marvels'. Melbourne *Punch* believed the play displayed 'hypocrisy'. *Table Talk* described it as 'old fashioned' and 'quite out of keeping for a modern age'.[9]

Management stress in the theatre business came in various forms. Tour managers suffered, but there was plenty of drama left for the non-itinerant staff.

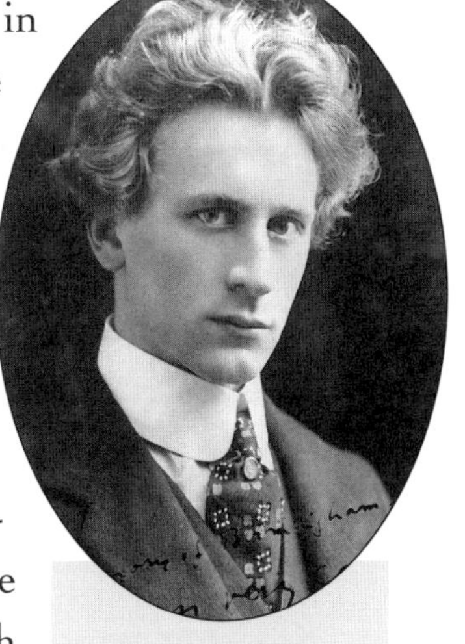

Percy Grainger

In 1908 the Australian pianist and composer Percy Grainger toured as part of the Ada Crossley company. Grainger was an especially difficult artist to manage. According to Percy himself, he was a shy, peaceable fellow!

The trouble may have started with the newspaper advertisements of his recitals. When the morning 'rags' arrived, he opened them with the pleasurable anticipation of seeing his name in blazing, black print. Not so! Percy Grainger was dwarfed by JC WILLIAMSON presents and, presto, the first walkout. But Percy prevailed, and he was moved to write, 'I have won, and not against one Australian. JC Williamson is Irish-American, Henry Bracy (an ex-tenor turned Williamson producer) is English and Tallis is a bloody Irishman.'

Matters went from bad to worse. In Sydney, Grainger had fallen in love with a three-pedal Steinway grand. But, by some appalling piece of mismanagement, what he referred to as the 'rotten Melbourne piano' went on the tour instead. Percy brutally kicked its pedals and thumped its keys at his recitals until he finally reached Melbourne. There, the pianist developed a full head of steam, raced to Her Majesty's Theatre and burst into Tallis's office. George was at his desk. He rose politely, and just managed, 'Do come in Percy, how nice to see you,' before Grainger vaporised.

When it was over, and the fuming pianist had stormed out of the building, George sat down and drew a deep breath. An order to immediately load the Steinway onto the train from Sydney had already been given. For a fleeting moment a fire flickered in his body, and then it died. He pulled out Grainger's card. Beside 'Percy Grainger, Concert Pianist' he added the note 'somewhat temperamental', and returned the card to the file.

A few weeks later, the subject of Percy's fee came up. It seemed too high for the amount of managing he required and news was sent to Adelaide that the services of Grainger were no longer required by the Firm. But the pianist had already gone. He was in Kalgoorlie attending to the cultural needs of the miners and their partners!

A perfectionist was needed to run a conglomerate such as Williamson's. In his book, *It Don't Seem a Day Too Much,* Claude Kingston, who joined the Firm in 1921 as a manager of celebrities, said that George Tallis was just the man:

He had come into the Firm and learnt his trade under JC Williamson; as well as that he was born with a streak of theatrical genius – a blend of creative perception, visual imagination, good taste, intuition, and courage.

To George Tallis, that quietly spoken, solidly built, well-groomed man of the world, near enough was never good enough. He was a perfectionist, everything had to be exactly right from the leading lady's gowns down to the lace of the youngest ballet girl's shoe. Watching a rehearsal, he would decide that the dresses of the chorus were unsatisfactory in some seemingly insignificant detail – perhaps the shade of the sashes or the length of the skirt.

'Scrap the lot', he would order.

When it came to a question of excellence or money Tallis never counted the cost. Excellence won every time.[10]

Tallis's presence was magnified as Williamson faded from the scene. How well was he suited to the cut and thrust of theatre management? With its customary lack of restraint, Melbourne *Punch* described the man in action:

And then [Tallis's] manner! He can vary it at will, with an ease that politicians envy and emulate, but fail to attain. To the public – the pleasant public – it is silky, genial and bland; but for the public which has to be rebuffed there is a curt iceberg manner which is insurmountable. To his refusals there are no answers, his 'no' serve is impenetrable. His long experience in the management of theatricals has made him a past master at the art.

When an hysterical lady star some months ago took umbrage at the stage manager's objection to her habits of arriving late for rehearsal, and threw herself a kicking, screaming mass of embroidery on the floor, it was Mr Tallis whom everybody rushed for. And it was Mr Tallis who persuaded the lady to forgive – temporarily at least – that 'dreadful man' who managed the stage, and thereby saved the show from collapse.

But when there is a reprimand to be administered, the delinquents march into Tallis's office in fear and trembling, for the velvet manner conceals a steel determination and his reproofs are things to be remembered. He knows the exact spot at which to apply the blister, and does it with an unwavering hand.[11]

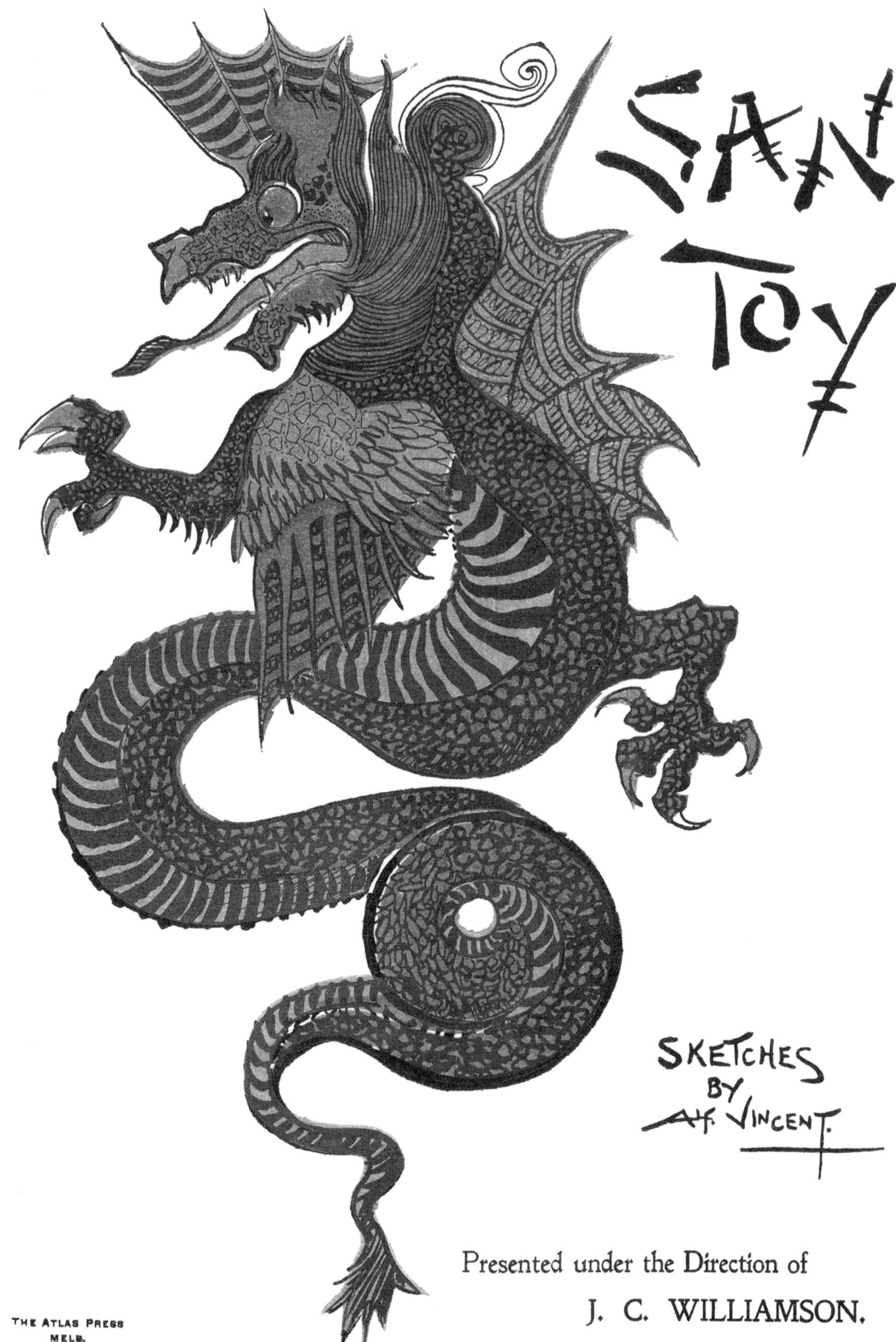

Presented under the Direction of

J. C. WILLIAMSON.

THE ATLAS PRESS
MELB.

CHAPTER EIGHT

Santoi George

Tallis was also expanding financially. By 1900 JC Williamson was once more on his own and George, even before he was invited to become a partner, had invested in the various productions. Syndicates were formed to underwrite the expenses of touring the larger companies, and he punted on those he fancied. He collected handsomely when the musical *San Toy* came in as a brilliant success, and as a mark of gratitude to the operetta, and as a concession to copyright laws, the Tallises named their first real home *Santoi*. By 1904, then, George owned the large house of his boyhood ambitions, and motor cars as well, while in the background the new junior of the Firm, Ted Tait, referred to him as 'Santoi George'.

Australia was growing and developing quickly. Choice real estate returned to favour after the 1890s crash, and so did the large commercial businesses in retail, engineering and mining. Despite the short-term roller-coaster rides of stock and property markets, the direction was ever skyward, and George was a passenger.

This last point was noted by the banks. George negotiated a large amount of business on behalf of the Williamson theatre enterprises, and his own investment requirements were growing. Impressed with his strong grasp of business issues, the managers of the leading banks in Melbourne received him well. They wove the first strands in a web of friendly contacts that were to extend throughout the city's business community. And according to the journalists, George's appearance and demeanour would surely have turned the heads of his bankers and business acquaintances:

The modern man – in Australia especially – seeks comfort rather than respectability: but if he is one who stands in the public eye he must beware how he seeks it. George Tallis grasped early the fact that respect for the well-dressed man is more than that for the man whose clothes fit him badly, or who is careless about his dress.

The average Irishman, while he delights in fine clothes, is utterly careless in his actual appearance. Tallis is not; his dressing is part of the day's work – a matter to be treated seriously and soberly. Therefore as with everything else, he takes pains with his appearance; his clothes are the latest in cut, the most perfect in fit. His neck-tie is a study, harmonising with the rest of his garb. He is point device in his equipment; his hair, his moustache, his watch chain, his boots, all play a part in the general effect, and help to make him what he is – the best dressed theatrical manager in Melbourne.[1]

George's commercial interests outside the theatre – real estate and equity investments – became as important to him as those directly concerned within it. For instance, as an ironical twist to his job interview of 1886 with Dr Cunningham, chief executive officer of Melbourne's *Argus* newspaper, George ultimately became joint owner of the Argus building as part of a widely diversified real estate portfolio.

By reputation, he had become one of the most astute business men in Melbourne. And it could not all be attributed to coincidence. George was a great listener. He knew who to consult on any investment opportunity that attracted him and he sought their opinions. A chance meeting would occur, and a friendly luncheon ensue. Half way through the *Poisson du Jour,* and significantly into the third glass of dry white, George would say that he was 'depressed' about the

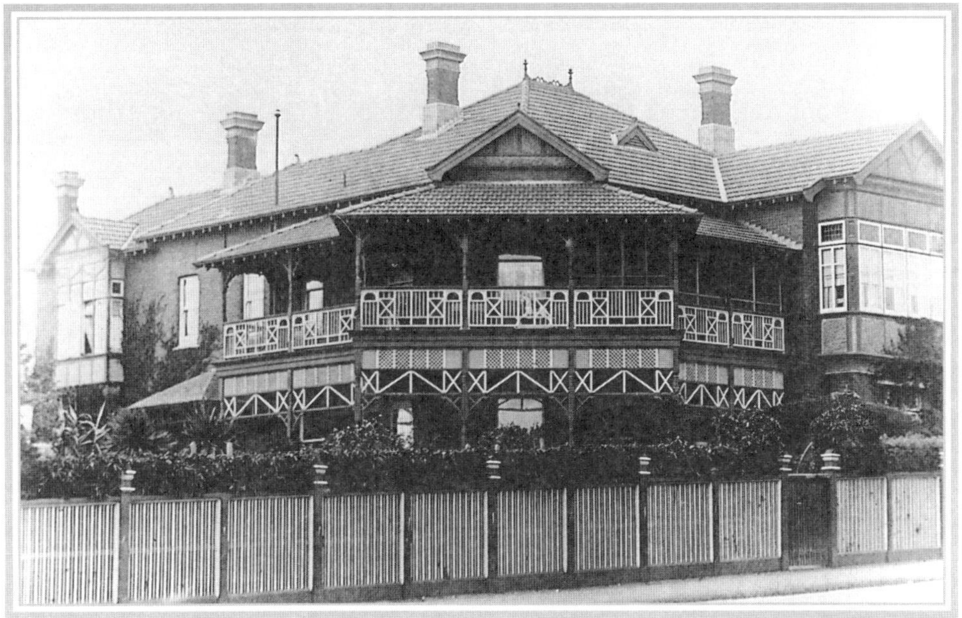

Santoi, ***1904–1920***

property market. This would bring a loud retort from his guest, a land expert, who was simultaneously trying to do justice to his profession and his fish. Both men left the table after an excellent meal, a robust exchange of ideas and favours, and an enhanced friendship. George would store the information until, by chance, he ran into another 'land man' of equal stature. When he had gathered the opinions of enough experts, he considered, and then carefully arranged to be in the right place, at the right time.

The purchase of the Melbourne Her Majesty's Theatre is a case in point. Real estate agents advertised the theatre in August 1914, just as the First World War broke out. The agents became nervous and moved to withdraw the property from sale. This was bad thinking. Any sign of a white feather would render the property unsaleable. So the billboards went up.

Tallis discussed the purchase with a realtor friend. 'I've got the wind up. The world looks shaky. Would you buy this theatre if you were me?'

The friend was an optimist and a counter-cyclical investor. 'If you don't buy it now, you may not get the chance again later on. Anyway, we are a long way from Germany, and if they ever come here they will wonder why they bothered.'

'Good advice,' said George.

Both knew that this charade only reinforced a decision already made. Her Majesty's went to the Firm for £35,000, and within a few years its value had quadrupled.[2]

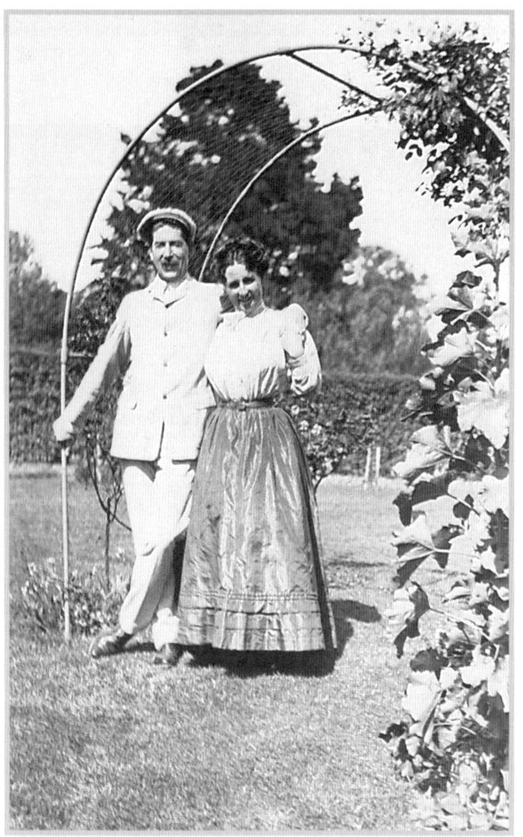

George and Millie in the garden at Santoi

The Tallis home, *Santoi,* was on the top of the hill at 17 Prospect Hill Road, Camberwell. It was a two-storeyed, Federation-style house with wide balconies, and it provided all that a growing family could wish for, and more. Among the less likely, but nevertheless legal residents were three wallabies, one kangaroo and two emus, all properly registered under the Game Act of 1896. The animals would escape from time to time, and join the passing traffic in Prospect Hill Road. They paced the cars up the slope, then tried to board for the downhill run. The amateur drivers, who were already fully occupied, failed to appreciate the *Santoi* escort.

Memories of those years are sketchy. A cyprus hedge separated *Santoi* from *Pottlerath,* the house George had built for his cousin Fred Nicholson, and named after the farm of their grandparents in County Kilkenny. Fred and his wife Delia had no children of their own, but they watched over the four Tallis children when George and Millie were away – there was a convenient access through the hedge. The children remembered long walks to the violet farms of Burwood, and foot races up and down Prospect Hill Road. For the two youngest, school was at Milverton, almost next door to *Santoi*. The two older boys went to Camberwell Grammar School, where they earned their nicknames, Pat and Mick, in the school playground. High from the balconies, flags flew on Armistice Day in 1918, when guns finally fell silent on the distant battlefields of Europe. These flags nearly marked the end of *Santoi* itself; the house was razed shortly after.

The *Santoi* days lie wedged between Melbourne's casual, colonial past and the time of its stiff urbanisation. There was a delightful informality about living in an outer suburb in 1904; the laws, by-laws and

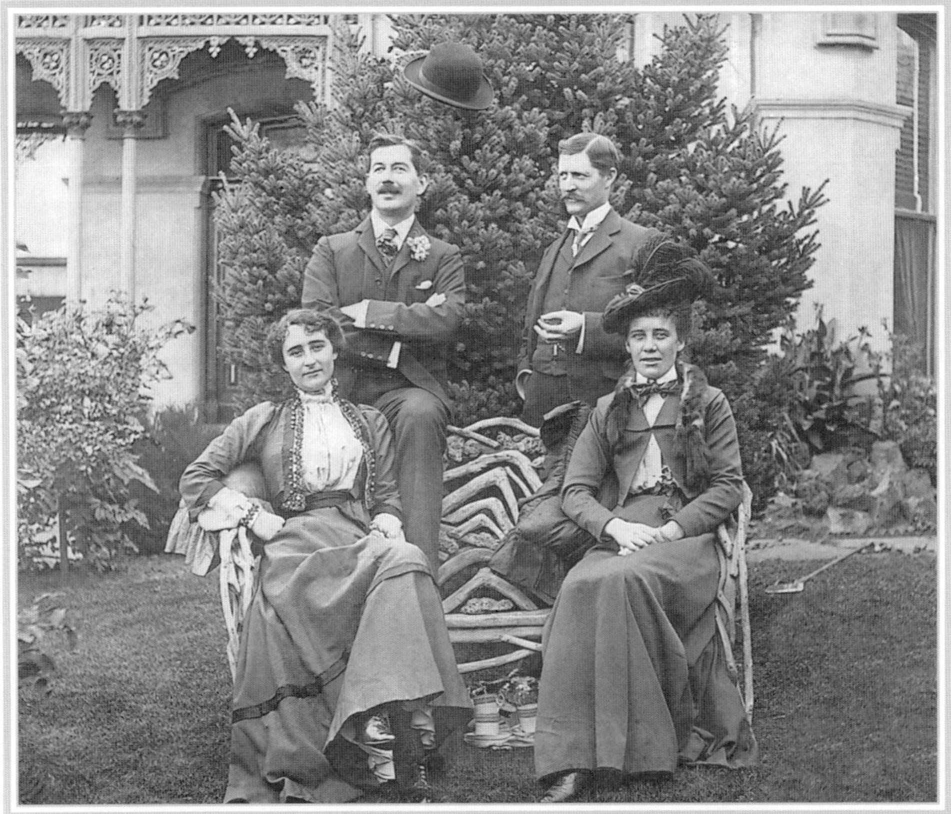

George and Millie Tallis and Fred and Delia Nicholson

bureaucracies were yet to come. Driving a car was exciting stuff, and a few kangaroos and emus only added authenticity to the experience. It was an age of mechanical innocence: litigation, black weekends and mounting death tolls belonged to the future. Those precious *Santoi* days remained among the happiest for the Tallis family.

They certainly were for George. His life was full of new challenge and responsibility. In the same year that he acquired *Santoi*, his hard work had been rewarded in the form of the partnership with Williamson. The future looked bright, and he welcomed it.

Innovation was the spice of life for George Tallis. When eventually the car displaced the horse and buggy, he *had* to participate and

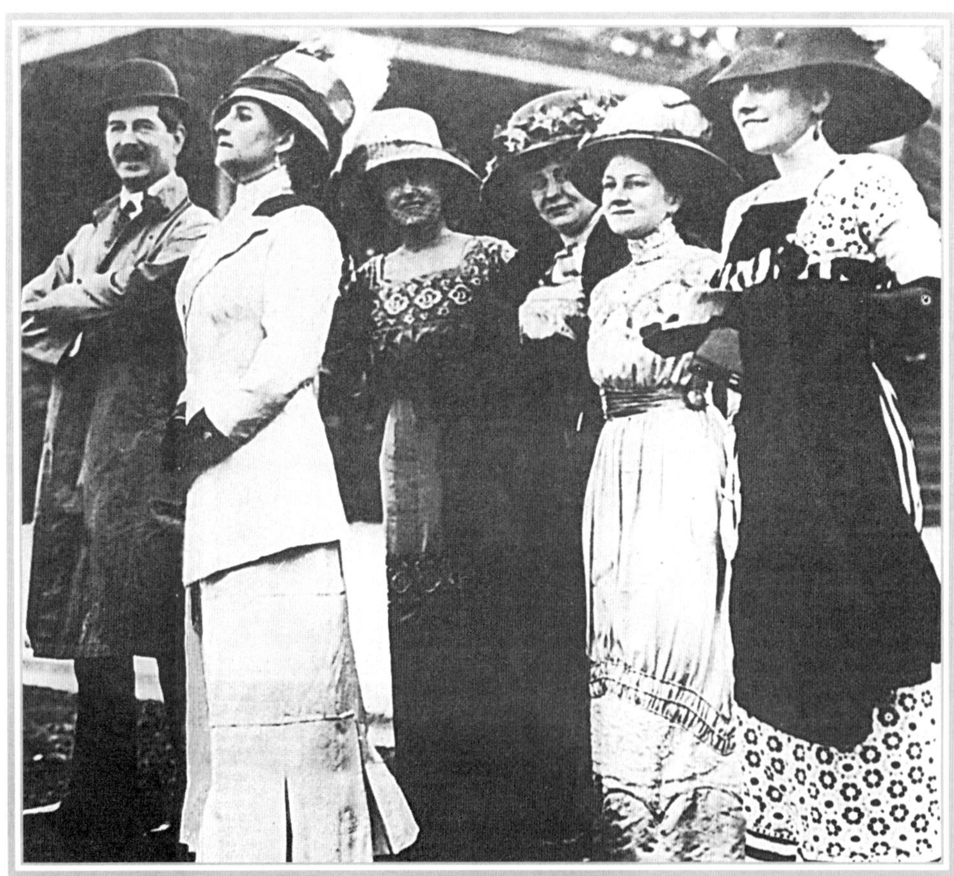

George with Millie and friends at the 1909 Melbourne Cup

an unpublished article written in 1905 describes his early response to the horseless carriage:

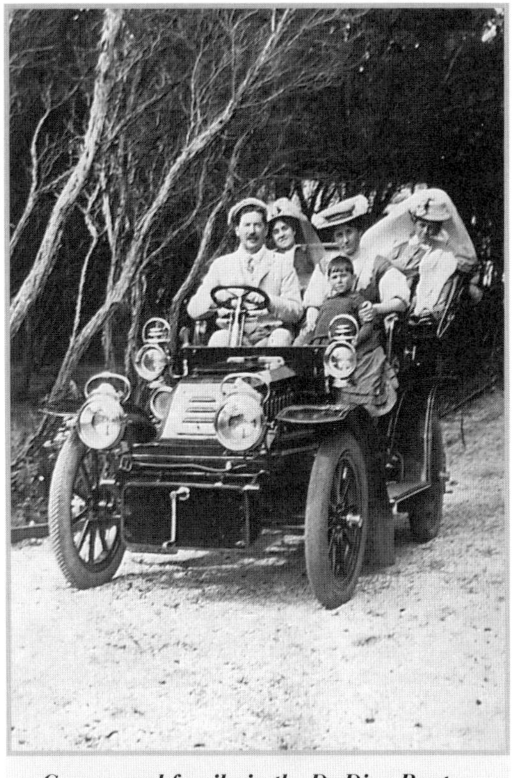

George and family in the De Dion Bouton

Mr George Tallis, manager of Her Majesty's Theatre, Melbourne, is one of the most ardent motorists in his home city. Early in 1904 he purchased a Little Humberette, but recently he went in for a more powerful and commodious De Dion, which he now uses daily to convey him from his home in Camberwell to the city. Mr Tallis says:

'Motoring is now my only pastime, and it meets all my requirements admirably. For one can get around so expeditiously and with such perfect freedom from worry about horses being tired. Motoring just suits me in every way, and I'm glad I took to it as a hobby, a pastime and a utility.'

The De Dion motor accommodates three passengers, and Sunday runs of 30 or 40 miles are normal. Among those who accompany the owner from time to time is Mr JC Williamson, who talks of buying his own car. They praise Mr Tallis's skilful management of his car, and so far he is the only motorist connected with the theatre profession in Melbourne.

It all sounds rather formal. In reality, away from work George shed his theatrical garb and applied himself to his diversions, of which motoring was one. With his cap perched on the back of his head to give the impression of speed and wind, he grabbed anybody who was available, and set off for a spin. His competitive spirit spilled over to his driving, and the lack of power in the early model cars frustrated him. Upon returning to *Santoi* with a full load, he would make some of the children walk up the steep incline of Prospect Hill Road, while he charged it with wide open throttle. As the older boys ran past the wheezing vehicle, taunting the driver and the remaining passengers, George would lean forward, straining to extract the last ounce of performance from the feeble engine. But this was one race he could not hope to win!

George was a competent driver, but he was the first to admit that he was no Syd Day. His friend Day, on 26 February 1910, established a record by driving from Sydney to Melbourne in twenty hours and ten minutes. Day could change wheels, mend punctures and fix his car when it stopped. Tallis, on the other hand, had no idea what made his machine work. He tackled the Melbourne to Sydney run and challenged his personal best times but, as the cars became more sophisticated, he preferred that others took the wheel. Even so, the anticipation of an early start to a long country run gave him purpose and excitement, and on the road he relaxed and forgot the woes of business management. He was an enthusiastic foundation member of the Royal Automobile Club of Victoria, and in 1947 he was 'delighted' to receive a letter from the club president making him a life member.

The Motor
15th March, 1910
VINOT
SYDNEY
TO
Showrooms—
20, REGENT STREET, LONDON, S.W.
577 miles over mountains, through rivers and bullock tracks.
On a 25 h.p.
VINOT
in 20 hrs. 10 mins. on a Standard Chassis driven by Mr. Syd Day, an amateur.
February, 1910.
RECORD BEATEN
By 1 hr. 9 mins.
Showrooms—
20, REGENT STREET, LONDON, S.W.
MELBOURNE
VINOT

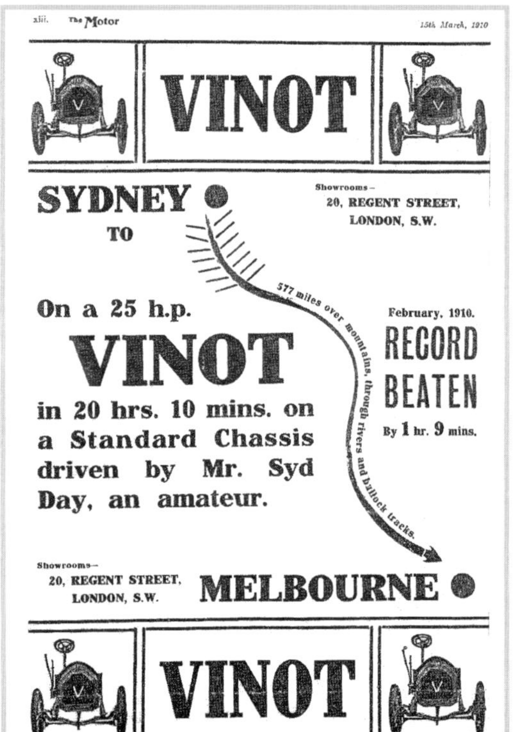

Syd Day was an interesting character. His friendship with Tallis, and his own rise to fame in the printing world, went back to 1900 when George chose him to print the program for *The Rose of Persia* when it opened at Her Majesty's Theatre in Melbourne on 27 October. The program was magnificent. It was the first printing in three colours, and as a consequence Day became the official printer for the Firm. Nicknamed 'Syd the Printer', he was a popular dinner guest with his stories of the bumpy rides his life entailed.

The years at the end of the century's first decade were lively ones behind the scenes at the Firm, especially for George Tallis. In a move that was overdue given its size, the partnership was incorporated on 25 July 1910. JC Williamson Ltd, the new company, had a capital of £180,000 divided into 140,000 fully paid one pound shares, and 40,000 contributing one pound shares paid to 10 shillings. JC Williamson held 50 per cent of the shares, Tallis and Ramaciotti 25 per cent each.[3]

Williamson, however, now sixty-five, wanted to lighten his investment in the Firm to accommodate his withdrawal into retirement, and he agreed to sell a quarter of his share holding to Tallis, and a further quarter to Arthur Wigram Allen, the company's Sydney solicitor. Ramaciotti also wanted to retire more or less immediately, and he sold his entire share holding to Tallis.

By 1911 Tallis had control of 62.5 per cent of the new company, Williamson 25 per cent and Allen 12.5 per cent. This was in line with Williamson's wishes to get on with his retirement and to hand over the reins to his closest business associate, George Tallis.

There was another major reshuffle in 1911. This was caused, in part, by the need to replace Ramaciotti, whose departure had left the Firm short of senior administration. It was also essential because Williamson was taking on even less of the day-to-day responsibilities, and the dearth of advanced theatre expertise was becoming obvious.

The comic actor Hugh J Ward, who was born in Pennsylvania, USA, in 1871, and trained with the tough stock companies of the day, was noticed by Williamson, who asked Tallis to check his suitability for joining the JCW Ltd board. Hugh had a peppery personality that often got the better of him, but he was experienced and theatre-smart.

In a letter to Tallis from London, undated but certainly early 1910, Williamson expanded on the problem:

The great weakness of our firm is [not] being able to make proper use of the splendid lot of material which we import. We are seldom able to get all out of a piece. Once a production is out it generally has to take its chances, and the stage manager leaves it while he takes up something else, or else lets his assistant run the stage [as] there is too much going on for one of the firm to personally supervise. This is why I advocated Malone [join] in addition to Ward thus giving three managers, one in Melb one in Sydney and one to generally supervise production.

Pat Malone, the Firm's London representative, was approached, but he made such excessive demands that the offer was withdrawn. He had undergone the usual hot–cold relationships with other producers, most noted of whom were Charles Frohman in America and George Edwardes in London and, on balancing the pros and cons, decided to stay put.

Negotiations continued with Ward. Williamson appeared keen, but Tallis seemed to drag his heels. As was his way with Williamson on most major issues, Tallis eventually came around and supported his mentor's view:

Re Ward [wrote Williamson from overseas on 16 September 1910] I am very glad you are discovering his good qualities. I felt sure you would do so, that is why I left you two to settle matters between yourselves without further interference on my part.

He then urged George to sign up Ward come hell or high water.

Difficult and protracted negotiations got under way. During these, Ward showed that he was well able to look after himself. He separated board members into two classes – experts and inexperts – and painted a picture of the latter riding to fortune on the backs of the former. He was offered an eighth interest in the Firm, demanded one-quarter and accepted a sixth. Then he kept raising other issues. Ultimately, on 24 June 1910 Tallis wrote a long and very interesting letter spelling out the bottom line to Hugh. From the new Articles of Association he simultaneously clearly identified Williamson's position in the new set-up and showed, by this example, how he protected the interests of the founder:

I know that all through the Articles of Association there are certain matters specified in which Mr Williamson's decision is to be final. I have acquiesced in everything that allows Mr Williamson the right to veto certain acts. I have been with Mr Williamson now for twenty-four years, and I am only too happy that so long as he remains with us, he will have the rights given him in the Articles. I hope he will live many years to give us the benefit of his advice.

In regard to JCW's position in the future, he is not obliged to take an active part in the management, but that has been the case for the last five years, and instead of taking an idle part, he has worked harder than ever. JCW is of great value to the Company, and his being in England and looking after things there is well worth all the money he will draw.

Hugh Ward finally joined the Firm on 1 July 1911. He bought his one-sixth interest from Tallis, who was probably keen to divest himself of some of his large shareholding.

The new partner was certainly a showman. It was his good fortune to be looking after the Williamson firm's business in Sydney when the Melba–Williamson Opera Company opened at Her Majesty's on 2 September 1911. Oddly enough, Williamson, who had plotted this season with Melba since 1909 to celebrate both the fiftieth anniversary of his own first stage appearance and the diva's fiftieth birthday, was overseas at the time. Ward appeared on stage with Melba after the opening night and gave a speech to great applause, as he did again after her final Sydney appearance in October. Characteristically, George Tallis, the Firm's senior managing director, took great pleasure in Melba's Melbourne triumphs but declined to share her spotlight.

The next year, 1912, both Williamson and Tallis were overseas. Shock waves hit when Melbourne *Punch* ran an article about Ward:

He began as a boy in a minstrel company in America. Now, at a little over forty, he is head of one of the most important theatrical organisations in the world. It is true that at present he shares his headship with others, but none who knows Hugh Ward doubts that in a very little while he will be the sole monarch.[4]

Not even Williamson could pick his man with absolute certainty. Enraged, he wrote to Tallis in London from Lucerne in mid-August 1912:

Re the Adventurous Career of King Ward . . . it is the biggest piece of cheek I ever read: and his ingratitude is only equalled by that of his predecessor General Ramaciotti. I should like to hear [your] opinion as to what should be done about it.

Williamson then explained that, as far as he was concerned, he would only do the work for the Firm that was required of him as governing director, and no more. He continued:

If King Ward is waiting for me to kill myself with work and worry for the benefit of the shareholders of JCW Ltd he may have to wait longer than he expects. There is no doubt he has the very worst form of enlarged cranium and needs pulling up.

On 21 August 1912 George wrote to lawyer Arthur Allen about the matter:

What has come over Hughie Ward? Is he trying to wreck the Firm of JCW Ltd, because he has certainly started the ball rolling and it is always difficult to see where it ends. He has been a valued friend of mine for many years, and I as you know was personally and solely responsible for his admission into the business . . . In the truly extraordinary Punch *article he has gone out of his way deliberately, it would seem to us on this side, to insult JCW, Meynell [by now the fourth director] and myself.*

I was very sorry to see our old policy of silent solidity which for so many years impressed the public of Australia and the profession in general violated ... This is so contrary to what has been our rule in the business. However, as it is now a matter seriously affecting the future welfare of our operation I would like you on behalf of JCW and myself to have a friendly chat with HJ on the subject as JC's personal representative, and solicitor for the company, and report result to us. I am writing this at JCW's request and he is also writing you by this mail.

What a pity this cloud should have arisen this early ... I cannot express how sorry I am over the whole business. You know personally I never care if my name did not appear from one year's end to the other.

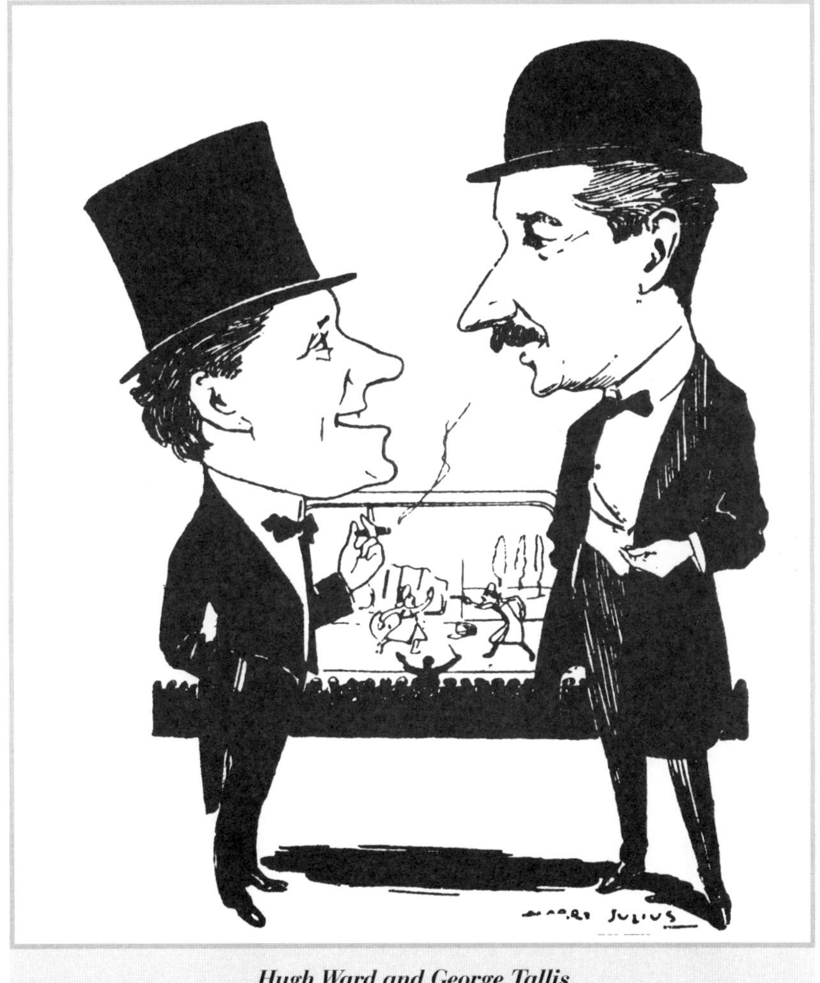

Hugh Ward and George Tallis

Three facets of George's personality are highlighted in this letter. First, Tallis assumed full responsibility for the Ward appointment, even though Williamson had leant on him to agree to it. Second, the matter was to be handled by a 'friendly chat', an approach which became a hallmark of Tallis's way of dealing with trouble. Finally, the last line expresses George's sentiment on personal publicity; a sentiment that would see him all but vanish from the annals of Australian theatre history.

This event set the stage for the uneasy Tallis–Ward relationship that would span more than a decade. The two were chalk and cheese and, although they maintained an effective working rapport, the 'valued friendship' George referred to in his letter to Allen had been tested to the limit. Sixty years later, in an article marking the Firm's centennial, Katharine Brisbane found that in some respects very little had changed over the years:

The Firm is famous for its private strife and its public unity and this has been part of its strength. Crisis is part of the JCW way of life, like every other theatrical management. That's show biz.[5]

In the case of the Ward affair it was the public display of disunity that hurt the Firm. It made Williamson and Tallis so incensed that they felt it necessary to have umpire Allen read the code to the new player.

The year 1911 had been a really momentous one for the Firm. As well as significant restructuring at the top, late in the piece a need arose to deal with the small Clarke–Meynell theatre company.

Clyde Meynell was born around 1867. After some preliminary experience with acting and managing, he and the Irish actor, John Gunn, arrived from England and leased the Theatre Royal in Melbourne for ten years, starting in November 1907. They also leased the Criterion in Sydney for one year. In April 1908, the Melbourne

Theatre Royal staged the newcomers' first London success, *Miss Hook of Holland*. Soon the critics were regarding the company as genuine competition in musical theatre for both Musgrove's business and the Williamson partnership.

Little seems to be known about Meynell. He wrote interesting and revealing business letters that suggest he was efficient and professional. He appeared to be strong on loyalty, but he was totally opposed to self-promotion. Meynell was a quiet man, and George was later to describe him as 'too much of a gentleman to be involved in boardroom brawls'.

Meynell and Gunn joined Rupert Clarke and John Wren as sole lessees of the Royal, with Clyde Meynell and John Gunn the managing directors. Over the next year or so, John Wren pulled out, and Gunn died of pneumonia. This left only Clarke and Meynell, and they combined to form Clarke–Meynell Ltd, which offered a mixture of popular light opera, comedy and drama.

Rupert Clarke, born in 1865, was a patron of the theatre. He was a good businessman, and his association with Meynell was but one of his many speculative ventures. Although he was not active in the theatre himself, he played his role well, providing money and financial advice, while remaining strictly in the background.

The leasing of the Theatre Royal in Melbourne by Clarke and Meynell turned out to be a cunning business move. It interfered with Williamson's bookings. When, in addition, some real theatrical competition followed, the Firm decided to push the merger button. There were negotiations, an agreement, and then celebrations all round.

Both Williamson and Tallis were involved in setting up the arrangements. To accommodate these, some changes flowed. The JCW Ltd capital increased from £180,000 to £300,000, there were alterations to the board, and Tallis sold more shares to the incoming directors. Most importantly, as George pointed out to the Melbourne *Age* in August 1911, the Firm became even bigger and more powerful:

Mr George Tallis explained the reasons that prompted the formation of the new company and the scope it would embrace. A directorate of four, namely, Messrs JC Williamson, G Tallis, Hugh J Ward and Clyde Meynell would control it. The cost of production had nearly doubled compared with what it was four years ago. The rearrangement, therefore, was made to meet the altered conditions.

The object of the amalgamation, Mr Tallis said, was to raise the tone of productions presented here to a higher artistic level and to regulate the production of pieces so as to avoid clashing. The new combination would take over Her Majesty's Theatre and the Theatre Royal, in Melbourne; Her Majesty's, the Theatre Royal and the Criterion in Sydney; the Theatre Royal in Christchurch; the Opera House in Wellington; and Her Majesty's in Brisbane. In all, the amalgamation would keep about ten or twelve expensive companies on tour. Theatres in Adelaide and Perth would be leased also. The new company would come into existence on 1st September, and the next night Madame Melba would appear in Sydney under its direction.[6]

The critical outcome of the amalgamation for the Firm was a permanent upgrading of its theatre circuit. The partners now had control of most of the important theatres in Australia and New Zealand. The new agreements left Williamson as governing director and made Tallis, Ward and Meynell managing directors, on condition that each held at least 15,000 shares. In exchange for the leases of the Melbourne Theatre Royal and the Sydney Criterion Theatre together with goodwill, Clarke–Meynell appears to have received between ten and fifteen per cent of the new capital structure of JCW Ltd.

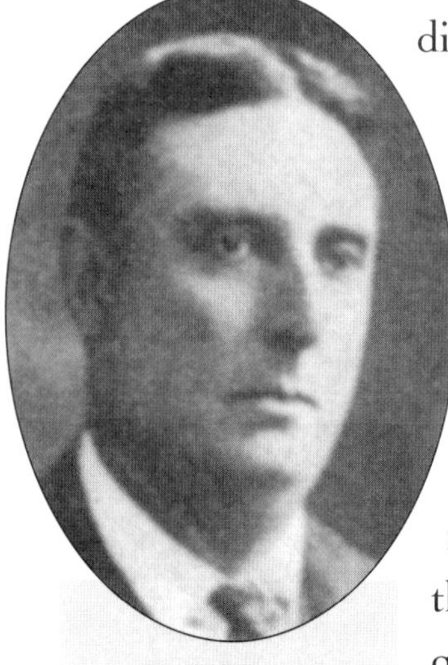

Clyde Meynell

A special clause gave Sir Rupert Clarke the right of appointment as a managing director in the event that Williamson, for whatever reason, relinquished his position on the board. This clause was never invoked.

As the skills of neither Ward nor Meynell lay in the direction of business, the load fell more and more upon Tallis. Melbourne *Punch* pointed out in 1913 that already, although the head office was nominally in Sydney, 'the headship was actually in Tallis's small office at Her Majesty's Theatre, Melbourne'.

George was now forty-four. It had been a long haul, but he had arrived. There was a rumour that he had modelled his public personality on that of his American acquaintance, Charles Frohman, the greatest theatrical manager of the day. Frohman was said to have watched the opening of a $100,000 production 'from the furthermost perch in the Gallery'.[7] That is what Tallis remembered; that, and the Frohman modesty.

Melbourne *Punch* completed its portrait of George:

He is a man who always works, but who organises his work so that it is made as easy as possible. He is a modest man. The public seldom hears of him. He never advertises himself. He knows that advertisement of a manager is good material wasted. The public are not to be induced to attend the show by any quality of the manager in it. His creed is that the proper place for a manager is the place he has always occupied – well out of the limelight, with all the glare thrown upon the wares he has to display to the public.

He is the ideal manager – cautious, bland, reticent, retiring – a man who, though engaged in show business, displays none of those blatant qualities which so often, unfortunately, go with a showman.[8]

Time out at Sans Souci in 1904 for four leading theatre personalities in Australia. Back, JC Williamson and Harry Rickards. Front, George Rignold and Bland Holt

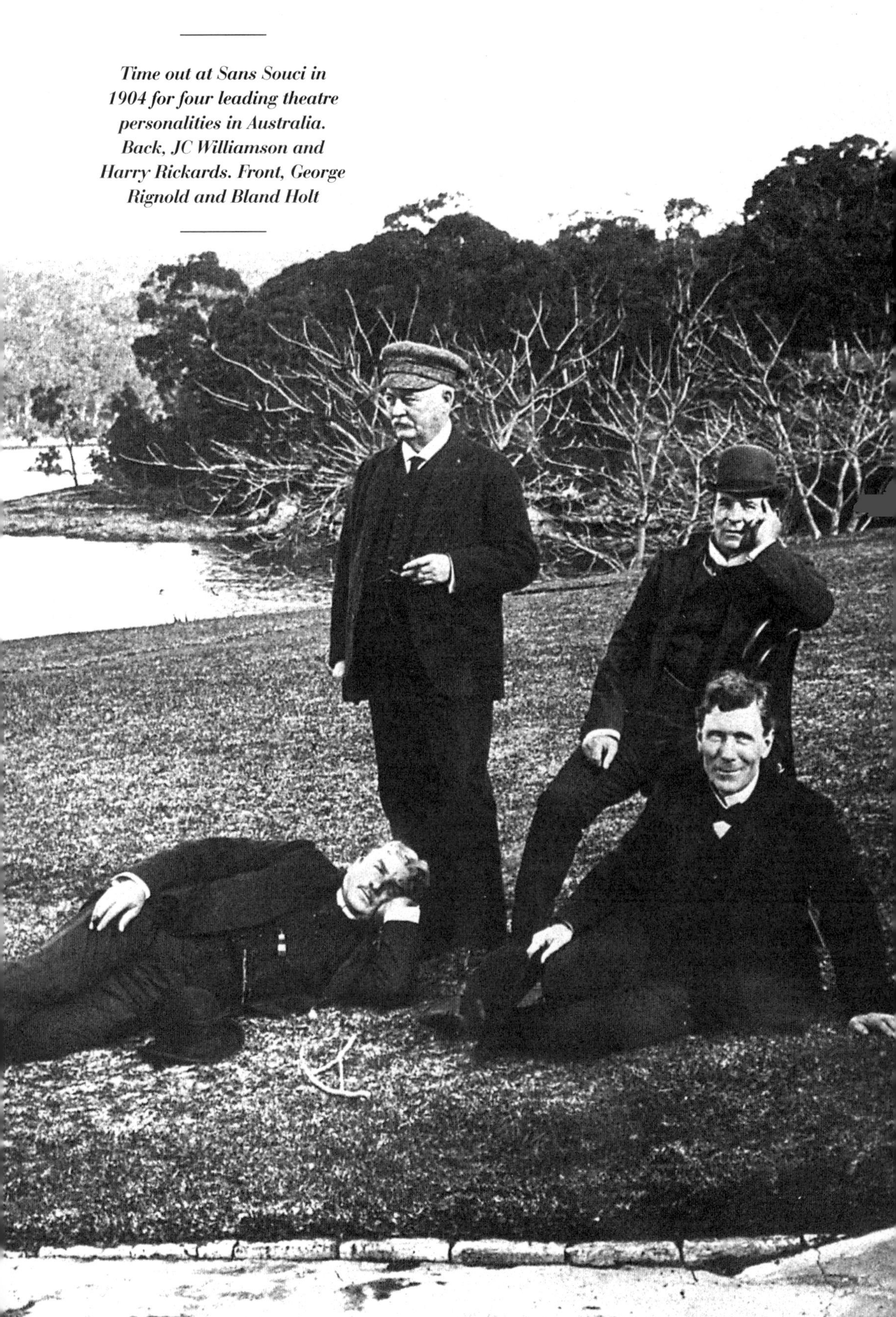

CHAPTER NINE

The Passing of Williamson

With the end of the Gilbert and Sullivan series at the Savoy and the Girl *series from the George Edwardes' Theatres, London, it was apparent that specially organised companies were necessary to adequately present the new types of musical plays now commencing to arrive from the American market. Thus, the Royal Comic Opera as a separate entity gradually faded out . . .*

So wrote George Tallis in his memoirs of Australian theatre at the turn of the century. New Williamson companies sprang up willy-nilly, and overseas touring companies travelled under the banner of one or another of a myriad of titles – The JC Williamson New Comedy Company, The JC Williamson Dramatic Company, or whatever was appropriate.

Searching for the shows and casts was no easy matter. It involved international scouting on the part of the Firm, although the New York and London agents took some of the sting out of the work. These were experienced and reliable men, and their referrals were well worth following up. Even so, the problems of finding and selecting theatrical fare remained, and all entrepreneurs had to face them.

Australian and New Zealand theatre-goers had capricious tastes. Shows that were raging successes overseas could fail abysmally in

Melbourne, Sydney or Auckland. To compound the problems, the public at various times favoured either British or American productions; exactly which should get the nod, and when, was the conundrum. Tallis wrote in his memoirs:

Although a visit by the well-known John L Toole in 1890 with his complete company from his London theatre proved very successful, we were unlucky in the main [in the early days] with our American importations. Six years later two of the most famous American stars, Nat Goodwin and Willie Collier, proved dismal failures.

Mr Goodwin had as his leading ladies Miss Blanche Walsh and Miss Maxine Elliot, then at her zenith. However, their season was cut short. Willie Collier, the most popular light comedian in America, supported by Jack Barrymore, then in his teens, and a brilliant company also unaccountably failed.

William Collier felt his failure keenly. During his Melbourne season, when business was particularly bad, one day a visitor went over to Collier's table at Menzies Hotel where he was lunching and, apologising for intruding, said he desired to congratulate him on his splendid performance the previous evening. Quick as lightning, Collier replied, 'Oh you are the gentleman who was present?'

Around 1908 theatregoers were becoming familiarised with American methods and subsequent attractions from the States were warmly received. In fact, from about this period onwards the United States gradually displaced England as the main provider of our musical dramatic fare in Australia.

The best that the managers could do was to brief themselves through the international press, correspond with their agents, and set up option agreements with overseas producers such as Charles Frohman and George Edwardes. Then, every two or three years, they had to travel to Europe and the States to assess the market for themselves.

Once all the possibilities were to hand ... well, Williamson once put it this way:

After collating all the evidence, the decision as to selection has to be taken, and it becomes a grave matter of judgement to choose something which will suit the public at that particular time.[1]

That was the first stage. Appropriate actors had to be found who could star in the plays, and who were also prepared to travel to the ends of the earth to do it. Because of these difficulties, some scripts were kept in reserve for years waiting for the right cast to appear; idle money that added to the costs of actually producing the shows.

Probably the greatest limitations were the small theatre-going populations in Australia and New Zealand, and the fact that there were not enough suitable local actors and actresses to fill the supporting roles alongside the overseas stars. This led to high overheads and large foreign casts. The small number of patrons meant much shorter seasons than in London, where essentially endless runs were achievable. So Australian managements had to mount – and fund – tours across Australasia to make up a season, rather than play just one city. The bottom line was that for the Australian theatre entrepreneur to survive, he had to be extraordinarily astute and business-conscious.

Punch summed up the situation:

No man is more constantly on the lookout for talent than the theatre manager. It is his business. He listens to bad actors. He tolerates awful singers. He hears dreary plays. And he does all these things to an extraordinary degree, because any time he knows he may discover a gem of great price, which will more than repay him for all the trouble and discomfort. One Australian entrepreneur through refusing once to make a journey of thirty miles to hear a conscript soldier sing missed the opportunity of engaging Caruso, the world's greatest tenor, and thereby missed a fortune. Every manager has had similar experiences, and they tend to make him keener than ever in the search for talent.[2]

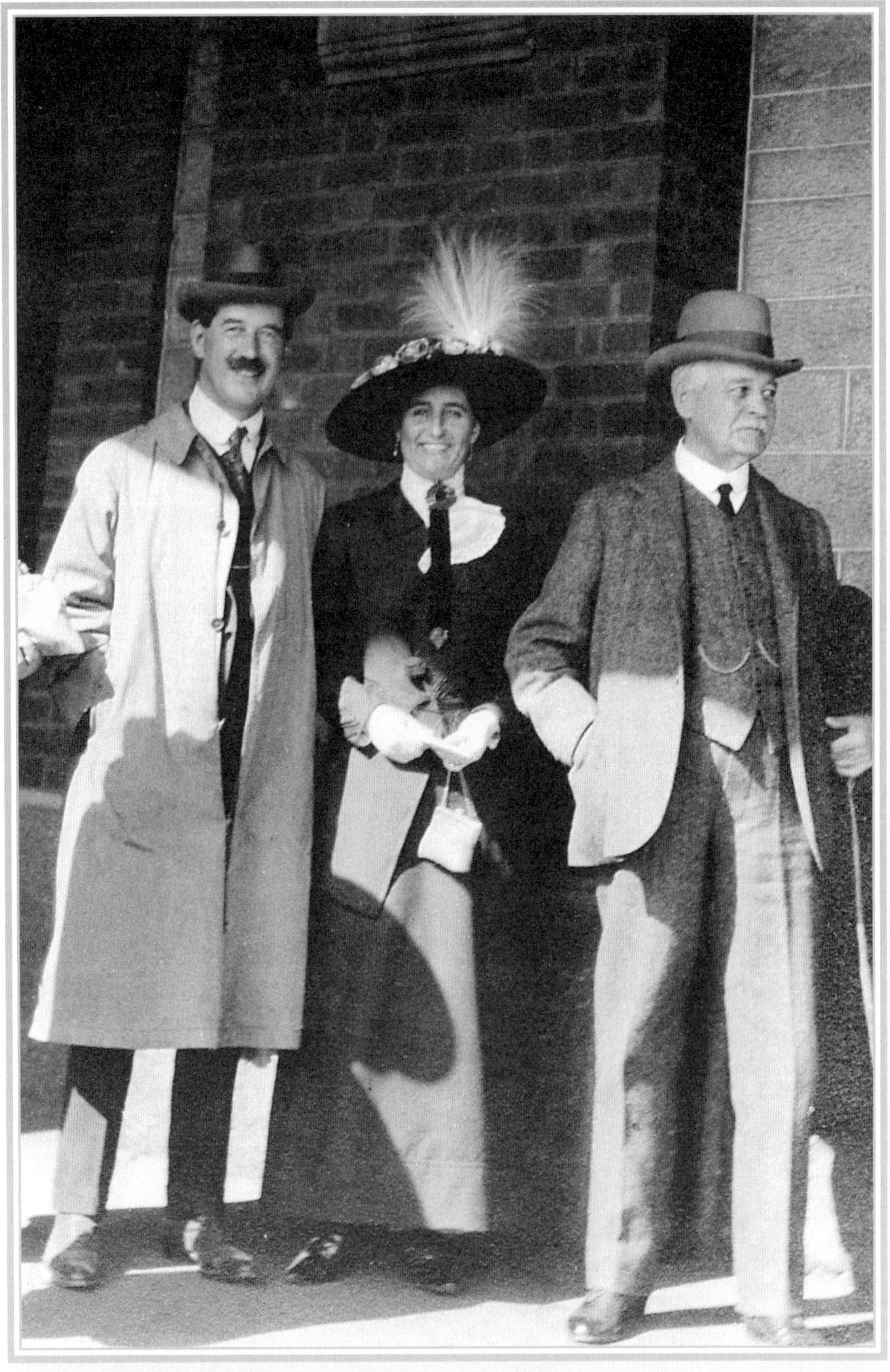

George and Millie with JCW before leaving for England on the SS Orama *in 1912*

During the busy days of establishing himself, George Tallis did not travel overseas extensively. The search for talent and shows was left to the early partners before 1900, with Tallis making his first trip in 1902. From 1903 to 1911 Williamson took on the task of rounding up the shows, while Tallis and Ramaciotti stayed home to manage the business. After 1912, Meynell and Ward did most of the travelling. For a long period, therefore, Tallis remained steadfastly in Australia, consolidating and expanding the Williamson enterprise.

In April 1912, however, George and Millie left for Europe, travelling on the same ship as Williamson, whose family was already there. This was a considerable undertaking for the Tallises. There was a full schedule of business in London as it was George's turn to select shows, do the rounds of the theatre agents for rights to new plays and find specialty acts for the coming Christmas pantomime. The pair also made the pilgrimage to Ireland to see George's eighty-four-year-old mother, Sarah, and other members of his family. In all, they were away from home for ten months.

Williamson spent most of his time in continental Europe, often in great pain while searching for cures for what doctors diagnosed variously as sciatica or bronchitis. But business was not overlooked and Tallis and Williamson communicated almost daily by letter. Unfortunately, George's letters are lost, but Williamson's to him are laced with insights into the kind of artistic, legal, financial and 'personality' issues that the Firm's directors confronted.

As an example, earlier, in 1910, George had written that he was unsure about the future of pantomimes in Australia. He knew that Williamson loved to be quietly requested for advice, and it was not long in coming. Williamson, who was in Europe looking for new attractions, responded by return mail:

I note that you are inclined to be pessimistic about the future of Panto productions. That is a pity as the Panto has really been the backbone of our business during the past four years. I think it is purely a question of being able to keep up the standard we have set for ourselves and vary the productions with novel attractions.

He then proceeded to discuss the novelties he had found to hot up the Firm's yearly big attraction. The 'fair scene' was to have a merry-go-round on stage, while a new film would distract the audience when the stage was being set for fresh acts. 'But you must keep the big turn for the second act,' Tallis was warned. 'So you see I haven't lost much time,' JCW boasted, also admitting to galloping insomnia as a result of the pace he had set himself.

Now, in 1912, George found that Williamson was relying heavily on him for business opinions about the Firm's affairs, and also for advice about his private matters. He never finished a letter without asking to be remembered to 'Mrs Tallis'. Williamson expressed complete confidence in George's theatrical judgement and his ability to produce high-quality, profitable shows. And why not – he had trained him! He wrote:

I hope you are getting on all right with the Pantomime. I feel confident that you will make a big success of it. Do whatever you think best and don't worry to refer anything to me.

But it was not all plain sailing. News of another of Hugh Ward's irritating activities interfered with Williamson's therapy. Her Majesty's Theatre in Sydney needed some alterations to improve its ventilation and seating. Before leaving Australia, Williamson had issued instructions about what was required. Ward disregarded the advice and rashly pushed ahead with renovations of his own devising. Hackles rose, and the Williamson pen went to work.

Not surprisingly, Tallis was immediately brought into the fray. From Florence, he received a fifteen-page letter that was amazing in its scope given that Williamson was so ill. In it the showman explored the business of altering Her Majesty's, and quoted figures and technical

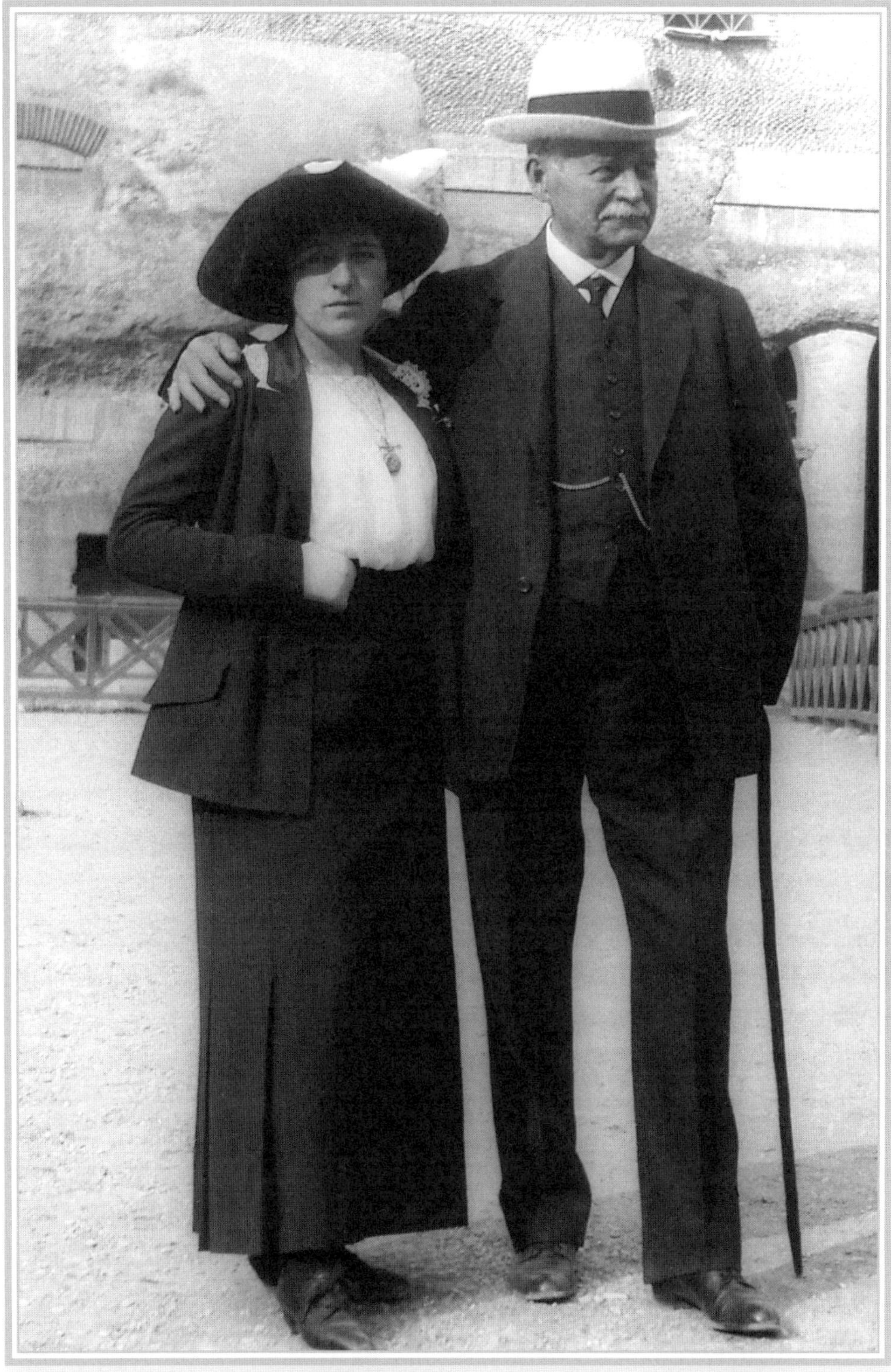

JC Williamson and daughter Marjorie in Rome – mid-September 1912

details that displayed exactly why he had been at the top of Australian theatre management for so long. As a main priority it had been proposed that the theatre should be properly ventilated, but Hugh Ward decided to extend the dress circle by one row. This is where he ran up against Williamson's intimate knowledge of theatre design. The extensions impacted on sightlines from various parts of the theatre, ventilation, structural soundness and access to exits. All this Williamson knew about, and Ward seemed to overlook:

Mr Ward . . . has taken it on himself to upset my decision and endeavour to finish through alterations according to his own idea by fitting an additional row of seats in the front of the dress-circle and gallery necessitating both circles being brought forward at least 2 feet 6 inches, altering the rake of the seats in circle and gallery to a very serious extent . . .

Neither [the architect] or Mr Ward can have the slightest idea of sighting a theatre when they make such a proposition – they have only looked at the matter from the back of the circle and gallery and have not considered the sighting of the sides of the two circles at all – had they done so, they must have seen at once that the view of the stage would be lost for everything except the front row – thus we would lose as many seats at the sides probably as would be gained from the enlarged circle.

I speak with the fullest knowledge as to the construction of the theatre, because before [The Princess] was rebuilt [in 1886], I spent weeks with [architect William] Pitt going through the plans and I know what the effect will be with the front-rail shoved out . . .

That the renovations were not delayed until his return was an insult Williamson never forgave. In further letters to Tallis he vented his feelings about Ward and also said that Ramaciotti had tied so many legal knots for the company that no one knew how to unravel them.

As his health continued to ebb, Williamson became pensive. He regretted that he could not meet George in London for a good old 'chin wag', and most of all he yearned to join him in Ireland:

I was much interested in your remarks about your dear old mother and her Irish homestead. I envied you the pleasure you must have enjoyed in fixing her up in a new house and bestowing on her the ease and comfort with which you are so well able to surround her. I tried to do the same for my poor mother, but I was too late as she died too soon.

I have often pictured a genuine Irish home such as you describe where the fire never dies out in the fireplace and the kettle is always boiling, either for tea, or something stronger. I wish I could have been there to join you in a sup and to taste whole meal bread which seems to be great breeding provender judging by the vigorous work your old uncle [Dick] has been equal to after his 72 years, though it seems to be in the blood as shown by your own record. I hope Mrs Tallis . . .

This warm association between Tallis and Williamson had brewed over such a long period, without double dealing or broken expectations, that the men referred most important theatre matters to each other. As new partners joined the Firm, and problems escalated, both found the complete trust they had built between themselves a comfort and convenience.

The friction generated by the Hugh Ward episodes was an example of an expanding sea of trouble for Tallis. Ward may have expected Tallis to support him against Williamson, and he may have been surprised, and miffed, at the outcome. Tallis had grown into the Firm, and all the long-serving senior staff were his friends. As he rose to the top, some of these people anticipated special treatment later. When they were dealt with in a way that reflected Tallis's responsibility to the Firm, they felt personally let down. There is no doubt that this conflict of interest weighed heavily on him, and some tried to capitalise on the quandary.

Williamson had a disastrous 'recuperation' in 1912. His health had been failing for some years, and his condition worsened during the overseas trip. He decided to seek a medical opinion in London. The diagnosis was an incurable kidney complaint. He returned to Australia, without his wife and children, to tidy up his affairs.

This took about three months of intensive work involving his solicitor, Arthur Allen, who was also the Sydney solicitor for JCW Ltd; Edward Major, the company secretary; and George Tallis, who had also recently returned home. Daily meetings took place at *Tudor,* Williamson's home in Sydney.

The great actor–manager made a final stage appearance on 22 February 1913, in a charity matinee at Her Majesty's Theatre, Sydney. He played a favourite role as a ninety-year-old Irishman in the one-act play *Kerry*. The audience, knowing that they were witnessing the last performance, greeted him with wild enthusiasm.

Williamson returned to France via the United States, but the rough seas of the Pacific aggravated his condition. By the time he reached Paris, he was desperately ill, and died with his family around him on 6 July 1913 – not 8 July as often reported. He was buried in Chicago.

Two executors to the Williamson will were Edward Major and solicitor Reginald Allen, brother of Arthur. The few JCW Ltd shares held by Williamson were sold to Arthur Allen and prominent Sydney businessmen Samuel and Anthony Hordern, thus disposing of the Williamson family's financial interest in the theatre industry.

Although the theatre world had known that JC Williamson was very ill, the news of his death in Paris came as a genuine shock. The Australasian press responded by publishing large obituaries. The JC Williamson theatres closed for one night as a sign of respect.

George Tallis wrote:

When you have worked in the closest daily association with any man for over a quarter of a century, the usual expressions of regret for his death cannot come readily from the tongue. My memories of Mr Williamson crowd too fast one upon the other – recollections of what he did in all that time and how he did it – all the associations that directly or indirectly were his. The whole story of the years is gliding before me, and I cannot set down in cold words what I feel.

A great personality has gone. In our theatres we shall all miss his acute perception, his large grasp of all that appertained to his business: we shall no less feel the loss of his friendship and his affection for his co-workers.

One hears a good deal nowadays about 'the personal touch'. I doubt whether any man had that in a greater degree than JC Williamson. He was pre-eminently a man to lead, a man to get always the best out of everybody associated with him; and I am confident that for long years his reputation and his achievements will loom large in the theatrical history of Australasia.[3]

Lindsey Browne, a theatre critic, later summarised Williamson's talents like this:

Probably many individuals can be named who excelled Williamson in one or another of his many attributes – in acting, in producing, in field-beating recognition of great talents to be, in star-building, in cleaving to the most rigorous artistic standards on all occasions, in evolving an exclusively home-grown Australian way of doing things. But probably no single person even nearly approached his place as a total all-purpose theatre personality whose every deed has had some vital bearing on the course of Australian theatre ever since.[4]

When the time came, Tallis was prepared to take on the role of chairman of directors of JCW Ltd. There was a smooth transition, and automatically he replaced Williamson as the most influential and significant theatre personality in Australia. In reporting the change-over, the Melbourne *Argus* wrote:

Mr George Tallis practically assumed control of the enterprise as far back as [1904], though for a decade previously his energies and his acute knowledge of Australian conditions had more and more to do with the framing of each successive year's operations. When the partnership terms expired in 1911 it was to Mr Tallis that Mr Williamson sold out quarter of his holding, retaining himself

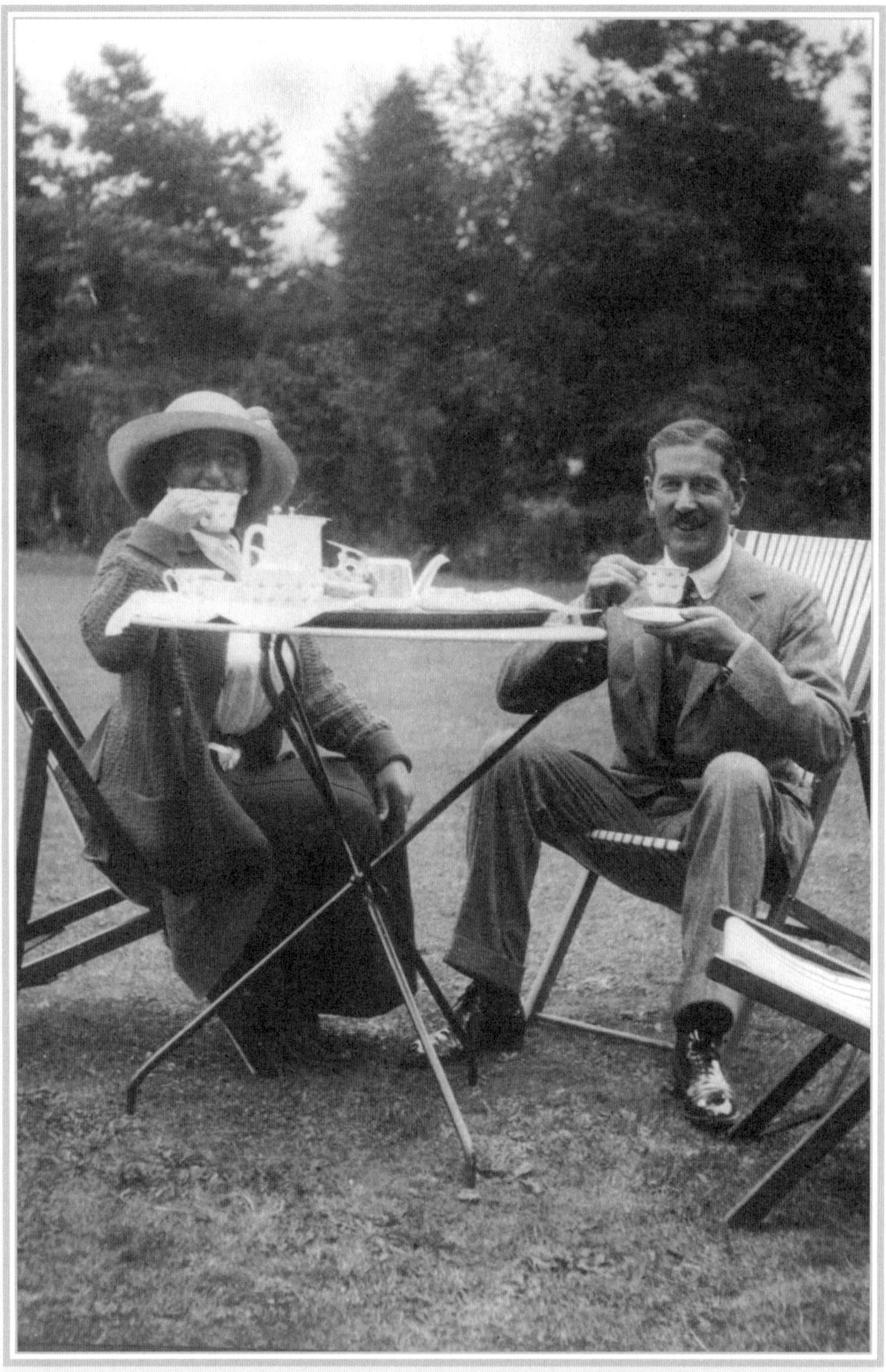

Tea for two – George and Millie, Hindhead, England 1912

only a very small interest in comparison to that which he formerly held. At the same time, Lieut-Colonel Ramaciotti also sold out his interest to Mr Tallis, who thereby became the predominant partner in the concern, holding the vast majority of the shares and becoming in fact, as he had been in deed, the controlling influence in the growing enterprises of the company.[5]

It is possible to surmise the nature of the long-standing relationship that existed between Tallis and Williamson. Although both men carefully guarded their own innermost feelings, leads can be found in letters, reported statements and actual events.

In his early days at the Firm, Tallis, who was twenty-five years younger than his chief, would have viewed Williamson as a stern, no-nonsense employer. Williamson had no children of his own at that time, and Tallis no immediate family in Australia. The two worked closely day by day and the barriers of reserve must have crumbled as Williamson became familiar with George's family background. A solid working relationship developed between the two men, replaced eventually by a very strong friendship.

As Tallis grew into the Firm, Williamson relied more and more on his advice, and the bond between the pair grew. Certainly there were the difficulties that relationships across generations experience, but if Tallis's approach to theatre management is examined carefully, it can be seen that he and Williamson shared many attributes. They differed markedly in two.

Williamson was firmly in charge and, although he listened to George, for better or worse, Williamson's conservatism overrode some of Tallis's ideas. This must have generated frustration in the younger man, as he realised that the entrenched ways of his employer could lead to difficulties for the Firm in the changing times ahead. Williamson did not worry about an opportunity missed. However, to Tallis, in the highly competitive and developing field of entertainment, an opportunity missed was an opportunity gone. It all came down to success rate, luck and personalities. Williamson could have claimed that he had already taken enough risks. But Tallis maintained that large profits required big risks, and the task of balancing risk and profit was a game that held his interest to his last day.

Secondly, as an actor, Williamson was comfortable promoting himself, his shows and his profession. Tallis, on the other hand, was happiest in the background. Bert Levy recalled that, to the best of his knowledge, George never made a public stage appearance. As the Firm grew, specialised businessmen such as Tallis and Ramaciotti, operating out of the stage spotlight, were needed to steer it through an evolving tangle of financial and managerial responsibilities.

In spite of differences, or even because of them, Williamson and Tallis collaborated well. When Williamson died, George lost more than a friend and a teacher. He lost his one source of comfortable, honest and totally professional advice on theatre matters and, in this sense, he was now alone.

In many ways, JC Williamson was fortunate. He had lived in relatively placid times, and his closest brush with an international conflict was the 1899–1901 struggle of the South African Boers for independence.

By contrast, Tallis and his contemporaries were also to experience the first two world wars of the twentieth century. They were only twenty years apart but firmly sandwiched between them, starting in 1929, was the greatest world depression of modern times.

In addition to these social, economic and military pressures, there was a technological revolution in progress. Stimulated by war, it gathered pace as the car and the aeroplane, merely curiosities around 1900, developed into fighting machines by 1918. The flow-on to civilian transportation was immediate.

Motion pictures, too, were evolving. The system Williamson and Tallis used for early film projections at the Princess was the Lumière

Cinematographe, developed in Paris. Shortly, these flickering, infuriating film debuts reached an acceptable level of viewing, and the live theatre industry was facing unwelcome opposition.

In 1899 the first wireless message in Australia travelled over a short distance in Adelaide. By 1901 messages were transmitted from ship to ship, and wireless transmission had come to stay. The wireless set would become common household equipment, and further stern competition for live theatre.

Change was everywhere as Australia matured socially and economically. George Tallis would certainly have to remain versatile if the momentum of JCW Ltd was to be maintained deep into the new century.

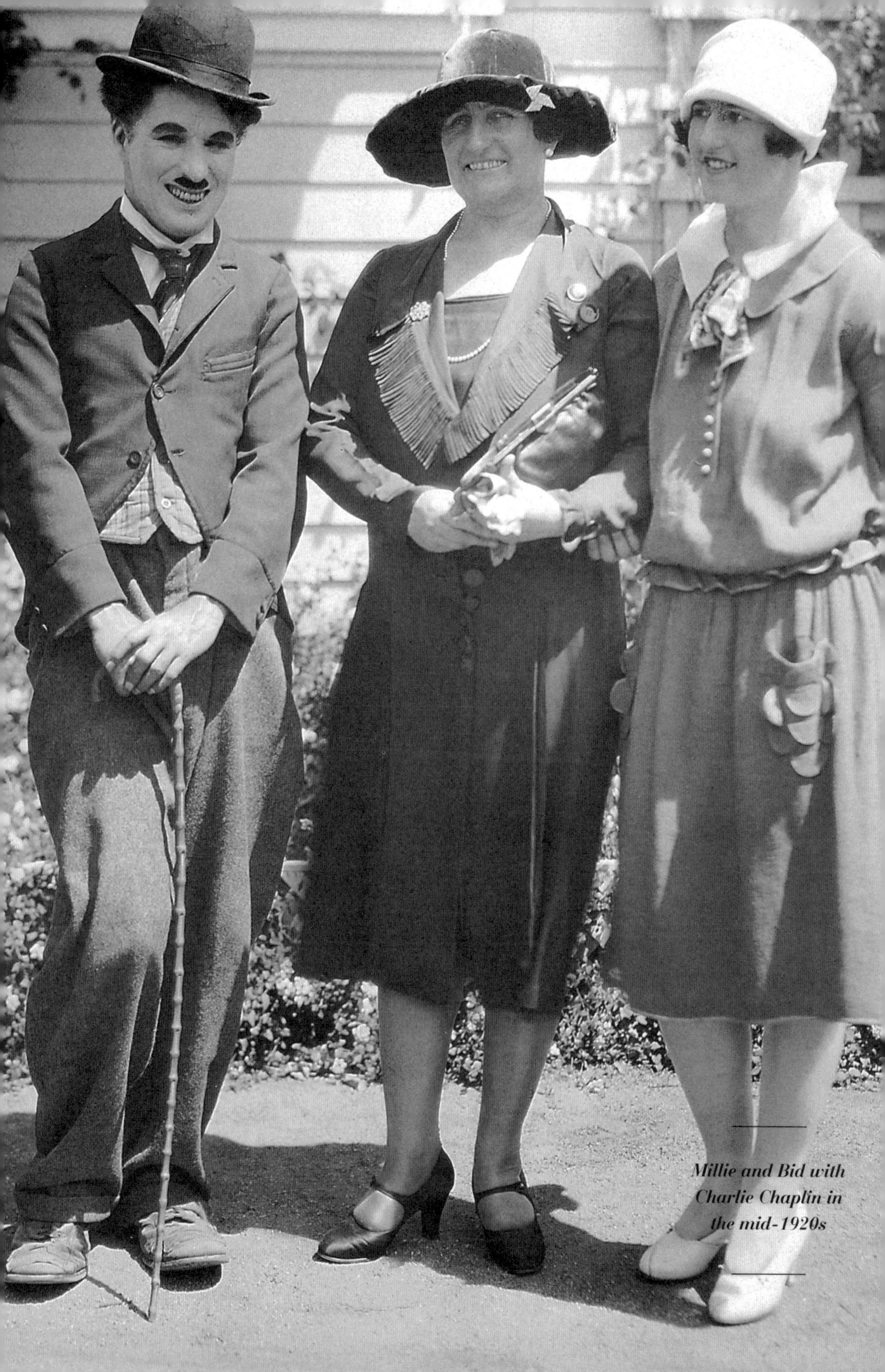

Millie and Bid with Charlie Chaplin in the mid-1920s

CHAPTER TEN

Faith, Hope and Charity

Ideas for profound expansions of the Firm appear to have been softly mooted around the corridors of power some time before Williamson's death. A short time after his passing, it was disclosed that the chairman of directors, George Tallis, had tentative plans for extending activities to South Africa. The New Zealand *Otago Witness* in July 1913 described this venture as 'one of the biggest deals of the day in the theatrical world'. To add fuel to speculations, some months later there were rumours that Williamson's would play the Adelphi Theatre in London with a performance of *High Jinks,* a lively American musical piece.

A strategy of international diversification was evolving at the Firm. Tallis would have remembered clearly George Musgrove's opening at the Shaftesbury in London and Williamson's refusal to become involved. But a hankering for the Firm to operate a theatre in London persisted. Before 1900, Williamson himself had said, 'Might not an Australian-made play also be welcome there?'[1]

A London base made good sense. For one thing, it would allow the testing of plays using Australian casts to discover if English audiences would receive them well. It was also an opportunity for such casts to informally audition before the London theatre industry.

Equally, perhaps high-priced artists who refused to undertake the long sea journey to Australia because of lost time and opportunity might consider engagements that embraced all three countries – England, South Africa and Australia. Such a triangular arrangement showed exciting potential, and now the planning that had been missing in the first attempt at lasting London success was gathering pace.

For some years the Firm had been sending tours to South Africa under the banner of B&F Wheeler Ltd, which controlled a major theatre circuit. Benjamin Wheeler was born in Ireland in 1835. He migrated to America, was naturalised as an American citizen and started an engineering career. He drifted into vaudeville, and set up his own troupe with himself as comedian and his wife as soprano singer. Their son, Frank, was a whistler, singer, reciter, impersonator and driver of the Wheeler Comedy Company coach, pulled by four horses.

In the 1870s, the Wheelers travelled the hinterland of Australia and New Zealand and then moved on to India, where they entertained British garrisons all the way to the Khyber Pass. They then went further west to South Africa, where the Wheeler company started up all over again. 'Mrs B Wheeler's Charming Ballads, Mr B Wheeler's Irishisms ... and Frank Wheeler's unapproachable impersonations and Negro delineations,' the advertisements proclaimed, were appreciated as the company crossed the Union by train, coach and ox-cart.

Small beginnings for a company that settled in Cape Town to eventually become a huge theatrical enterprise and importer of 'some of the most famous dramatic and musical performers in Victorian and Edwardian times'.[2] Benjamin Wheeler, worn out, died in 1908. He was publicly mourned, and praised for having 'purveyed wholesome entertainment abreast the times'. Frank and his son soldiered on until 1913, when B&F Wheeler was clearly near the end of its days.

In an article on the English theatre in South Africa, DC Boonzaier recalled:

There must always be reserved a special niche in my storehouse of theatrical memories for the Royal Australian Opera Company, which appeared, under Wheeler management, at the Good Hope Theatre on 4th May, 1903, and numbered in its ranks that dainty and sprightly actress Miss Gertie Campion, and Dan O'Connor, a young baritone of much promise. The piece selected for the opening night was a fairy-tale of Japan entitled Djin Djin, *by Bert Royle and JC Williamson, music by Leon Caron. The fairy-tale turned out to be something between a pantomime and a musical comedy, but what did that matter when the ladies of the chorus, with their pretty faces and extremely shapely limbs, proved to be something altogether in advance of what we had hitherto been accustomed to see.*

Yes, such girls had never been seen before and the young men in town went crazy over Djin Djin, *and flocked to the theatre every night. I remember the piece went with great swing each night owing to the enthusiasm of the audience.*[3]

Here was opportunity to build on. George formulated a masterplan that embraced Britain, South Africa and Australia. The first step was to take over the Wheeler circuit in a formal way that would not put JCW Ltd at risk should things go wrong. A new company was formed, JC Williamson (South Africa) Limited, which was incorporated on 12 November 1913. It had a nominal capital of £50,000, and the same directorate as JCW Ltd, but expanded to include Pat Malone and Harold Ashton.

Ashton, one of the Firm's tour managers, was moved to Johannesburg as the permanent resident director in South Africa where his task was to supervise the main touring circuit, which took in Johannesburg, Pretoria, Durban and Cape Town. Other towns booked included Port Elizabeth, Bloemfontain, Kimberley and Pietermaritzburg.

GEORGE TALLIS
HUGH J. WARD } MANAGING DIRECTORS
CLYDE MEYNELL

J. C. Williamson, Ltd.

CABLE ADDRESS: "STOFEL."
A.B.C. CODE (5TH ED.) USED.

AUSTRALIA AND NEW ZEALAND
— THEATRES —

HER MAJESTY'S, SYDNEY. HER MAJESTY'S, MELBOURNE.
THEATRE ROYAL, SYDNEY. THEATRE ROYAL, MELBOURNE.
CRITERION THEATRE, SYDNEY. WILLIAMSON THEATRE, MELBOURNE.
THEATRE ROYAL, ADELAIDE. HIS MAJESTY'S, BRISBANE.
OPERA HOUSE, WELLINGTON, N.Z.
THEATRE ROYAL, CHRISTCHURCH, N.Z.
HER MAJESTY'S THEATRE, AUCKLAND, N.Z.

SOUTH AFRICA.
H.M.T., JOHANNESBURG.
THE FOLLOWING TOWNS ALSO BOOKED AND VISITED BY J. C. WILLIAMSON, LTD'S COY'S:
CAPETOWN. DURBAN.
BLOEMFONTEIN PRETORIA.
KIMBERLEY. PORT ELIZABETH.
PIETERMARITZBURG.

EUROPE—DIRECTOR: J. A. E. MALONE, ADELPHI THEATRE, LONDON.
SOUTH AFRICA—LOCAL DIRECTOR: HAROLD ASHTON, HIS MAJESTY'S THEATRE, JOHANNESBURG.
U.S.A. AND CANADA—REPRESENTATIVE: WALTER C. JORDAN, EMPIRE THEATRE BUILDING, 1428 BROADWAY, NEW YORK.

REPLY TO:—
"DEWAR HOUSE,"
11, HAYMARKET,
LONDON, S.W.

CABLES & TELEGRAMS:—
"ENOLAMA," LONDON.

TELEPHONE:—
REGENT 4237.

February 12th, 1915

The takeover was an act of faith by the Firm; faith in its own abilities to master a specialised market at long range without the help of the Wheeler family, who were masters of the game. Good management was needed and, most of all, good luck.

JCW (SA) Ltd commenced operations in Johannesburg on Boxing Day, 1913, with Gilbert & Sullivan pieces, using a company direct from London. The chorus came from Australian ranks and again we read that 'the body of our boys and girls astonished the natives'.[4]

The next successful venture was a call-in on the way home to England of Lewis Waller, Madge Titheradge and their company at the completion of an Australian tour. Following this the Firm dispatched their own Minnie Everett, assisted by Fred Young (Millie Tallis's brother) to produce *Puss in Boots*. A string of light shows followed: *The Girl from Utah, The Girl on the Film, Cinderella,* and more serious productions.

Very early on, however, Tallis had become aware that all was not as well as it seemed, largely due to the problems of communication and a growing economic depression in the Union. The information flow between London, Johannesburg and Australia was slow and confused. Pat Malone in London had his own views about what was required in Africa, and these clashed with those of Harold Ashton, who was, after all, on the spot and better able to assess local conditions.

George and his colleagues soon learnt that touring theatrical companies around South Africa was a vastly different proposition from taking them through Australasia. Certainly there were the same problems of long circuits, sparse populations and high transportation costs, but the prime difficulty was a lack of knowledge in how to manage theatre the South African way. Added to this, poor and

His Majesty's Theatre
Johannesburg - South Africa.
Sole Lessees J.C. Williamson (S.A.) Ltd
Resident Director Mr. Harold Ashton
J. C. Williamson. (S.A.), Ltd.,
have the honour to present
Englands finest romantic actor Mr.
Lewis Waller
— and Miss —
Madge Titheradge,
Together with Mr. Waller's Complete London Company.
"Ring up the Curtain"!
Tuesday, March 24th, 1914,

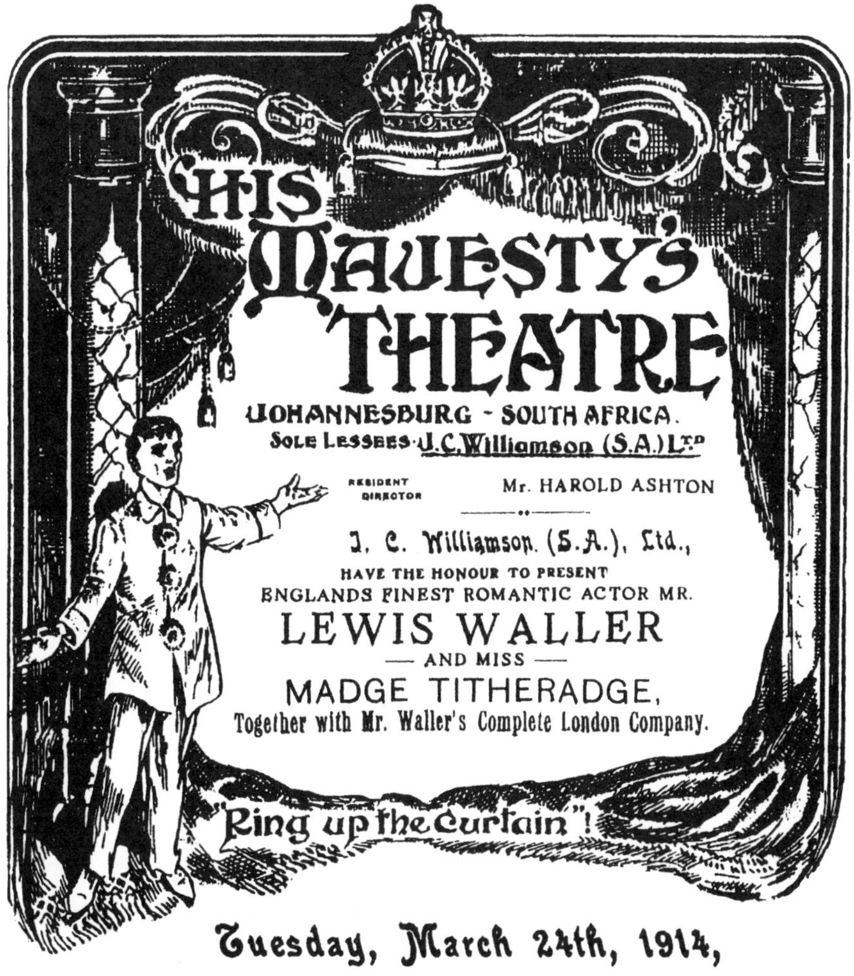

Theatre program for A Marriage of Convenience

inappropriate advertising campaigns resulted in the shows being slow to catch on during the first week of a season. The best advertising, the Firm discovered, was by word of mouth, and takings were invariably low until the news spread that the Firm was in town. By Saturday of the first week the seats started to fill, but this was often too late for a short season to be profitable.

The original aim was to tour one or two companies a year. Scripts were sent from Australia accompanied by instructions for making the scenery. It was all too slow, although pantomimes were an exception and often toured well. Attendances generally were consistently poor during the growing recession in South Africa and JCW (SA) Ltd was left with unexpired contracts and the problem of working out redundancy packages for entire casts. Sometimes wages were cut instead. Economies were everywhere as the Firm realised how badly it had misjudged the South African market.

George received letters from Ashton and Malone informing him of the state of affairs at each end of the business. It dawned too slowly that touring entire foreign theatre companies was unsustainable. The only way to handle South African touring under the existing conditions was by stock companies with wide repertoires. Such companies could be built around a number of versatile actors who delivered drama, farce and musical comedy. This acting core, consisting of English and Australian imports, would work with local South African supporting casts to further reduce costs. Economically nimble, they could stay on the road for a year or more, individual seasons being kept short, sharp and tailored to particular audiences.

With Britain, South Africa and Australia at war with Germany in 1914, Malone at the London end had magnified the Firm's woes by signing contracts with touring companies without the benefit of a clause to protect against contingencies of war. Malone considered such a clause too drastic, but drastic is what George Tallis thought of the South African situation.

Then Harold Ashton came up with the idea that perhaps active dramatic and comedy companies would do the trick. He proposed the formation of a Farcical Comedy Company. In Australia, Tallis was not so sure. The war, political troubles and martial law in South Africa were muddying the waters in that country and he was worried. In October 1914 he wrote to Hugh Ward, outlining his reaction to Ashton's plan and his general concerns about what was going on:

I immediately cabled to Ashton asking him whether, if martial law had been proclaimed, he still thought it wise to send a comedy company. Of course, it would be utterly ridiculous to think of sending one if there is going to be any serious rebellion there and martial law proclaimed for any length of time, as it would be just a repetition of the strike period in Johannesburg earlier in the year when all the theatres had to be closed and everybody in doors by eight o'clock. We certainly are having a joyful time down there.

The war induced depressions in Britain and South Africa, and thereby increased the prices of rights for plays from America. The bad news from London was that the Gaiety, Adelphi and Daly's theatres had closed. Nor was there anything new coming from the Continent. 'We will have nothing for our musical people as soon as we have exhausted our present material' a Melbourne director had written to the Sydney office in 1914.

Harold Ashton wrote to George Tallis an unhappy man:

It is so cold here I can scarcely hold the pen . . . I took this position in the hope and belief it might lead to an appointment on the Australian directorate, and unless I receive some assurance of that, I would not dream of remaining in a country away from all my relatives, friends, lifelong associations, and any materialistic interests I have.

George, once again, had to decide a friend's future.

The South African initiative had seemed a good idea at the time. No doubt the very experienced Ashton made the most of an extraordinarily difficult job as he fought to extract profits from a stream of shows that the local theatre market could not support. But he was in his mid-forties and his main aim was to get back to Australia and a job on the board. His morale was fading fast.

When litigation against the Firm started to flow from disgruntled theatre companies that had been financially compromised by some Williamson South African touring contracts, George had palpable evidence that his first major initiative as chairman of directors had come unstuck. He was grateful that he had set up a separate company to limit the liability.

The South African adventure raised thorny questions about the benefits of overseas expansion but there was not time to dwell on them. The plans for London were reaching fruition. As promised, *High Jinks* eventually opened under the Williamson management at the Adelphi Theatre in August 1916. Produced by Pat Malone, its 383 performances, interestingly enough, made it at the time the longest-running American musical in London since Musgrove's importation of the *Belle of New York* in 1898.

The show was popular, of that there was no doubt, but the possibility of JCW Ltd producing any further pieces in London was blown away by the war. The time of the armistice saw the company, and George Tallis, occupied with other, more urgent business. For the time being, expansion into London was postponed.

By 1916 the position in South Africa had not improved either. The Firm was looking for a way out; in fact for a buyer of the complete South African circuit. The going price was £20,000, just forty per cent of the initial capital of JCW (SA) Ltd. Was there a buyer? We only know that the Firm continued to tour South Africa on an irregular basis long into the future; details of the later managements, and their local arrangements, remain buried.

Harold Ashton was back in Australia as an associate director of the Firm. He became critically ill, and although the company engaged the best doctors to treat one of its most loyal employees, he died in 1917.

The Firm had been beaten by bad luck, slow communications, poor management, war and the unknown. A company takes over a business situated thousands of miles from its head office and which no longer has associated with it the senior administrators who made it work. Fresh brooms move in, and the learning starts anew. How often does it happen that way?

Another move that George made during the war years was to have more lasting consequences for the Firm. He took decisive steps to ensure that JCW Ltd would not be left behind, or mown down, by the advancing cinema industry.

The first primitive motion pictures flickered in Australia in August 1896. By September of that year there was a 'Salon Lumière' in Pitt Street, Sydney, followed closely by a 'Salon Cinematographe'. Both used French equipment patented by the Lumière brothers in 1895. In November, one of the Lumière cameramen filmed the Melbourne Cup – putting the Australian future of films beyond any doubt!

From his first viewing of a Harry Rickards' film in 1896, George Tallis had been 'worried'. Called 'Photo-electric Sensation of the Day', it was screened at the Opera House in Melbourne. Tallis foresaw the time when more finely developed versions of the cinematographe would compete for live theatre audiences and immediately debated this issue with Williamson.

One theatrical entrepreneur after another began jumping onto the band-wagon, among them Williamson and Tallis. In that first year, they imported some movies, and showed them as a supporting attraction to a pantomime. Modestly, they toured the films as the Wonderful Williamson Biograph, but later changed the name to the Anglo-American Bio-Tableau.

For some years, the Firm continued to tinker with the screening of films as the new medium went through the necessary stages of evolution. In the beginning, films enhanced the interest of other forms of entertainment, such as vaudeville and concerts, and the latest newsreels kept the people in touch with world affairs. With time, feature-length films became the main attractions and live entertainment the side-show.

In 1914 JCW Ltd became alarmed at the prospect of American companies making film versions of the plays they were presenting. In retaliation the Firm decided to exploit the lack of a copyright agreement between Australia and the United States by making its own films of the plays. Hired for the job was an American actor–producer, Fred Niblo.

Niblo had been producing some of the Williamson plays, but he was a newcomer to screen directing. His first attempt was *Get-Rich-Quick Wallingford* and it suffered from a slavishly theatrical production technique that was to affect all his Australian films. Niblo's second effort was *Officer 666*, and it was no more successful than his first. In due course he gravitated to Hollywood and, with most of his mistakes already made at the expense of Australian entrepreneurs, he became a very successful movie director of the 1920s.

JCW Ltd persevered by commissioning the production of four more films. They all failed, and in 1916 the company's two-year flirtation with film production ceased.

The First World War halted the making of films in Europe, and by 1918 eighty-five per cent of all films produced were American. These were distributed by the American companies Fox, First National, Metro and Paramount. Westerns took over from the Australian bushranging sagas after they were banned by the New South Wales police in 1912. Perhaps the police had been losing too many celluloid shoot-outs!

With the genius of Charlie Chaplin came a whole new era of comedy. In about 1916, Harry Musgrove, who was George Musgrove's nephew and general manager of Australasian Films, recognised this.

He made a trip to the United States to secure the rights to the Chaplin films, and, not surprisingly, they inspired a generation of Australian comedians.

The film industry was moving rapidly, and the Firm was starting to lose patrons to the 'flicks'. There was no time left for further dilly-dallying. Something had to be done and Tallis raised the problem with the JCW Ltd board on many occasions. His proposal was that the Firm secure the franchise to one of the Hollywood stream of films as well as suitable cinemas. Apparently he met stiff opposition, especially from Hugh Ward. Although Ward vacillated, he mainly argued that the idea was too expensive and that live theatre could be better served with the capital injection needed to get films off the ground.

Tallis felt frustration and foreboding. This was not like the good old days when Williamson, who may have been conservative as an investor, was the first to face all competition and business problems fairly and squarely. Had he been alive there is no doubt that he would have insisted that the threat of films be tackled now and not later.

To avoid further fruitless discussion, in 1916 George put up £60,000 of his own money and approached an acquaintance, Frank W Thring. Thring had shown entrepreneurial skills with early films and Tallis made him a proposal: JCW Ltd would set up a film company to be called JC Williamson Films Ltd, bankrolled by the Firm via Tallis, and he and Thring would run it. Done!

Even though he was using his own money, Tallis felt rumblings from the board. One of the directors had heard bad reports of Thring, yet Ward wrote 'but I always notice that you [Tallis] speak well of him'. Hugh thought that Thring could run the film end of the Firm's Sydney operation, but George had far bigger plans in store for the man.

Frank Thring was born in 1882 at Wentworth, New South Wales. He had roughed around as a young man, but by 1911 he came to the notice of Tallis as a projectionist at Kreitmeyer's Waxworks, a popular entertainment spot in Bourke Street, close to Melbourne's Theatre Royal. Thring had strong ideas about the future of films, and these coincided with those of Tallis. This was the beginning of a congenial and profitable partnership that lasted for fifteen years.

Tallis and Thring set up the Paramount Cinema, Melbourne, and secured the rights to screen Paramount films from Hollywood. They started showing them under the Williamson banner in March 1916, and during the first year more than eighty different films were screened. By 1917, two or three different movies showed per week. Additional space, such as the Town Hall and the Victoria Theatre, was pressed into service when needed.

The Paramount was in Bourke Street, next to the Tivoli variety theatre. It ran continuous shows during the day. Evening shows, with special orchestral effects, started at eight. JC Williamson Films Ltd was the governing director, and FW Thring the manager.

This tilt at the film business was timely. The war had made it difficult to book foreign theatre companies to tour the usual Australasian circuit. Paramount, however, had Adolph Zukor as one of its main directors, and he had built his studio around the concept of filming great plays using the famous theatre stars of London and New York. During the First World War, clearly the next best thing to touring live shows with international talent was to tour the Zukor films.

To add realism to these 'theatrical' films, in 1916 Tallis booked the Theatre Royal in Sydney for some of the screenings. This raised the eyebrows of the purists, who felt that theatres such as the Royal were for stage performances only. Although live music and singers supported the films, this only partially countered the objection. Tallis announced 'a new era in entertainment – a grand combination of high class concert artists and supreme motion picture photoplays – twice daily at 2.30 and 8'. With Gustave Slapoffski, the Firm's senior conductor, holding the baton how could such a venture fail?

The Royal provided entertainment that the public appreciated, and it screened films continuously from 1916 until it returned to the live theatre mainstream in 1919. At the time, the combination of good quality films and Slapoffski musical arrangements was unbeatable.

THEATRE ROYAL

Direction . . . . J. C. WILLIAMSON LTD

BRIEF PHOTO OPERA SEASON.

29 July 1916

Unique Combination of Orchestral
Score and Story of the World-famed
JAPANESE TRAGEDY
MADAME BUTTERFLY
Presenting
MARY PICKFORD AS CHO CHO SAN.

Selections from Puccini's Beautiful Score will accompany the subject. For the Orchestral Direction of this great musical work Gustave Slapoffski has been specially engaged.

The favourite aria from *Butterfly*, 'One Fine Day', also 'The Garden of My Heart' will be sung by MADAME SLAPOFFSKI.

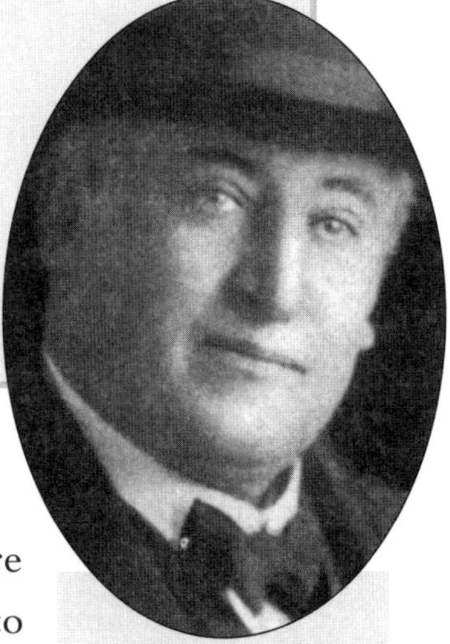

Gustave Slapoffski

They opened the doors, and in flu enza! Not funny now, and much less so in 1919, when there was an influenza epidemic. All motion picture theatres and halls were closed from January to March. When they reopened, only three-quarters of the seats could be used. Continuous running of films was prohibited. There were day sessions with a two-hour break for airing before the evening session, and only theatres with adequate ventilation were allowed to operate. In those days, no one trifled with the flu, an ever present problem to be overcome in bringing entertainment to the masses.

This early investment by Tallis in the film industry was an act of hope; hope that it would help catch 'disloyal' live theatre patrons as they defected to sample the wonders of the screen. It was a great strategy, and most of the big theatre managers were following suit.

During the war years, George, Millie, JCW Ltd – indeed the whole of the Australian theatre industry – threw their weight behind patriotic charity drives. Although charity may begin at home, in the early part of this century theatre people carried it a lot further under the umbrella of their industry. Here were the entertainers, and theatres in which to unleash them. Theatre managers, friends and relations all pitched in to organise countless drives, and the 'running order' at the end of this book shows the sheer diversity of them.

At a glance we see the time and effort devoted by the Williamson organisation to charity. Add in the support of other managements, and the immense scope of the theatre's contribution is revealed. The theatre industry was filling a role since taken over by professional charity organisations and governments.

The least formal affairs, advertised as Theatrical Café Chantants, were held at the leading hotels 'under the patronage of', or 'in the presence of', some dignitary. Leading singers and performers turned foyers into makeshift theatres, and staff and patrons found themselves singing along. This intimacy of the audience with popular stars established a bond that encouraged public generosity. The cost of a cup of tea had risen, but who cared? The amusement section of the *Argus* carried advertisements like these:

THEATRICAL CAFÉ CHANTANT,
At the
ORIENTAL HOTEL,
Under the Patronage and in the Presence of
LADY STANLEY,
In Aid of the Children's Charities, Wattle Day Fund
NEXT FRIDAY, SEPTEMBER 1, 1916 at 3 o'clock

Informal charity performances often took place in the lounges and foyers of theatres. For example, on 1 May 1911 Flo Young held her own show at Her Majesty's with all the bubble and drive for which she was renowned. For two and six, the people were getting a bargain.

Miss Florence Young and the Ladies and Gentlemen
of the Opera Company will give an
At Home
in the Lounge of Her Majesty's Theatre in aid of the Funds of the Alfred Hospital. A Splendid Musical Program by all the Favourites.

Considerably more ambitious was the combined bridge party and café chantant organised by her sister Millie Tallis and held at the Theatre Royal. How patrons played bridge on stage amongst the hubbub, and under the critical eyes of the dress circle and stalls, is not explained.

During the afternoon leading actress Muriel Starr also worked for Belgium by donating a 'kiss for the cause' at a cost of five guineas. The Melbourne *Argus* of 12 March 1915 reported:

The most entertaining episode of the afternoon was yet to come. For the sum of five guineas, Mr Hugh McIntosh [proprietor of the Tivoli vaudeville circuit] has been allowed to plant a 'long and fervent' kiss on the lips of Miss Muriel Starr. It was for the sake of the Belgians that Miss Starr permitted the trespass. It would be ungracious to say she endured it, and impertinent to say she enjoyed it; but as to the enjoyment of Mr McIntosh there can be no doubt. He made a good bargain, and two or three Belgian families can be supported for a week on the five guineas.

A Belgian flag was spread on the stage, and on this the money fell with the strength of a hailstorm. It came from dress-circle, gallery, and stalls in such

THEATRE ROYAL

Under the Patronage of the GOVERNOR GENERAL

March 11, 1915

THIS AFTERNOON, at 2

In Aid of the

BELGIAN RELIEF FUND

BRIDGE AFTERNOON and CAFE CHANTANT

The whole of the stage will be given up to the Bridge Tables, and while play is in progress a Magnificent Programme will be presented by the BEST PROMINENT ARTISTS in MELBOURNE.

THREE SHOWS IN ONE:-

THE BRIDGE PARTY ON THE STAGE,

THEATRICAL WAITERS and WAITRESSES,

THE MAGNIFICENT PROGRAMME.

---

quantities that it kept half-a-dozen collectors busy for at least ten minutes picking up the gold and silver coins. There seemed to be no limit to the generosity of the audience.

This event was part of a giant effort to provide food for the starving victims of war in Belgium. It was an ongoing commitment. Newspapers reported on contributions and compared the figures with the monthly target for Australasia of £75,000. Considering that this was just one of the many supported causes, the size and persistence of the community help was enormous.

According to the *Theatre Magazine* of 1 June 1915:

Belgian Day should bring home to the public more than ever before the part the theatrical profession plays in this country in relieving stress. It should also acquaint those in power of the place the profession occupies in popular esteem. The way theatrical forces can influence the public in missions of mercy was never more clearly demonstrated than on this day. That those forces should have been directed so as to raise 120,000 pounds in the day is a matter worthy of marked recognition.

Sometimes the great stars helped by featuring in the bigger charity programs. Madame Melba made herself available when she could, pulling in the customers and raking in the patriotic takings. As an alternative to mega-stars, there were monster-programs. At these, many well-known performers played the whole day for free. They were leading actors, comedians and singers, supported by equally generous lesser lights.

It is difficult to convey in a few words the enormous size and diversity of the 'Monster Matinees', or the effort of their staging. Whole columns, even pages, in the newspapers gave details of the events, their location and the participants. All the major theatres and companies became involved. At sporting arenas displays of acting and dancing headed the list, followed by three-legged races, tugs-of-war,

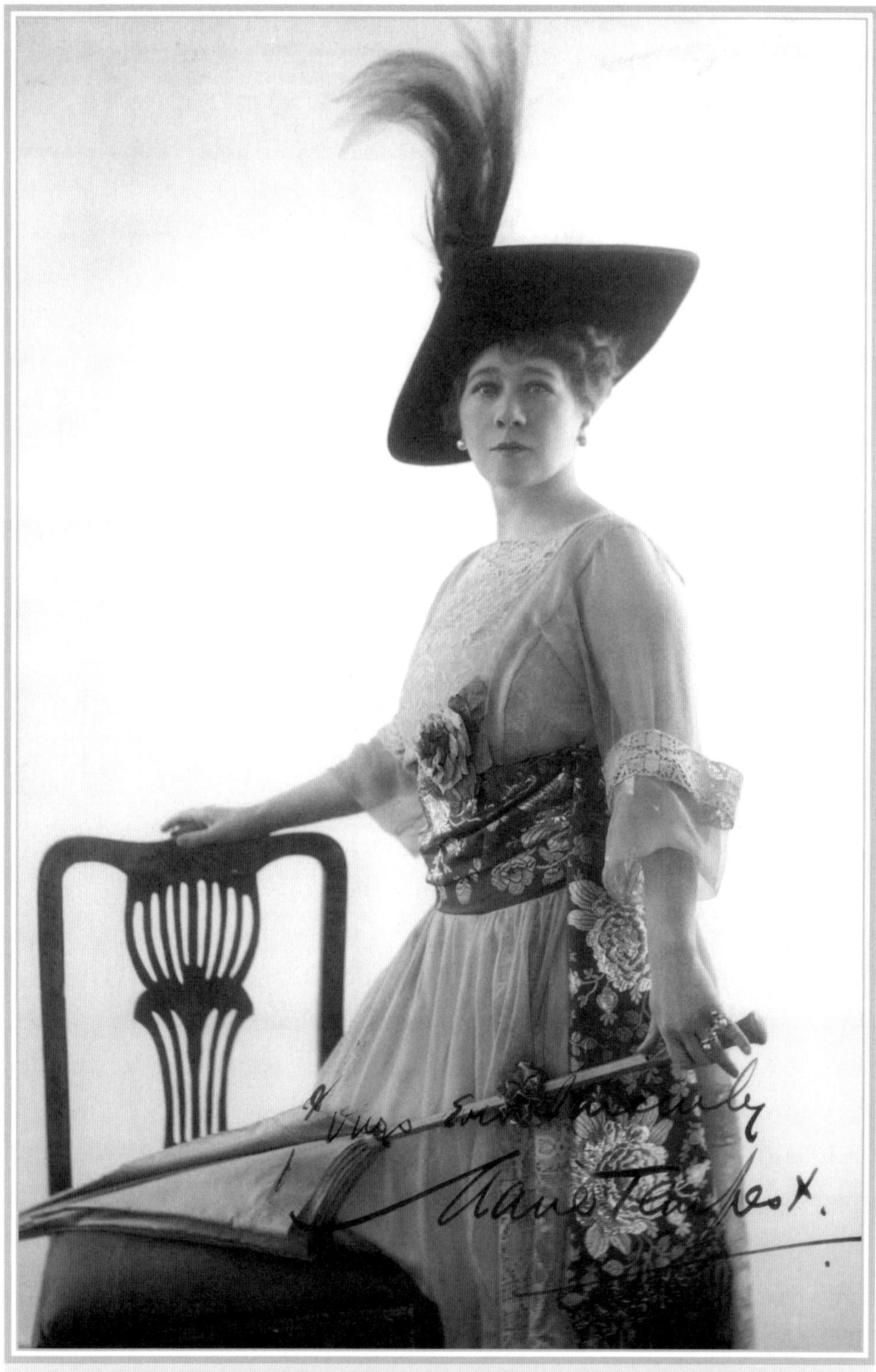

Marie Tempest, English star, played the Theatre Royal Melbourne in 1917

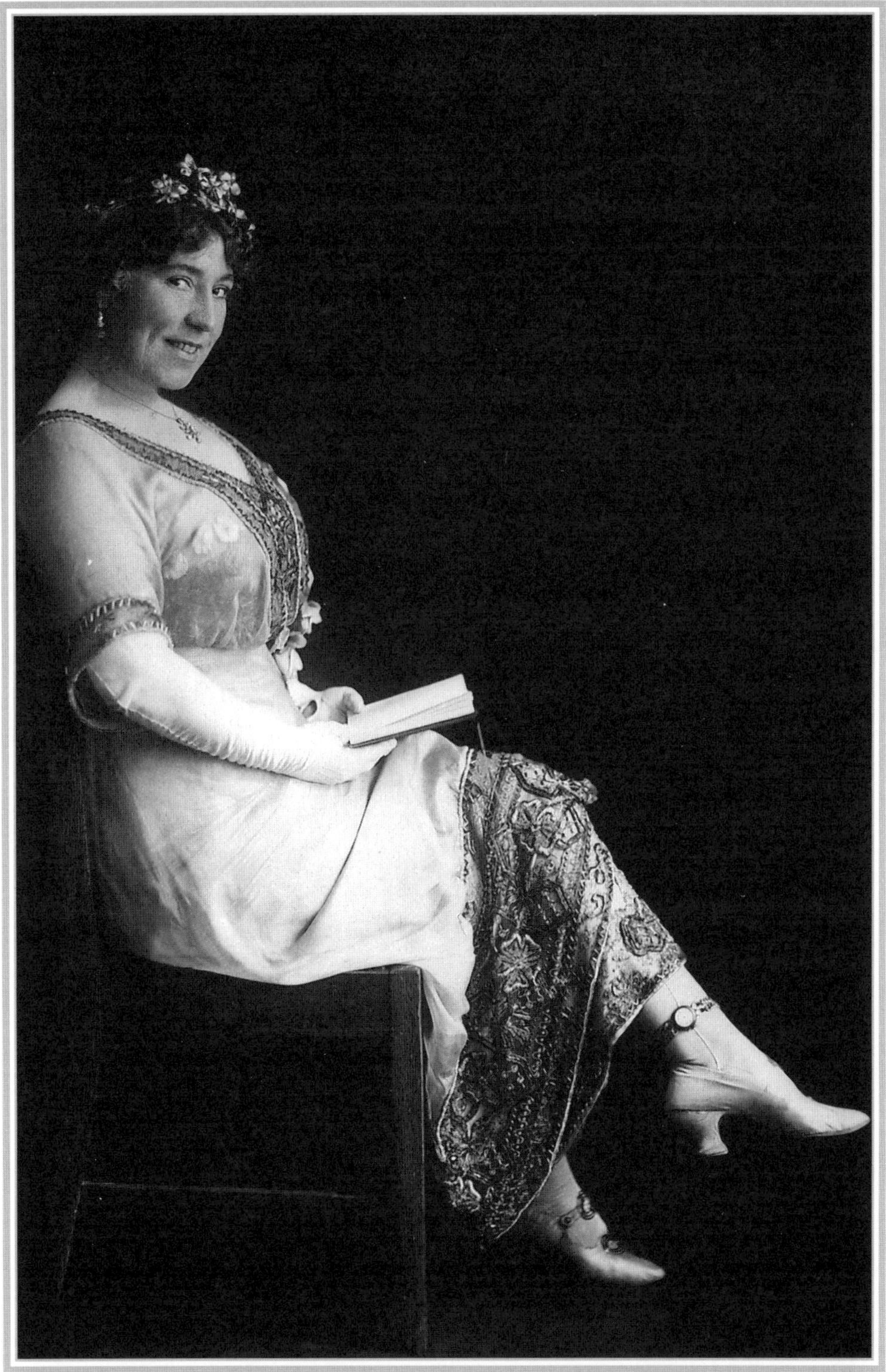

Florence Young, Australia's queen of comic opera

camel races, and other spectacular novelties. The pavements filled with 'button ladies', and the streets sported huge pennants and armies of marching bands. Proceeds supported individual causes, groups of causes and, from 1914 to 1918, the war effort.

For years George and Millie worked for these and other charities. Millie organised and shaped the various events while George worked behind the scenes to provide theatres, honorary performers and management staff. George joined Hugh McIntosh, Hugh Ward, Ben Fuller and many other entertainment managers in supporting the various drives with his own money. It wasn't easy come, but it was easy go. As fast as money flowed from his regular theatre business, chunks of it were redirected to the community through charities and war loans.

Tallis's personal generosity was wide. He received countless letters of gratitude from people he helped. Hospitals and institutions also benefited from a quiet appeal to his community spirit. By his response to others' needs, George was perpetuating a JC Williamson tradition.

The First World War brought America and Australia closer together. Australians were seeing plenty of American films, and they were intrigued by the strange mannerisms. On the other side of the Pacific, the 'Yanks' had heard of the military exploits of the Australian and New Zealand soldiers at Gallipoli and in France. Against this background, George Tallis visited the United States in 1918 to seek celluloid and theatrical attractions. On his return he gave an interview to the *Argus*:

The Americans think Australia is magnificent. The very name Anzac stirs them deeply. New York is full of Australians and of people Australians know. It is just like going down Bourke Street.

The secret of the success of Australian artists in America is that they have a vigorous style that suits the Americans, they are good workers, and owing to the frequent changes of bill in this country they obtain experience that tends to make them versatile. They are not one-type artists, as so many of the British players are nowadays! [5]

America was beginning to replace Britain as Australian entertainment's major feeding ground. George went on to announce that among the prizes he had secured was the 'greatest film DW Griffith had yet produced', *Hearts of the World* – a propaganda film financed by the British government – as well as American musicals, comedies and pantomime acts.

What a difference a decade makes. American shows were now in favour in Australia, and JC Williamson's warning in 1905, that managers courted disaster by importing American productions, no longer held true. The burgeoning American silent film industry had seen to that.

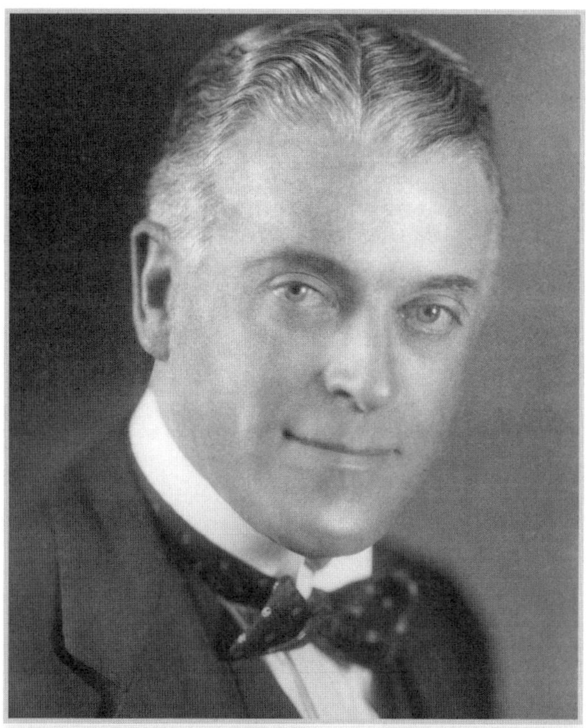

Cyril Maude organised fund raising shows in 1917 with Dame Nellie Melba

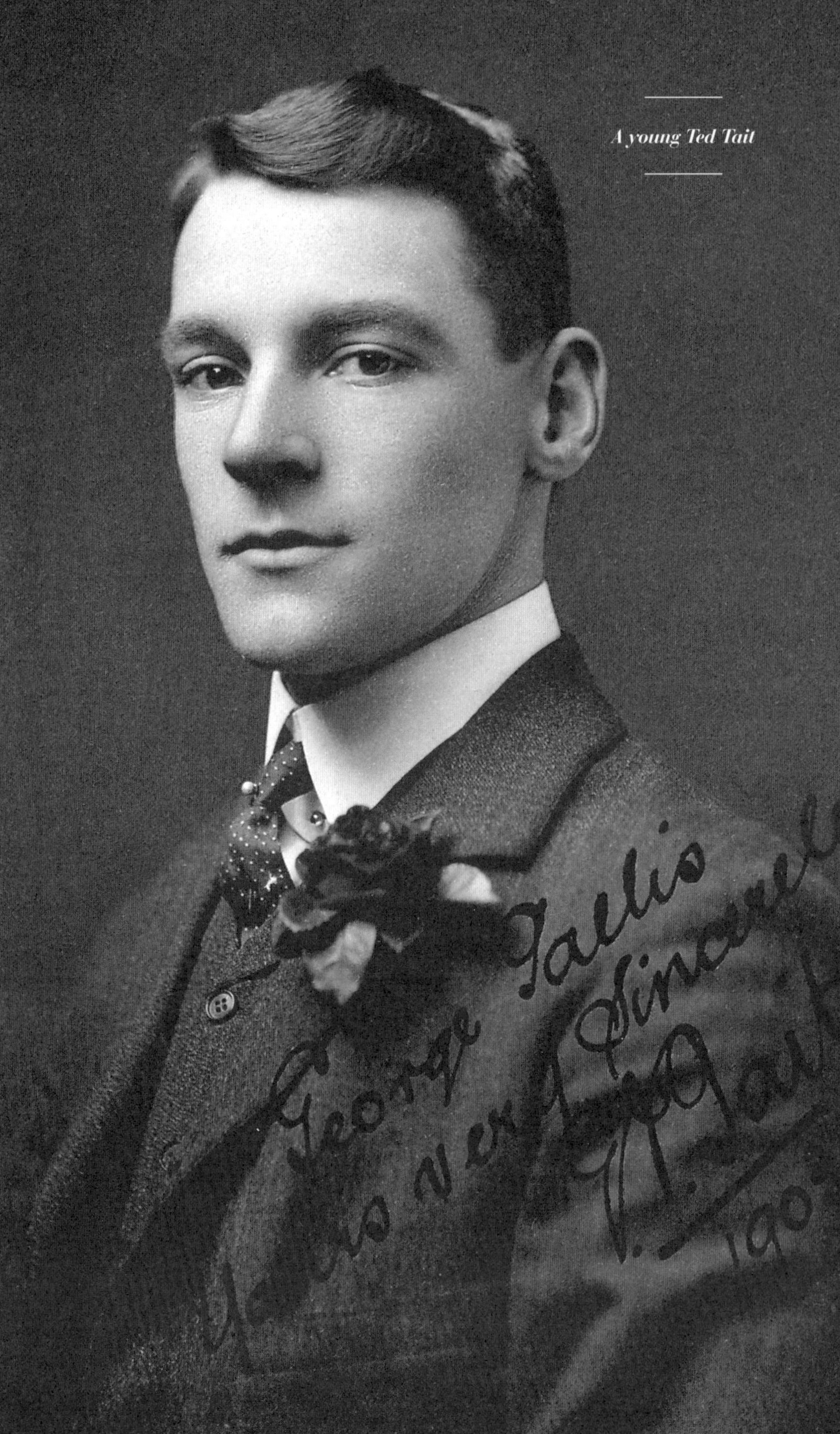

A young Ted Tait

CHAPTER ELEVEN

Amalgamation

As we have seen, despite the problems posed by the war, in its early years under George Tallis's leadership the Firm continued to look for ways to expand its operations. To merge with rival managements was an option and at the time there were three main possibilities.

Harry Rickards, the king of Australian vaudeville, had set the style of popular entertainment from 1895 until long after his death in 1911. He opened his first Tivoli theatre in Sydney in 1893, and built the business into one of the most important vaudeville circuits in the world. When he died, it was purchased by a syndicate led by Hugh D McIntosh, an ex-boxing promoter and hotelier. McIntosh had absolutely no theatre training, but what he lacked in stage-craft he compensated for with an extraordinary entrepreneurial flair. Under his ownership small changes were made to the Rickards format, but the stream of international attractions for the Tivoli circuit was maintained and improved.

The trans-Tasman showmen Ben and John Fuller were also contenders for a possible Williamson merger. In partnership with their father they had launched John Fuller and Sons, the pioneers of permanent vaudeville in New Zealand. In 1912, the brothers moved to Sydney and took over the James Brennan vaudeville circuit, which was second only to that started by Harry Rickards. Fullers rapidly enlarged the Brennan enterprise and began to give the Tivoli some real competition.

A third management, J&N Tait, was also gathering strength. Formed in 1902, its first steps were into concert management, although films were soon added to the list. Around 1911, the Auditorium, a short distance west of Russell Street in Collins Street, became the nerve centre of the Tait operation; it was also the main venue for Melbourne's concert and musical programs for many years. But the careful observer would have sensed an interesting shift in the direction of J&N Tait during 1913–1916. The company began to produce theatrical shows as well as concerts and films.

George Tallis and the Firm might have been busy with their programs to take South Africa by storm, tackle the film industry and raise money for the war effort, but it can be seen that they were not alone. Other entrepreneurs were also going about their business of entertaining Australia. Vaudeville would be an attractive addition to the Firm's portfolio, if for no other reason than to provide an outlet for all the contracted actors walking the streets at the Firm's expense, victims of failed shows or miscasting by overseas agents.

A merger with McIntosh or Fullers, however, would have to wait. Neither encroached seriously on the Firm's traditional fishing grounds and they were therefore no immediate threat to smooth cash flows. But J&N Tait was much more of a danger. This enterprise was starting to act like the Clarke–Meynell partnership of old. Surely they weren't about to rock the boat and disturb Tallis's plans for the Williamson company?

In the history of Australian entertainment, the story of the five Tait brothers, who for over seventy years made contributions to the music, concert, film and theatre worlds, is unique. The eldest of them, Charles, was born in 1869, and began work as an office boy at Allan &

Co.'s Music Warehouse. Under the eye of George Allan, Charles made his way by streamlining the sheet music operation of the store, and by his flair for concert management.

The other brothers were John Henry (Dick), born 1871; James Nevin (Jim), born 1876; Edward Joseph (Ted), born 1878; and Frank Samuel, born 1883. They were Australian-born sons of a father from the Shetland Isles, Scotland, and a mother from London.

As Charles became more experienced, he coached his brothers in the ways of concert administration. In 1902 John and Nevin founded J&N Tait, Concert Directors. Charles and Ted were also foundation partners, and Frank joined soon afterwards.

John, Nevin and Frank worked for the family company and specialised in the celebrity concert business, with Nevin later posted in London to secure artists. Ted Tait, on the other hand, had been invited by George Tallis in 1900 to join JC Williamson as assistant treasurer and he stayed on with the Firm. He was promoted to business manager in 1911 and then to general manager in Sydney in 1913, but resigned in 1916 to join his brothers in J&N Tait. He spent most of the following four years overseas.

Of the five, Charles was the elder statesman and John the business brain. A prime example of John's eye for an opportunity is described in Peter Game's book *The Music Sellers*. Early in 1900 a bank manager, who was aware of John's business leanings, had apparently mentioned casually that he knew of a shareholder in Allan's Music Store who wanted to sell preference shares. Charles worked at Allan's, and so John knew of the company's potential. He bought the shares, and by so doing the Taits gained not only a large shareholding in Allan's, but also a strong representation on the board, much to the discomfort of the Allan family.

This business move was important for other reasons. It alerted Ted, and perhaps all the brothers, to the immense advantages that accrue from smart share acquisitions. The Allan affair was a corporate manoeuvre that was never far from Ted's mind as he toiled to learn his craft at JC Williamson's. A decade later, the Clarke–Meynell and JCW Ltd amalgamation afforded a much more immediate model for Ted to ponder, and he watched the moves carefully. When he eventually finished his sixteen years with Williamson's, he had been given the best schooling of its kind that Australia could provide. He regarded his time with the Firm as invaluable. Repeatedly he pointed out that he knew more about theatre than the rest of his brothers collectively, a fact that they readily conceded.

In his last few years with the Firm in Sydney, Ted learnt about the contracts that JCW Ltd negotiated with American and English managers, the price of plays and terms and conditions. He said once: 'Oh boy, what a lot there was to learn from November 1913 to January 1916. Two years and two months, but I got it all.'

Ted Tait was a workaholic, with driving ambitions for himself and J&N Tait as a whole. He was excitable, and referred to himself as 'highly strung'. He was prone to deep bouts of depression when he was under stress and away from home, and psychological problems later dominated his life. This worried his brothers, especially when they received long letters from him endlessly reviewing injustices, real and perceived. A massive correspondence built up between the five brothers over the years, ventilating all disagreements. Yet in spite of headstrong disharmony, they managed to unite on important decisions that directly affected them. Indeed, as Ted once put it, they were 'stout fellows'.

Everyone who worked closely with Ted Tait had to make allowances for his mood swings. George Tallis was in close contact with him over a period of forty years, and he, too, was subjected to Ted's darker moments, especially through Ted's letters. Correspondence from Ted raised every perceived injustice that clouded the 'best-of-friends' relationship Ted claimed for himself and George. As time passed, the list grew longer, as did the letters bearing the tidings. George seemed to absorb the news as Ted's brothers advised him to do, and he either wrote an expansive letter of praise in reply, or remained silent. Neither strategy suited Ted, who regarded the friendly letters as 'insincere' and the non-responses as an abdication of responsibility. Expecting George to counter-attack, Ted's frustrations often boiled over.

The telephone would sometimes ring for George when he was at work, at home or on holiday: 'Who is your best friend, George?' Ted would ask ominously. When George dutifully replied, 'Ted Tait', the other end would erupt, 'No, he's not . . .,' and George was informed in strong words of a surprise downgrading of their relationship. Ted kept George on edge, more or less continually, and perhaps vulnerable to his point of view. As the bad patches became more frequent and protracted, this barrage took its toll, and George sought escape. In the short term though, the only recourse was to ride out the volatility, and make the most of a relationship that, often enough, worked well.

Ted Tait was nine years George's junior, but in terms of theatre and business experience he was much further behind. He soon appreciated the magnitude of the Firm, and its potential, and saw what hard work, application and talent had done for Tallis. This gave him his goal.

Apart from age and seniority, there was another major difference between the two men. George handled personal conflicts with courtesy and circumspection, fending off damaging and senseless rifts. He avoided capricious confrontation, and his easy manner made him uniformly popular. Ted, on the other hand, was brash and his intemperance resulted in unnecessary hardship for himself and others.

A good deal of the trouble caused by Ted at the Firm was ultimately referred to a reluctant Tallis – as was one tricky, unavoidable problem. J&N Tait was continuing to grow, and the Williamson board had noticed that Ted, as their employee, was developing a conflict of interest. Although he officially distanced himself from his brothers' activities, his direct involvement with them was clear enough.

Believing that more senior responsibility under managing director

Hugh Ward might refresh him, render J&N Tait more remote and lessen Ted's conflict with the Firm, in 1913 George had him promoted to business manager and posted to Sydney. Once there, though, Ted found blemishes in some of the Williamson company's departments, and he attempted rather forcefully to improve the systems. The entrenched department heads became restive, and referred Ted to Ward.

Ted Tait and Hugh Ward was not a good pairing from the start. Although the association had potential, Ted being clever with money and Ward with theatre, it was a combination that would never work. Both had fiery personalities, both were ambitious, jealously eyeing off the Firm, and each was suspicious of the other. This was in spite of the fact that Ward was senior, a respected actor and generally very experienced in theatre matters. One might have thought that Hugh had no need to feel threatened and yet, as it turned out, his instincts did not let him down.

He suspected that Ted was passing confidential JCW Ltd information on to J&N Tait, and he used this, in part, as a reason for refusing Ted's repeated applications for a senior promotion to the board. He also expressed his view that Ted had very little aptitude for theatre. Ted, in turn, thought that his desk had been rifled, and he held Ward responsible. These two complaints hit Tallis's in-tray. George filed the letters carefully, no doubt wondering if Ted's move to Sydney had actually solved anything.

Then there was the *Peg o'My Heart* debacle. The Firm had been stalking this very promising musical since 1914, but had somehow been unable to tie the knot. When Nevin Tait, who worked the London and New York markets for J&N Tait, mysteriously snatched the rights to the Hartley Manners show from under the very nose of Hugh Ward and JCW Ltd in 1915, a state of war arose between the two companies. At the Firm, it was all over for Ted Tait. His position became untenable, and early in the following year he resigned to formally join his family company full time – a move that perhaps should have taken place considerably earlier.

Despite occasional difficulties besetting the personal relationship between George and Ted, on work issues at the Firm they had collaborated effectively, enjoyed confidence in each other's ability and socialised well. It was unfortunate that George stood in the way of Ted's overriding ambition to control JCW Ltd, and that he was therefore in Ted's sights. George had to act for the board in matters relating to Ted, and fend off any efforts to gain financial control of the Firm. To do this without fracturing a friendship was a tricky balancing act requiring all the skills of the Irish.

J&N Tait's production of *Peg o'My Heart* was successful, and it played for twelve weeks in Sydney and eight in Melbourne. To turn up the heat, in 1916 the Taits introduced more importations. JCW Ltd came out swinging, and between 1916 and 1917 there were about eighty shows under the Williamson banner. Although there was no *Peg* among them, stalwarts such as Julius Knight and Florence Young, as well as rising new stars kept the flag flying. John West in *Theatre in Australia* claims that:

The Firm deserves real credit during those war years for fostering young Australians as leading ladies for musical comedy, to complement and replace long-established favourites. The new stars were young peppy girls – Dorothy Brunton, Minnie Love, Maud Fane, Madge Elliott . . . But the biggest star-to-be of the whole Williamson's crop was Gladys Moncrieff.[1]

The Tait assault continued into 1918–1919 with modern plays, including some by Bernard Shaw and Henrik Ibsen. Their success was mixed. Tallis and his Firm responded by presenting a higher proportion of popular shows, such as the play *Lightnin'*, and musicals *Katinka* and *Going Up*. Altogether, competition had freshened up, and from the public's point of view, that was good news indeed.

In the years preceding 1920, Ted Tait dreamt up many proposals to take over JCW Ltd. One story relates that while overseas Ted had sent some plans home disguised in a series of coded cables, but there was confusion due to decoding errors, Ted's clandestine wording, and a mixing of the correct sequence of the cables. But mostly the trouble was that Ted had sent half the cables to Sydney and half to Melbourne as a security measure, and that cable five ended up in the wrong hands.

It seems that the essence of all the schemes was to somehow acquire enough shares in JCW Ltd, or to get sufficient friendly shareholders on side, to allow J&N Tait to control the company. While Ted was still a member of the Firm, he tried to work from within the company, but after he left he worked to apply external pressure.

For most of the four years from January 1916, Ted scouted in America for J&N Tait. This was a huge assignment as it involved seeing literally hundreds of shows, and he chased all over the country to view them. Finally, when he found a gem, he would approach the agent for the Australian rights, only to be told he was just too late. JCW Ltd had beaten him to the punch. Who was in the States doing business for the opposition? It was, of course, Hugh Ward, and since Hugh was an American with plenty of contacts, he knew his way around and slammed the door in his competitor's face as often as he could.

The game was such that Ted could not hope to win, although he must be awarded eleven out of ten for effort. In 1917 he complained that Williamson's and the Taits were such terrible enemies, it was just like the Great War – a fight to the finish. Each time Ted ran second to Ward, which was too frequently, Ted warned the agent concerned that Hugh was bad company.

American agents are not renowned for being slow. They soon realised that the number of Australian bidders for their products had doubled from one to two. So it was that whenever Hugh called on his circle of agents, he found that the price of the shows had risen. This was noticed by Ted, who said: 'The Australian field cannot stand the opposition of two Australian managers wanting the same material from New York and London managers. This opposition has got to stop.' But there was not the slightest indication from Ted that he might set a good example by being first to give in.

All this fuss and confrontation had done nothing to improve the relationship between Hugh and Ted. In fact, antipathy had matured into a violent chemical reaction. This animosity was noted in New York, especially after the Lambs Club affair.

George Tallis described the famous New York Lambs Club as a place 'where they never go to bed'. It was a venue used by theatrical people to conduct business and pleasure. In the days of the Williamson partnerships, Williamson and Musgrove used this club during their American trips, and many a good deal had been struck within its walls.

Hugh Ward also availed himself of the Lambs Club during his visits to New York and occasionally, by invitation, so did Ted Tait. It seems that it was during one of Ted's club visits that he heard of JCW Ltd's negotiations for *Turn to the Right*. This was a play that J&N Tait ultimately signed up, and with which the company did very well. With all the disaffection that was about town, the *Turn to the Right* deal, and unpleasant rumours around the Lambs, it was inevitable that something would explode between Ted and Hugh.

Ted wrote an undisciplined letter to Walter Jordan, the Williamson New York agent, concerning Ward and the Lambs Club. Since Hugh was 'family', Jordan passed the letter on to him, and Hugh kept it for the time when Ted would apply for guest membership. When Ted finally wandered into the club with refreshment and a visiting membership on his mind, the bomb went off. 'Very sorry, sir, but your request for membership is denied.'

The ensuing conversation between the club secretary and Ted was not recorded, but he further tested his luck by applying for full membership. His letter to Jordan got in the way again, and members of the club suggested that he might have more luck at less salubrious establishments. Fuming, Ted whipped around to the Friars Club, which was similar to the Lambs. But Ward had pre-empted him there as well. Ted was now persona non grata in two clubs, and counting. The simple sum was that Lambs plus Friars equals Hugh Ward – EJ Tait's suspicions precisely.

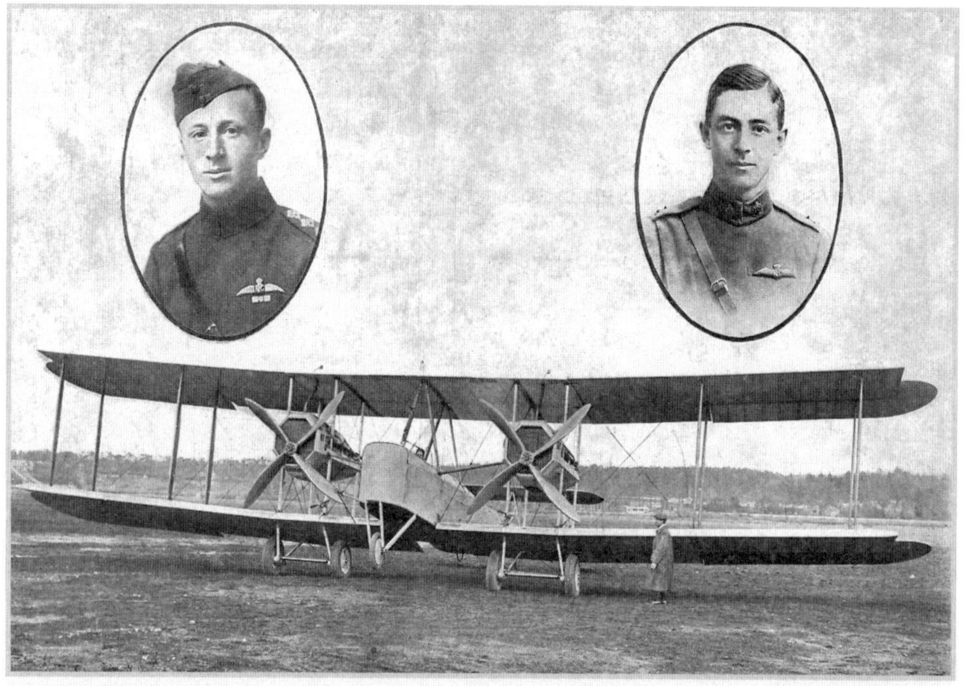

Aviators Ross and Keith Smith who made the first flight from England to Australia in 1919 in their Vickers Vimy biplane

This piece of theatre added fuel to the flames of a growing fire. It also further soured Ted's feelings for JCW Ltd, although he knew that the Lambs Club affair was strictly personal. His health deteriorated as he became obsessed with Ward.

On his own American home ground Hugh Ward played unbeatable hard ball, but Australia was Ted's native turf, and the game was far from over. For the moment, however, life in New York was looking up. Ward's comfortable existence at the Lambs, which had briefly been under threat from Ted, returned to normal and he felt that this

HER MAJESTY'S THEATRE

Sole Proprietors - - - - - - - J. C. WILLIAMSON Ltd.
Managing Directors - - Messrs. GEORGE TALLIS, HUGH J. WARD and CLYDE MEYNELL
Associate Director - - - Mr. CHARLES A. WENMAN

WEDNESDAY NIGHT, FEBRUARY 25, 1920

In Honor of, and in the Presence of
Captain SIR ROSS SMITH, K.B.E., M.C., D.F.C., A.F.C. (Australian Flying Corps)
Lieutenant SIR KEITH SMITH, K.B.E., (Royal Air Force)
Sergeant J. M. BENNETT, A.F.M., M.S.M. (Australian Flying Corps)
Sergeant W. H. SHIRES, A.F.M. (Australian Flying Corps)

THE ALL-BLUE ROUTE

Blazing a trail across the sky from shore to distant shore,
They win their victory in Peace, as once they won in War;
The birds have made their homeward flight along the all-blue route—
And as they flutter down to rest Australia gives salute!

Into the blood-red skies of war they flew all unafraid,
Not theirs to shirk the lone patrol, barrage or bombing raid—
And now they flutter back to us across the boundless blue,
Flying into a world unknown to find the land they knew.

In other days and other ships there came across the sea,
Spaniard and heavy Hollander, Frenchman and Portugee.
But, conquerors of the clouds above, we take it as our boast,
Australia's sons were first of all to sight Australia's coast.

A message from the motherland they brought to us on high,
To bind us with a triple bond of earth and sea and sky;
And show to all the wondering world Britannia rules the air—
When the first flight is made to Mars, Australia Will be There!

"ORIEL," in "The Argus."

GALA PERFORMANCE
...OF...
J. C. WILLIAMSON'S GORGEOUS PANTOMIME
"THE SLEEPING BEAUTY"
"THE KNIGHTS OF THE AIR"

Left London—
November 2nd, 1919.

Ross Smith.
Keith Smith

Arrived Darwin—
December 10th, 1919.

From the gala performance program for Sir Ross Smith and Sir Keith Smith

would be good for Williamson's. It certainly seems that business started to improve as Ward indulged in club life away from Ted's critical gaze.

At home, Ted's problems in New York bothered his brothers. They told him to calm down, and to attempt to be civil to the Williamson staff. All the confrontation had been damaging. Ted's answer to this was that if they wanted to be friendly with any of the Williamson

HER MAJESTY'S THEATRE

Sole Proprietors: J. C. WILLIAMSON LTD.

Managing Directors:
GEO. TALLIS, HUGH J. WARD, CLYDE MEYNELL

Associate Director: CHARLES A. WENMAN

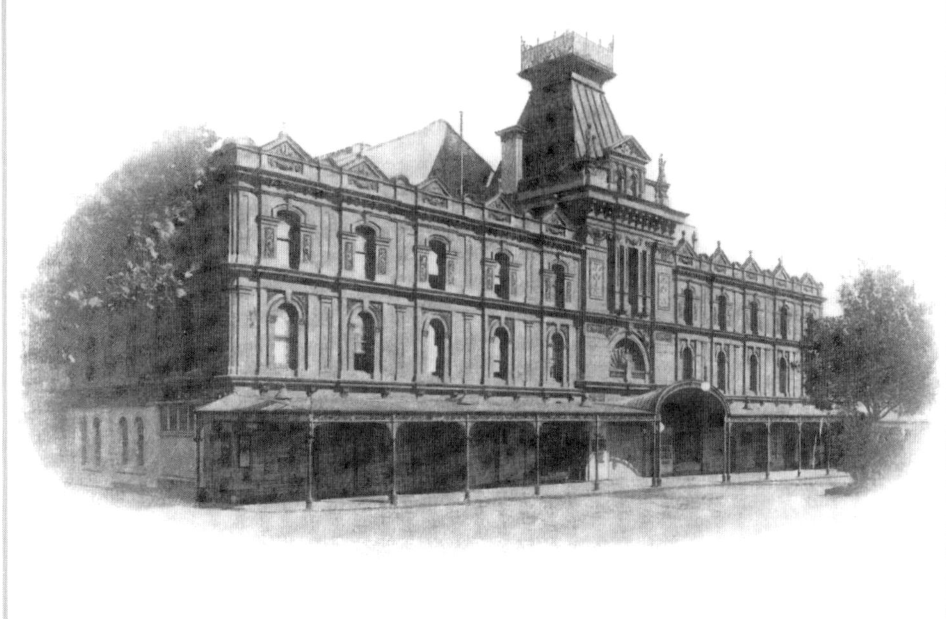

HER MAJESTY'S THEATRE, MELBOURNE

From the gala performance program for the Prince of Wales, 1920

organisation, let it be Tallis and not Ward, for 'I have great respect for Tallis's ability and I can handle him when I'm with him. It's only when he gets away from me that he slips'.

Early in 1918, Tallis was in his office at Her Majesty's Theatre. He had slipped away from Ted alarmingly since 1916, and had enjoyed every moment of the process. The number of confrontations had dwindled pleasingly, although George noted impatiently that most of the Williamson departments were fighting. Ward had written that it seemed that 'all the heads of departments not only seem to give offence to each other, but are insisting on ... criticising each other'. What was wrong with everyone? Was it sheer ego that made people neglect their jobs and not mind their own business?

Then Tallis remembered that Ward himself could be self-promotional, obstructive and difficult, and he felt the familiar twinge of irritation that he usually was able to suppress. Not to worry! He would have a friendly chat with them all shortly, and he immersed himself in the business of theatre that for years had been his refuge from the ugly side of management.

The mail arrived, and among the mass of local and international letters he noticed two from the United States: one from Ted Tait and one from Ward. With apprehension he opened them, and read two versions of the Lambs Club affair. The small irritation he had just subdued returned, tenfold. This time it started in his feet, swept up his legs and totally engulfed him. He stood up and went to the window, took deep breaths and swore quietly in Gaelic for almost a minute without repeating himself. He sat down and re-read the letters. What on earth were these clowns up to in New York? Australian theatre would be the laughing stock of the town for years to come, and the purchase price of shows would never come down again. What did they expect? Both men were quick to chide and slow to bless, yet as soon as things went wrong he was called in to arbitrate. Uncharacteristically angry, George stuffed the letters in a drawer, and walked out into the sunshine.

As he strolled towards his club in Collins Street, Tallis realised that something would have to be done about J&N Tait sooner rather than later. So far the Tait assault had cost both sides money for shows, inefficiencies and lost opportunities. Most of all, it had caused him aggravation that he didn't need.

He walked into the reading room of the club, and one of his friends said, 'What's up George, why so pensive?' Tallis looked up and became aware that a group of men was looking at him. George mumbled, 'I must be getting old', and hoped that it was explanation enough. It was for him.

Over 1918–1919, work continued on the idea of a Tait–JCW amalgamation. Whenever George bumped into Frank or John, they raised the question. When Tallis made one of his frequent business trips to Sydney, he occasionally ran into Ted, who always had new plans for a merger. Tallis listened, expressed great interest, and then vanished. Efforts to locate him at his regular Sydney hotel failed; he had moved to Manly. Moreover, his travelling arrangements, once the model of precision, had become vague. At random he travelled by train, boat or car, and his arrival and departure times became blurred by 'inevitable delays'. In brief, there was a period in 1919–1920 during which he was enormously difficult to find. In Melbourne or Sydney, the Taits were having trouble contacting him for discussions on an amalgamation.

Part of the problem was that Tallis knew that his evasions simply made the opposition keener, and more vulnerable. The other, and perhaps more important part was his realisation that he had come to a critical crossroads in his life. His usual ploy of ignoring the difficulties in the hope that they would go away had failed. The problems were still there, and an extensive shake-up was inevitable – even, perhaps, desirable.

He quickly eliminated the option of doing nothing. Selling out his interest in the Firm would also be foolish with brighter post-war prospects on the horizon, although he had long talked vaguely of retirement. The positives of an amalgamation were clear. The injection of new managerial blood into the Firm was overdue and, anyway, some extra pressure on the Williamson departments might help stem the bickering. The time was surely right for expansion.

HER MAJESTYS

Direction - - - J. C. WILLIAMSON LTD.
Managing Directors - - Messrs. GEO. TALLIS, HUGH J. WARD, CLYDE MEYNELL
Associate Director - - CHARLES A. WENMAN

SATURDAY, SEPTEMBER 7 1918

FIRST TIME IN AUSTRALIA

J. C. WILLIAMSON'S

ROYAL COMIC OPERA CO.

Including **FLORENCE YOUNG**

In the Musical Comedy in Three Acts

Oh! Oh!! Delphine!!!

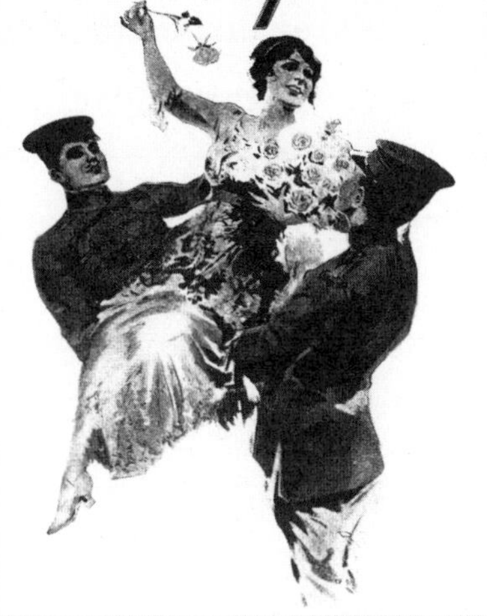

Book and Lyrics by C. M. S. McLELLAN; Music by IVAN CARYLL
(Author and Composer of "THE PINK LADY")

A BRILLIANT CAST OF FAVOURITES
INCLUDING

FLORENCE YOUNG	PHIL SMITH
OLIVE GODWIN	REGINALD ROBERT
JACK RALSTON	ADDIE LENNARD
JOHN FORD	KITTY DOWNES
NESTA BARRY	CYRIL RITCHARD
EVA WEBBER	CLAUDE BANTOCK
PHYLLIS AMERY	OLIVER PEACOCK
WINNIE HOOD	HARRY RATCLIFFE
HAROLD REEVES	RUBY ARMFIELD
EILEEN SHETTLE	ANNIE SEDDON
WYONNE HAYBITTLE	LEAH PRITCHARD
GLADYS MONCRIEFF	GEORGE WELCH

The Play Produced by - GEORGE A. HIGHLAND
Dances, etc., Arranged and Invented by - MINNIE HOOPER
Musical Director - - - VICTOR CHAMPION

Music with a Swing; A Story with a Tangle;
A Host of Lovely Girls—and Such Dresses!

Above all, Tallis needed help with the business side of JCW Ltd; his managing directors, Ward and Meynell, were theatre-strong and business-weak. The Taits were the reverse. George had been at it for nearly thirty-five years, and he wanted a break. It was time to regroup, and to assess the future of the entertainment industry. When it came down to it, the Taits were the only way forward. And it would not be prudent to invite just one or two of them to join: the brothers worked as a team.

There were potential disadvantages. The four Taits could vote *en bloc* and cause trouble if they ever crowded JCW Ltd board positions. Yet they all seemed reasonable men, except for Ted, who was sometimes the reverse; and perhaps he still haboured takeover aspirations. George remembered previous experiences only too well. Surely the family would prevail upon Ted to maintain his composure . . .

George Tallis had these matters on his mind in 1919, when a letter arrived from Ted marked URGENT, PERSONAL AND PRIVATE. He was writing from America and he blamed the tone of previous correspondence on recent events in New York. Now he wanted to bury the hatchet. There was room for all, he said, and he was anxious for JCW Ltd and J&N Tait to coexist happily. Ted referred to the good old days when he and Tallis were 'practically as brothers', and explained how he had written to Millie . . .

Tallis thought long and hard, and balanced the past against the future. What the hell, nothing in business has an iron-clad guarantee! Let's look at a Williamson–Tait amalgamation!

In 1920, the JCW Ltd board consisted of six members. They were Chairman of Directors George Tallis; Managing Directors Clyde Meynell and Hugh Ward; and Directors Arthur Allen, Fred Smith and Theodore Fink. We have already mentioned Arthur Allen. Theodore Fink was the Melbourne solicitor for JCW Ltd,[2] and Fred

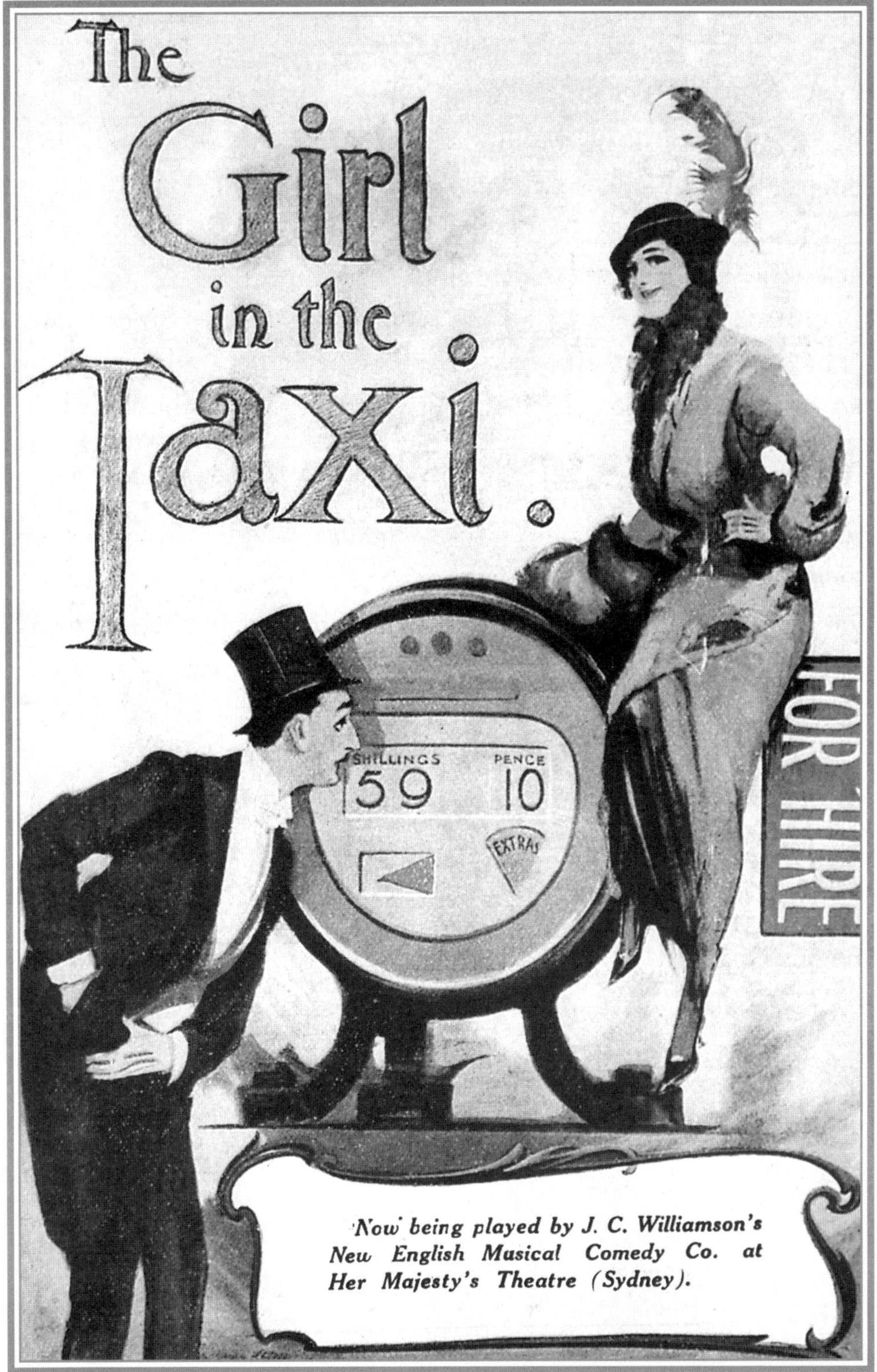
The Girl in the Taxi.
SHILLINGS
PENCE
59
10
EXTRAS
FOR HIRE
Now being played by J. C. Williamson's New English Musical Comedy Co. at Her Majesty's Theatre (Sydney).

Smith of Smith and Johnson Pty Ltd Sydney was the Firm's accountant. Both had been around for a very long time.

Meynell and Ward were the new boys on the block, and the old guard of Tallis, Allen, Fink and Smith were part of the furniture. Meynell had lost interest in the business side of the Firm and Ward, by means of word and deed, had made himself unpopular with the rest of the board. This fact was to determine his future.

With the psychological stage set, only the bartering remained. The Taits wanted one-quarter of an expanded JC Williamson Ltd, but Tallis responded by asking what they were bringing to the party. The answer was three building sites, the lease of Auditorium Hall and the Palace Theatre, part lease of the King's Theatre and all the concert business, future contracts and goodwill. Tallis remained silent.

At a later meeting George said that Allen and Smith were wavering, Ward was against a merger, and he 'didn't see how he would pull off anything unless the agreed figure [for the Taits] was a one-fifth interest and not a quarter'. The Taits conferred, came up with an agreement and it was game, set and match at the next board meeting. Hugh Ward's stocks took a tumble, and perhaps he rued the days of the Lambs Club incident. It was all too late. The Taits were in, and it was get-even time for brother Ted.

The number of ordinary shares increased from 300,000 to 375,000, 75,000 going to J&N Tait, which maintained its name under the merger. Tallis and the Taits bought the 12,800 shares of Mr Gillett, a managing director of Hordern Bros., and the 35,700 shares of Sir Rupert Clarke, as a joint fifty–fifty holding. Major share holdings now were approximately:

Taits 82,000; Tallis 60,000;
Tallis–Tait 48,500; Allen 42,300;
Ward 33,400; Hordern family 21,000.

Ted became a managing director of JCW Ltd, and Frank became an ordinary director, giving the Taits a representation on the board of two out of eight. John, Nevin and Frank were all managing directors of J&N Tait, and these arrangements suited everyone except Nevin, who wanted a board position.

The major details of the amalgamation were finalised on 3 July 1920. A reshuffle of Australian theatre management had taken place to form the biggest theatrical company that this country had seen. The Firm expanded, and it had the capacity for further growth. With proper attention to the prevailing JC Williamson standards of excellence, the sky was the limit.

The new concern was known as JC Williamson Ltd and J&N Tait. The arrangement put the Tait name before the public, and left the most senior man in the company to occupy the shadows of anonymity. Tallis had already occupied that position during the Williamson years; it seemed that he had now settled for the same role again.[3]

After the amalgamation George was sitting in the bar of the Riversdale Golf Club. He needed time to think. He felt vaguely unsettled. Where on earth was his old mate Wasley? His eye caught the honour boards, and under the heading of President he saw: *1916 G Tallis*. That pleased him.

For many years now he had been playing golf regularly. Anyone conducting a futile search for him at the usual haunts in the city concluded, with some justification, that George was 'playing golf again'. At the club he pushed aside the worries of theatre, and exchanged anecdotes with old friends.

He was a keen, middle-handicap golfer and, as was the custom in those days, he used a caddy. Caddies were cheap and efficient. For Tallis they were a boon. While his caddy dashed off after his ball, George could socialise with his playing companions.

It was the membership contacts that he prized most. After golf,

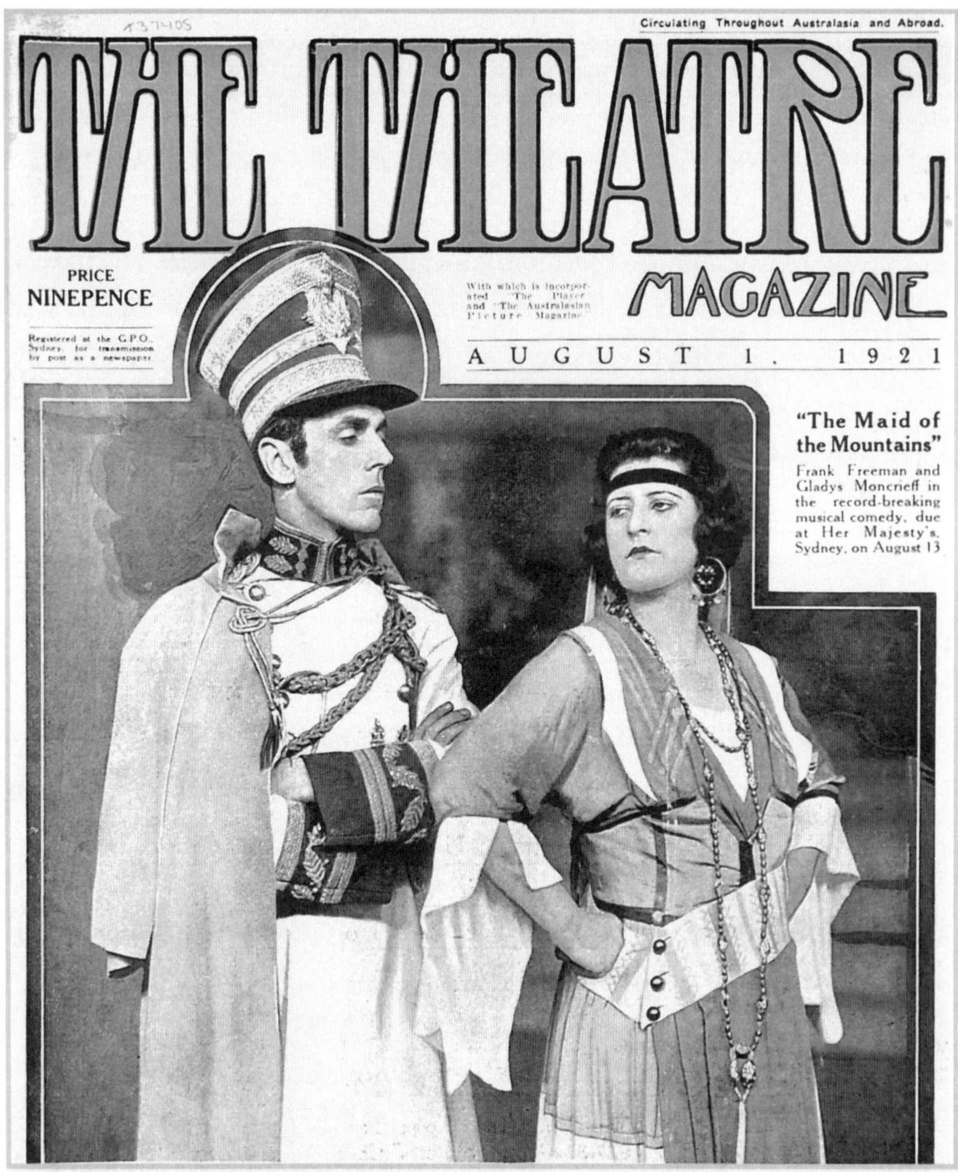

In spite of managerial shake-ups the show goes on

before golf or instead of golf he would also play bridge and, although he was delighted to play with anybody, he had his favourite groups.

George was musing when his playing companion and neighbour, Judge Josiah Wasley, startled him. Wasley was a supreme court judge and a man of great intelligence. He played golf off a handicap of thirteen and was also a ferocious bridge player. Mostly, people liked and respected him for his keen analysis of problems, and his free legal advice. Now he was looking at Tallis with concern.

'We're all worried about you, George. What's up?' Wasley walked to the bar, and returned with two drinks. He continued his interrogation: 'Is it the amalgamation?'

Tallis looked at his friend, and felt exhausted. ' It's a long story, Jo.'

Wasley was quiet. He had not seen Tallis like this before. Usually, his companion carried business worries without a sign. He made major decisions and didn't turn a hair; he never embarrassed his colleagues by discussing his own affairs. If George asked for an opinion, everybody knew that he had already made up his mind. Today was different. 'Tell me about it.'

Tallis described general aspects of the amalgamation, the personalities and the new constitution of the Williamson board. Wasley listened, and when George had finished he said, 'It sounds all right to me. You have some new blood at Williamson's now, there's a ton of potential. It must stack up on paper. You've got virtually no competitors, and there's an open field in front of you.' Wasley paused, 'Unless ...'

'That's right Jo, unless.' The two looked at each other briefly, stood up and went to the first tee.

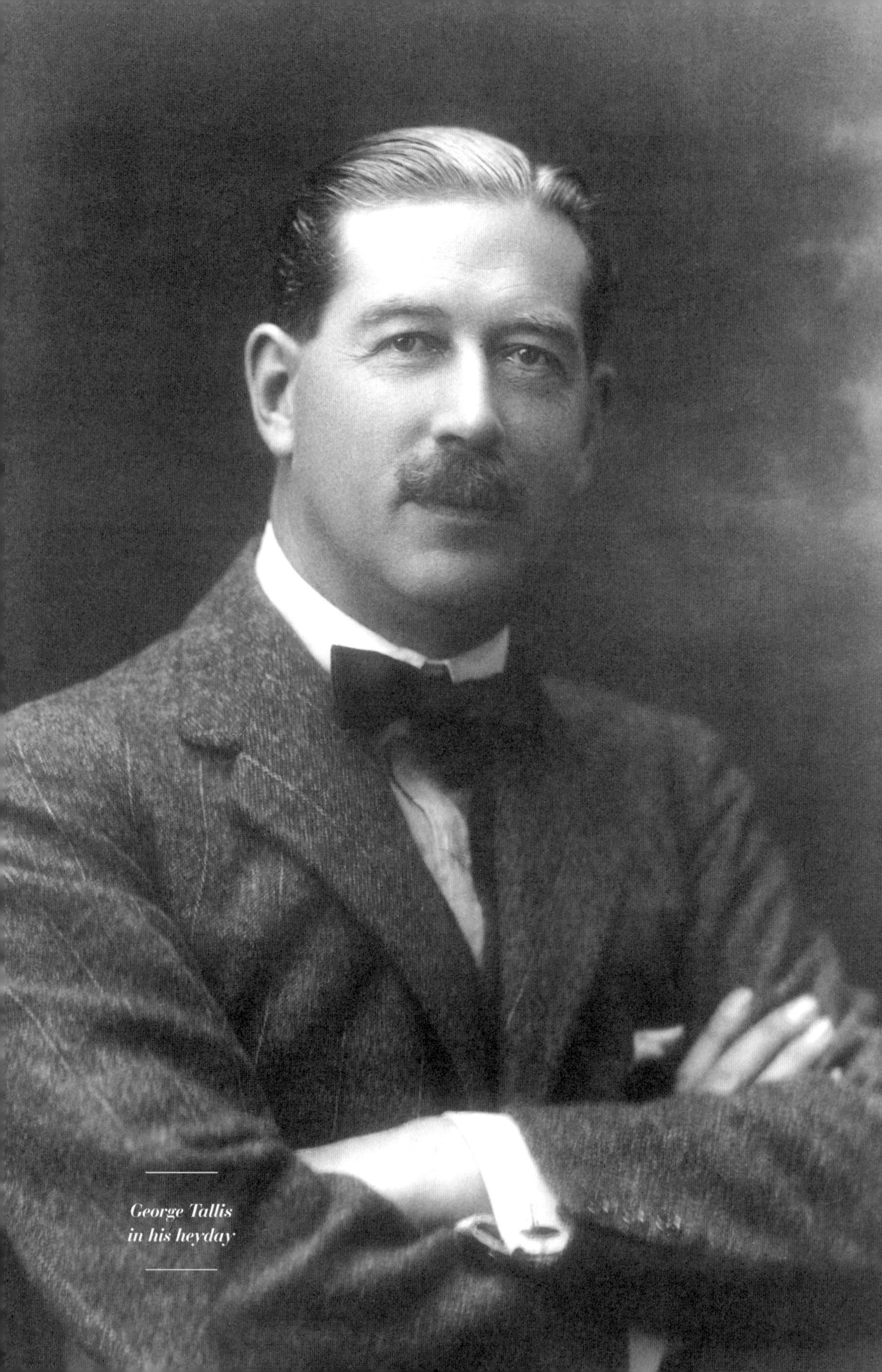

George Tallis in his heyday

CHAPTER TWELVE

What's This I Hear?

Around 1920, while settling the Williamson–Tait amalgamation, George Tallis finalised his arrangements to change houses. *Santoi* had served its purpose well, but for some time past the house had proved inadequate to handle the rounds of official entertaining that he and Millie were obliged to undertake on behalf of the Firm.

If George had been looking for a grand house, he surely found it on the corner of Toorak and Glenferrie Roads in what was originally the suburb of Malvern, but later became Toorak. *Grosvenor,* as the house was called, was an enormous, two-storeyed Italianate mansion on a five-acre block. In order to make the most of the sun it had a northerly aspect. Both floors had wide, airy porches, and graceful arches set off the parapets. The windows were large, and the overall feeling was of spaciousness, light and ventilation. The house, according to *Australian Home Beautiful* in 1926:

commands a fine view of the Dandenongs and an all-round outlook over the surrounding districts. The park-like grounds are effectively screened from public gaze by dense plantations of trees and shrubs; and the restful green sward that stretches away on every side is dotted with sheltering trees and massed

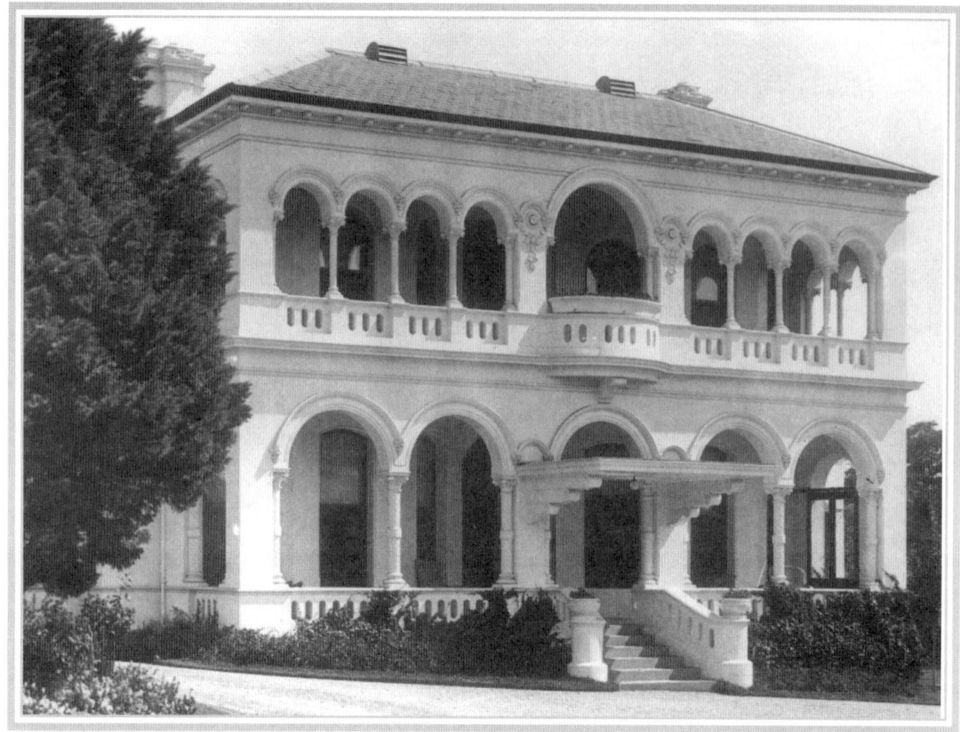

Goodbye Santoi, *Hello* Grosvenor

flowers ... It stands today a stately white residence replete with modern comfort and convenience.[1]

The article failed to mention a tennis court, croquet lawn and meandering accesses to both Toorak and Glenferrie Roads. The most serious omission, however, was the lack of a description of the wide driveway, which started at the apex of the corner of the two main roads and wound gracefully through the trees to the front entrance. Even then the great iron gates, giving as they did onto this busy intersection, were difficult to negotiate.

During his time of active management, George's regular routine was demanding. After a day in his office, he went home to 'modern comfort and convenience' to prepare for the evening theatre sessions. From four to six the Tallis house was under curfew. Banned were children, dogs, noise and any other impediments to the rest of a recumbent theatre manager. Refreshed, George dined with his family, then returned for another round in the city to supervise the running of the theatres, handle behind-curtain dramas, and assess audience reaction in front of the curtain. By the time he came home for the second time, *Grosvenor* was in darkness, and the milk was on the doorstep.

It was just as well Tallis enjoyed travelling. Between 1920 and 1940, he was overseas on various trips for a total of about five years. Of the remaining fifteen years, he was away from home for another five, mostly in Sydney. Conservatively, then, George was absent from his Melbourne base at least half the time. 'Is Mr Tallis still alive, I haven't seen him for years,' people would say. In reply: 'Oh yes. He's very well, we just don't know where he is.'

In truth, George loved to travel. He often sailed into Melbourne after a long absence, then within a few days headed for Sydney by

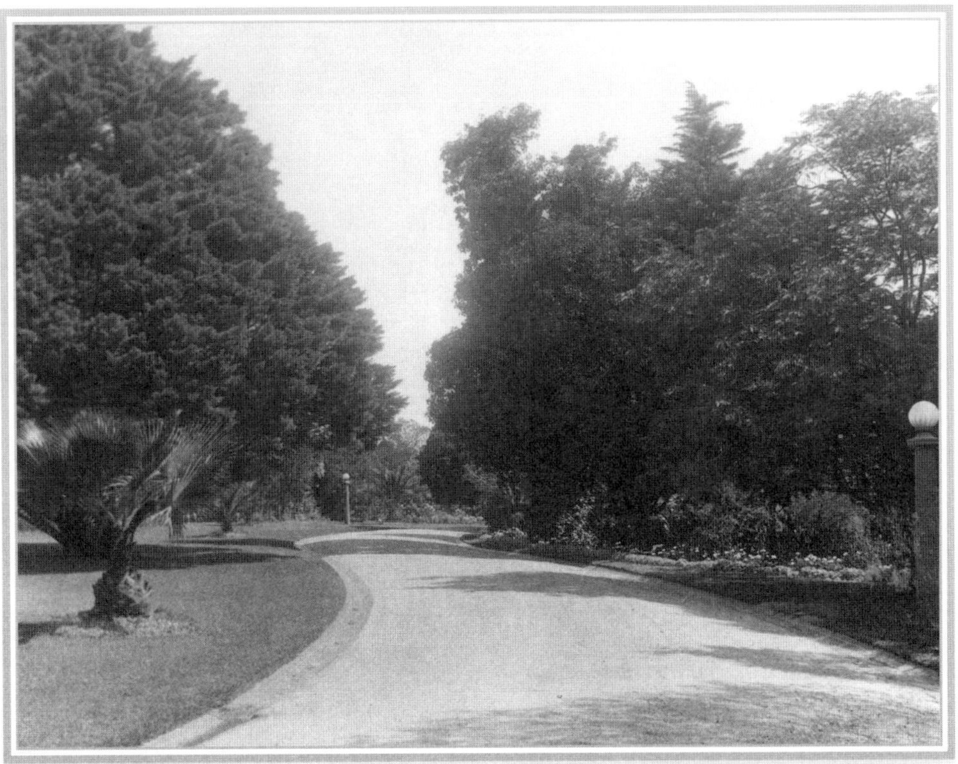

The **Grosvenor** *driveway*

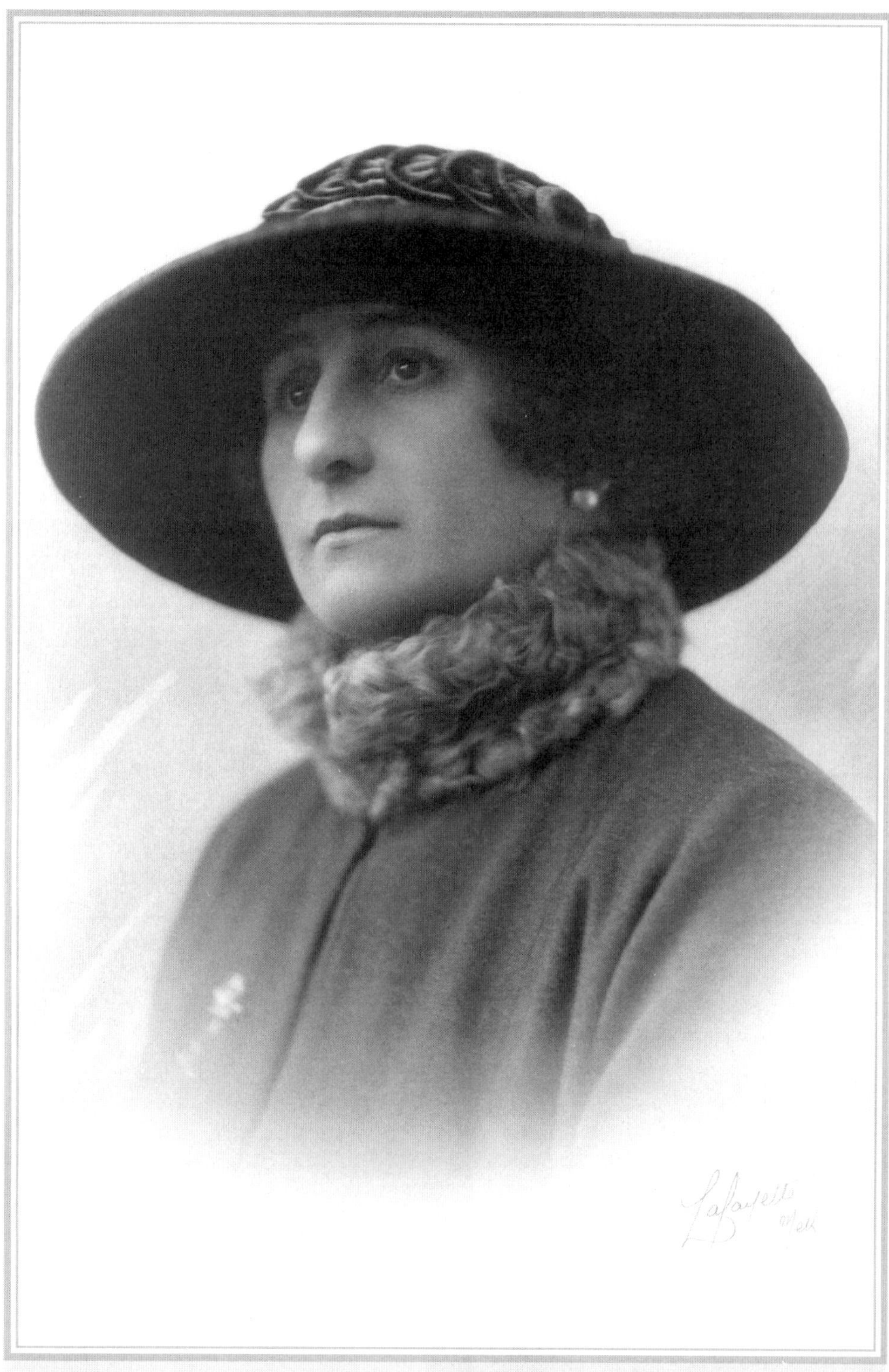

Amelia Tallis in the mid-1920s

car, train or boat. Long, rough voyages did not trouble him and he never seemed to complain about the incessant commuting between Melbourne and Sydney. These were periods of relaxation and contemplation.

His schedule in the twenties probably did not allow him to gain full value from his investment in *Grosvenor,* but the house was always on his mind as he roamed. He bought a grandfather clock here, a painting or two there, and somewhere else he acquired Venetian glass, silverware, linen, antique furniture and marble mantelpieces. Then he shipped the lot back to Melbourne. In the end, *Grosvenor* was groaning with artefacts and the house became a combination museum, gallery and family home.

Table Talk magazine remarked in 1925 that Tallis was one of the first in his business to discover that an artist may be 'some talented, but neglected fellow deeply attached to a paint brush or etching needle'. The writer noted that George had one of the finest collections of Australian, English and foreign prints in the Commonwealth, and that he was also the proud owner of numerous oils and water colours by the Australian masters. Added to this were the vices of collecting old clocks and breeding competition-winning Ayrshire cattle. *Table Talk* concluded that it was a pity that TALLIS, GEORGE was tucked into a 'chink between the Who Aren't' in *Who's Who,* and that 'a person who is a theatrical manager, art connoisseur, collector of old clocks, and cattle breeder, deserves a whole page to himself!'[2]

According to George's youngest son, Jack, life at *Grosvenor* was orderly. One fixed routine involved Mr Straub, the horologist, who came once a week from Camberwell to wind the many clocks in the house and test the chimes. Behind the scenes, there were shades of 'Upstairs Downstairs'. After each staff upheaval, Millie would phone Miss Allpress, who ran the local hire-and-fire service. Fresh new faces magically appeared, but not a word was uttered. It was poor form to notice.

Grosvenor parties were affairs to remember. They centred around the huge ballroom, where hundreds of guests swayed and glided, eager for supper. In this way, notable visitors to Melbourne from inside and outside the theatre were entertained at the Tallises' in a manner befitting the setting.

A frequent visitor was Dame Nellie Melba. At times she and George walked some of the way into the theatre together. Melba's chauffeur kept pace in the auto at a discreet distance; not too close to suggest that the pair was tiring, but close enough in case they were.

Another highlight of these days was the visit of Anna Pavlova, the great Russian ballerina, who was touring Australia in 1926. She arranged to make a film of some of her shorter dances in the gardens of *Grosvenor*. Carpenters from Her Majesty's Theatre built a low platform on a lawn at the side of the house and, although a bedroom was at her disposal, she changed in a tent made from sheets strung between shrubs. She danced without music, no doubt hearing the orchestra in her mind. Unconscious of a growing audience, she moved lightly and gracefully around the platform in a brilliant display.

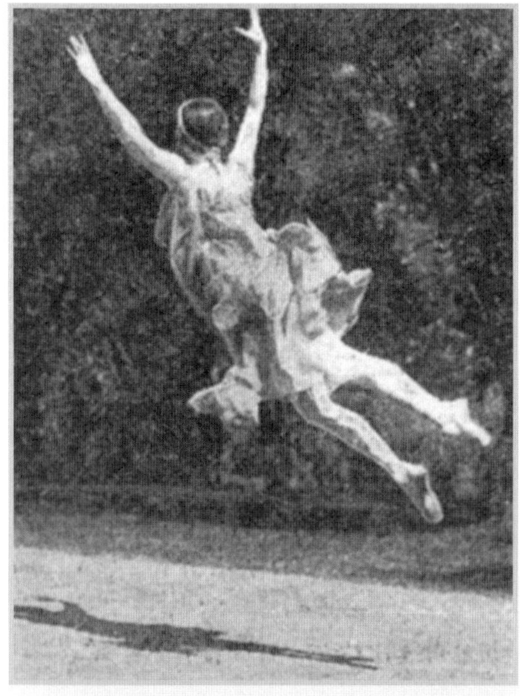

Pavlova in the garden at Grosvenor

Then, disaster! The ballerina staggered on the slippery boards. There were gasps from the viewers as she slowly regained her composure. 'Resin, more resin for Madame,' they called, and cars sped off to Her Majesty's for more supplies. The forced respite brought the crowd of onlookers to Pavlova's attention, and she showed her dismay at their intrusion.

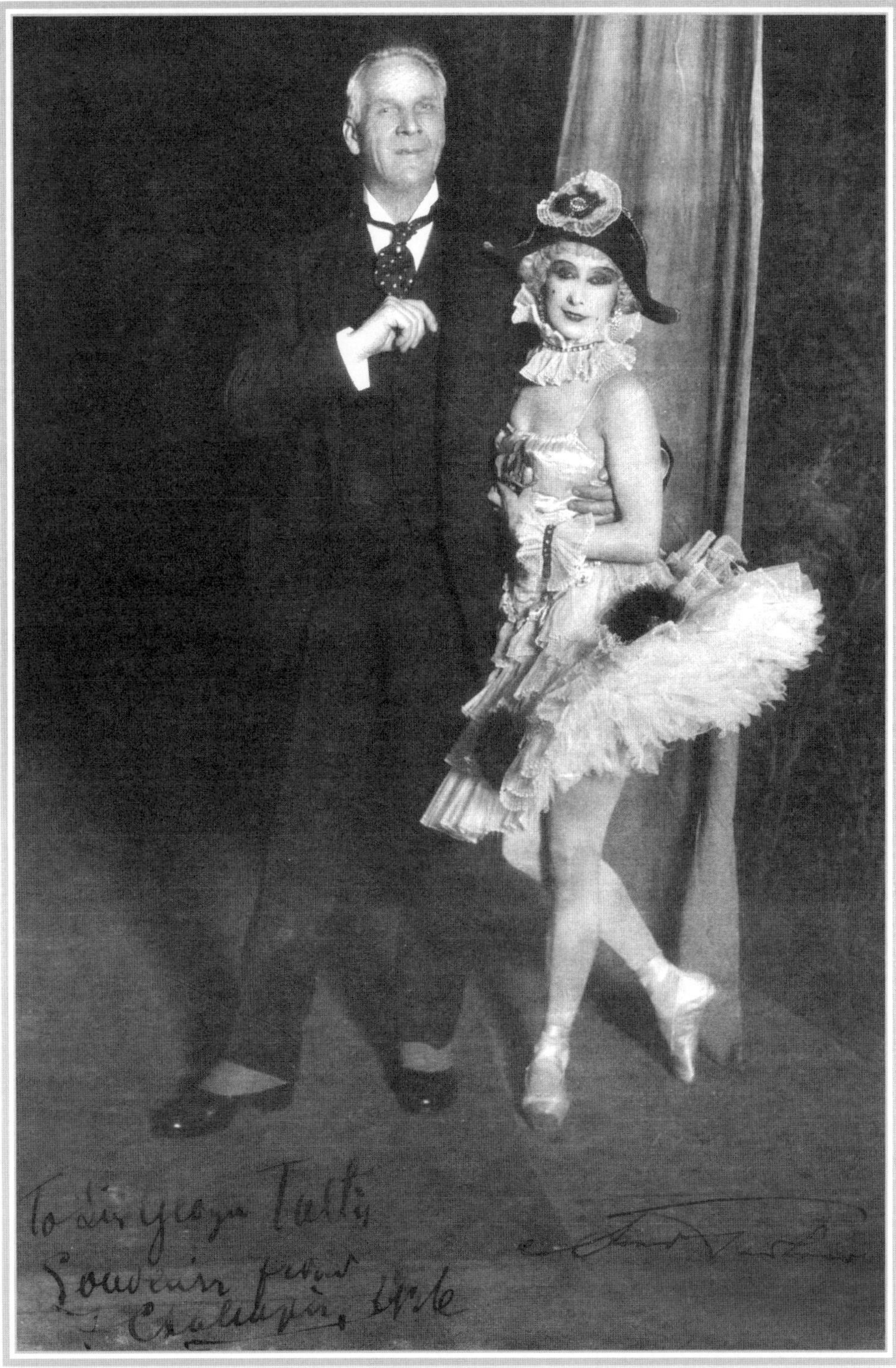

Pavlova with Fyodor Chaliapin, great Russian 'Basso', 1926

In spite of his comfortable city existence, George found Melbourne oppressive in the summer. He joined the stream of holiday-makers to the Mornington Peninsula for healthy sea dips, and enjoyed the drive from the city to his current beach resort as much as the break itself.

To Tallis the sea was a cure-all. It really did not matter which physiological system was playing up, a good swim in turbulent Port Phillip Bay, preferably in freezing water, did the trick. This was usually such an unpleasant cure that George's guests suffered in silence, lest he drive them to some desolate beach and personally supervise the therapy.

For a time, family holidays alternated between two big houses only a few miles apart. The first was a gloomy place at Mount Eliza named *Sunnyside,* and the second appeared in 1916 after Tallis noticed the following advertisement:

BELEURA-ON-THE-SEA

RAILWAY TICKET, FIRST CLASS

MORNINGTON RETURN 2/-

SPECIAL TRAIN LEAVES FLINDERS ST STATION

12.28 PM DAY OF SALE

PICNIC ON THE ESTATE

(HOT WATER PROVIDED)

BUY A LOT

And George Tallis did! He bought the house *Beleura,* surrounding blocks, and 2000 acres of open farm-land nearby.

Here at last was the holiday refuge the family had craved. *Beleura-on-the-Sea* the agents had called the house. Well, the sea *was* visible from the house; a distant view. But the township of Mornington was just a walk away, and the property would suit George's penchant for farming.

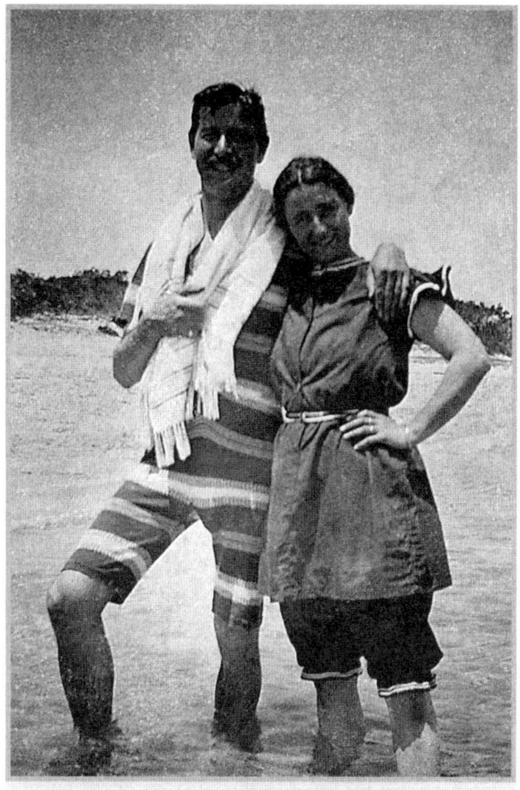
Millie and George on the beach in earlier days

Then the question arose: which house should he keep, *Sunnyside* or *Beleura*? One event settled this issue beyond doubt. Two of the Tallis boys camped one night at *Sunnyside* with their large canine companion, Brutus, while the rest of the family slept at *Beleura*. Around midnight, the huge bell in the *Sunnyside* belfry started to toll, although it had been silent for decades due to a broken chain high in the tower. Brutus was not impressed, and quickly took off for *Beleura* with fur up and ears back, emitting a blood-curdling howl. The boys considered the position momentarily but could not fault Brutus's strategy. They ran too, pausing to look back. Was that a round, leering face at a top window; or was it a reflection of the moon? What moon? It was cloudy!

The next day George listened carefully to what his sons had to say. There was no ridicule, and no debate. There was not even a suggestion of a re-run of that ghastly night, using adults as the guineapigs. Within a week, *Sunnyside* was up for sale.

During the days of *Sunnyside,* George had considered turning the grounds into a golf course. There was the potential here for a hilly eighteen holes, with sloping lies, a big gully to gobble up errant balls, and plenty of wind. Similar, perhaps, to an Irish course, perched on the Ring of Kerry. But the theatre was too demanding, and the dream hung in the air until sixty years later Jack Nicklaus inspected the property.[3] You can imagine the conversation between Nicklaus and his entourage. 'Hey guys, this would make a marvellous course.' 'Fantastic, Jack. Why on earth didn't somebody else ever think of that?'

The Nepean Highway runs north-south for the full hundred kilometre length of the Mornington Peninsula. The highway links Melbourne with Portsea, dropping in at most of the towns and bay-side resorts along the way, but bypassing Mornington itself. In the early days, it was a long, sandy driveway that connected *Beleura* with the main road.

Built in 1863/64, the house is on top of a small hill and faces south-west. Like *Grosvenor* it was designed in Italianate style, and it was built to last. The walls are massively thick, and the front entrance is part of a wide, tiled, colonnaded verandah. The exterior is white, and the overall impression is of a squat, solid villa with spacious grounds.

In the 1920s, a short climb to the roof allowed a 180 degree view of Port Phillip Bay, with the Mornington pier at centre stage. Bluffs, headlands and beaches rounded out the picture of a comfortable

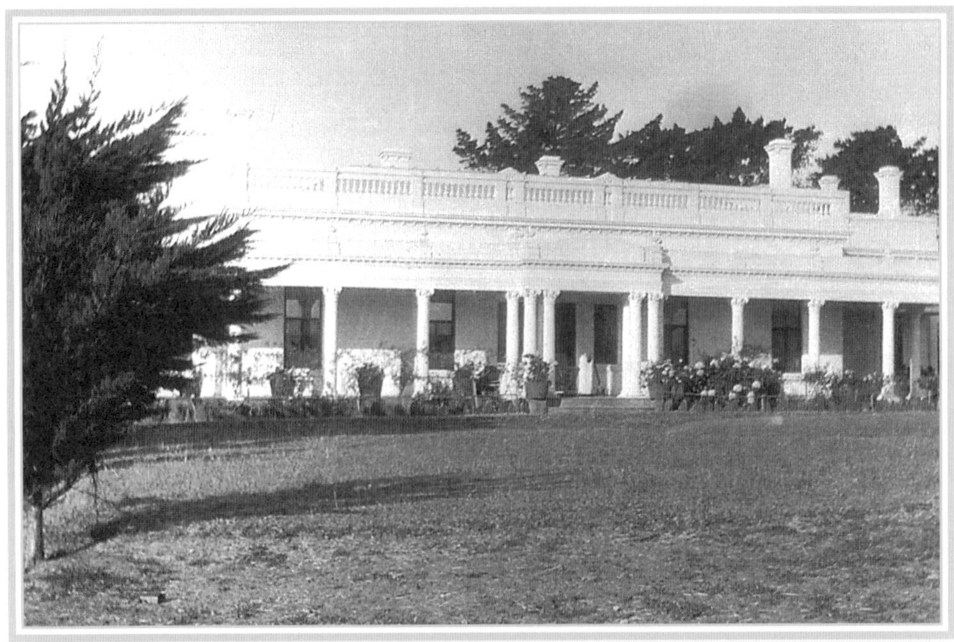

Beleura-on-the-Sea

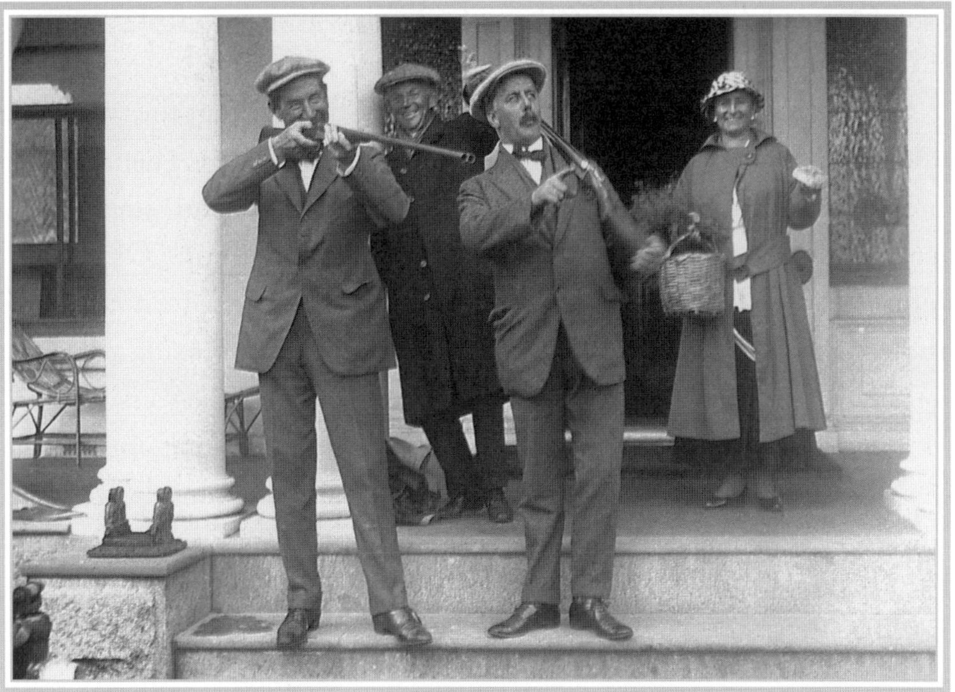

Good shot, Sir!

holiday resort. On calm days, small boats and yachts bobbed near the shore, while international shipping slid across the horizon. The scene extended on all sides: sea, scrub and some open country. This expansive view has since been permanently lost thanks to a forest of tall gums and pines.

Almost from the moment George bought *Beleura,* he used it for entertaining and relaxation. Close friends and theatre personalities visited for weekends or summer holidays. Mornington may have been far from the footlights, but it had good beaches, fishing and enticingly long, lonely walks.

Melba often escaped her onerous schedule to relax at *Beleura,* just as she did at *Grosvenor.* She was friendly with the Tallis clan and enjoyed the informality of a family holiday. She mentioned once how therapeutic it would be to take hot, sea-water baths. George was listening. He arranged to pipe water direct from Port Phillip Bay, heat it to a comfortable warmth, and reticulate it to a central bathroom in *Beleura* for Melba's pleasure.

The bath was popular with everyone. With a twist of the wrist, the balms of a sea water immersion were instantly available. There was no interminable walk to some windswept beach; no sand, flies or icy arms of a choppy sea. 'Have you had a swim today?' 'Of course, before breakfast,' went the charade. No one seemed to notice that 'the sparkling play beaches' of the Mornington Peninsula – as they were advertised – had just been made redundant by progress.

Florence Young was not only popular with her comic opera fans, she was also a family favourite. Flo visited her sister and brother-in-law whenever she could, and as the Tallis children grew they encouraged her to act out her exuberance with her repertoire of song and comedy. *Beleura* became part of her circuit.

Late in 1920 Flo and her friend, actor Reginald Roberts, were involved in a car accident as they drove down the *Beleura* driveway on their way back to Melbourne. Although no one appeared badly hurt, within a few days Flo suffered a sudden seizure. Three weeks later, on 11 November, Florence Young died of a stroke at the age of forty-nine.

Flo had been so well and full of energy that everyone thought she was indestructible. Retirement had been casually mentioned, but the suggestion wasn't taken seriously. Her short life was abruptly over, and her legions of fans and friends felt cheated.

Among the many tributes paid to Florence Young during her life, one in the *Theatre Magazine* accurately pinpointed her hold on the theatre-going public:

There is an unaffected cheeriness about Australia's queen of comic opera that cannot be resisted. Brimming over with good nature, incapable of pettiness of mind, Miss Young's bright outlook in life has become part of her personality. She carries this happy optimism on to the stage and transmits it to the audience in a breezy wholesomeness.

> *No Australian artist has ever won greater recognition from the public than she, and success has not spoilt her. Anyone who wants to discover how firm her hold is on the affection of playgoers need only attend a first night production of an opera in which Miss Young is appearing. Hers is always the reception of the evening. The gallery boys call her 'Flo,' and there is no surer sign of popularity than that.*[4]

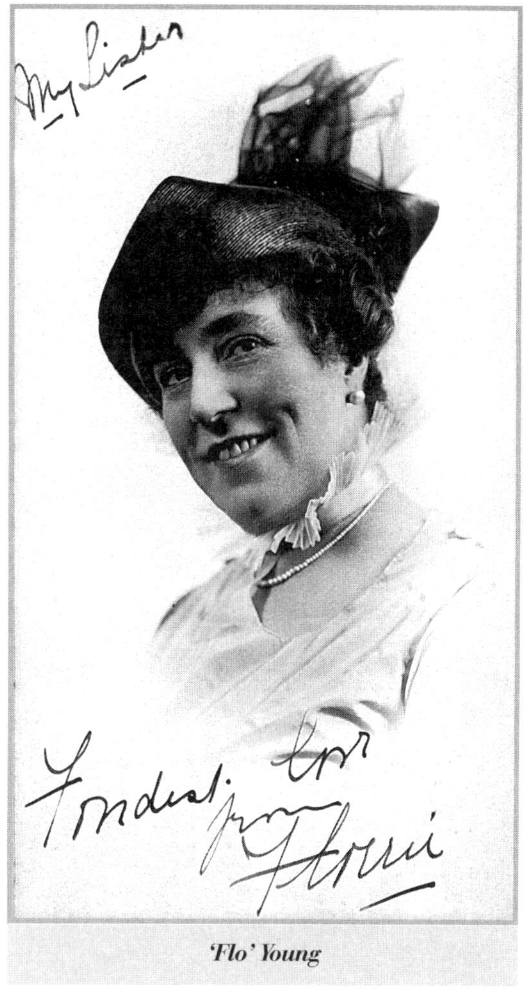

'Flo' Young

The year 1922 was probably George's best, although it had a shaky start. He and Millie headed for London in March, but Millie became ill on the ship. She was rushed into hospital at Colombo, where the diagnosis was appendicitis. An emergency operation followed, and the ship left without the Tallises. A month later George and Millie joined the *Orvieto* and continued their trip to London.

In May, a letter arrived for George from Downing Street. Mr Churchill wanted to recommend his name to the prime minister for submission to the king. The honour of Knight Bachelor was mentioned. Was this Honour acceptable to George? An early reply was requested so that the king could deliberate the matter.

Would George accept? John Tait was worried about Tallis's egalitarian ways, and with good reason. He knew that George had once refused a previous approach for a knighthood, and theWilliamson London office received an urgent cable from Melbourne:

Our chairman will be offered knighthood: make every effort to persuade him to accept; great benefit to prestige firm against opposition.

Whether or not George found this argument convincing, he thought the honour indeed acceptable, and by a miracle of coincidence he was on the spot to attend the investiture ceremony in person. He and Millie had left Australia as Mr and Mrs Tallis; they returned as Sir George and Lady Tallis, and people who thought that this had not dramatically changed their lives were deluding themselves.

Suddenly doors previously closed to George were opened. The British press sought his opinion on all manner of topics, and from then onwards Sir George was never short of an opportunity to talk about the Firm and its latest acquisitions. He used interviews to promote Australian productions and Australian actors. In time he became known to the newspapers as an 'ambassador for the Australian theatre'.

Tallis received literally hundreds of congratulatory cables. A particularly generous one was from John Tait:

Nobody more delighted than me at your richly deserved and unsought honor. Congratulations to both of you and long life and happiness. It certainly won't spoil you or your game. Dick.

Bert Royle captured the general feeling among George's old working colleagues with his cable: 'DEDAB NEMWA GOUMWFULEC = ROYLE. In other words, 'Hearty congratulations old friend sincerely, Royle.' The telegram from his eldest son, Mick, spoke for the family: 'What's this I hear?'

Although Ted Tait wrote, 'Dear George, No – I will not address you as Sir George even though the King does,' as the mantle of formality descended, George and Millie lost some of the easy contacts they prized so much. There is a price for everything.

Jealousy among some of George's peers was one of the costs. Hugh Ward was apparently very upset, and stories of his resentment trickled down through the years so that even as late as 1956 – fifteen years after Ward's death – the Melbourne *Herald* carried an article that said:

[Ward's] ambition was a knighthood. Nobody could have been more deserving of it . . . Something went wrong with Hughie's plans, and for the war effort for the theatrical profession Tallis was knighted instead.[5]

Officially, the knighthood was conferred on George 'as head of the theatrical profession in Australia, and in recognition of the profession's constant efforts in the cause of charity, and for service rendered on behalf of the various patriotic funds during the war'. Of course, he accepted with pleasure a tribute to the profession he had served for more than thirty years.

George was delighted by the good wishes he received. Newspapers in Australia, New Zealand and Great Britain ran glowing articles, and these reflected how influential he had become. This was a popular award, and the writers stressed George's early beginnings, achievements and rise to prominence. Most of all they emphasised his courteous nature, humility, generosity and integrity. The Williamson theatres interrupted their performances to drink to 'Sir George', and to 'jolly good fellow' him in song.

In a lively piece by theatre commentator Frank Morton, the *New Zealand Herald* encapsulated George Tallis's contribution to the entertainment industry:

There is no member of the big theatrical firm of Williamson of whom you in New Zealand know less, and yet in that firm he is the man who counts most. More than that, he has been for years in that firm the man most influential for good. And as that firm is the oldest and most important theatrical firm in Australasia, Mr Tallis was quite properly chosen as the man through whom the whole enterprise of theatrical management in Australasia might most be honoured. For that reason, I hold that he merits congratulation on his knighthood.

If he had been knighted for political services, or because he had given large moneys to a political party or social cause, I should not have esteemed his knighthood worthy of passing mention.

But Sir George Tallis is in many ways a very remarkable man. To start with, he has never schemed or bothered about a knighthood at all, and if it were by some inexplicable freak of nature now taken away from him he wouldn't lose an hour's sleep over the deprivation. Modesty with him is not an affectation. He was the leader in all the Firm's patriotic enterprises during the war, but his name was seldom mentioned. He is knighted, but his name is still George Tallis simply on all the Firm's advertising matter and business forms, and so it will remain. He is just the sort of nice, quiet knight I like, a knight to be happy in. And the business of theatrical management on the big scale is honoured by its association with the name of such a man. So that's that.[6]

George and Millie returned to Australia in mid-December 1922. They had motored 17,000 miles through Britain, France, Germany, Austria, Italy and America. Interviewed by the Melbourne *Herald* Tallis said that 'Australians do not fully appreciate their blessings ... Expenses in London and New York are appalling. In America, prohibition has meant a big loss for most of the hotels, and they are making that up by charging more for meals and accommodation'. Prices were better for the visitor on the Continent, where a few pounds bought a night of luxury at any leading hotel.

There was bad news, though, for actors heading to England. It had been a poor summer there, and thousands of actors were unemployed. In London, many of the chorus girls were working in tea rooms, or as models. Business in New York was fair, but companies on the road were doing badly. 'Of the seventy plays I saw while we were away, very few impressed me,' George said. The exception was *If Winter Comes*, which was having one of the most sensational successes on record.[7]

In future years George was to be interviewed by the press many times, not only about the theatre but also for his observations on the economies of various countries, and the behaviour of their peoples. He was a fascinated observer of events and, in days when overseas travel was less common, newspapers sought him out as a commentator. He loved world travel, but was not always so keen on the interviews after a long trip and at times he would give news-hounds the slip.

This was something he did not find at all difficult. He would simply disembark when the ship reached Port Adelaide and vanish into the city. There he boarded the first train to Melbourne, and by the time the journalists discovered that Tallis was not among the throng descending the gang-planks at Port Melbourne, it was too late. He had already passed through the gates of Spencer Street Station, mixed with the other jaded interstate travellers, and dropped out of sight.

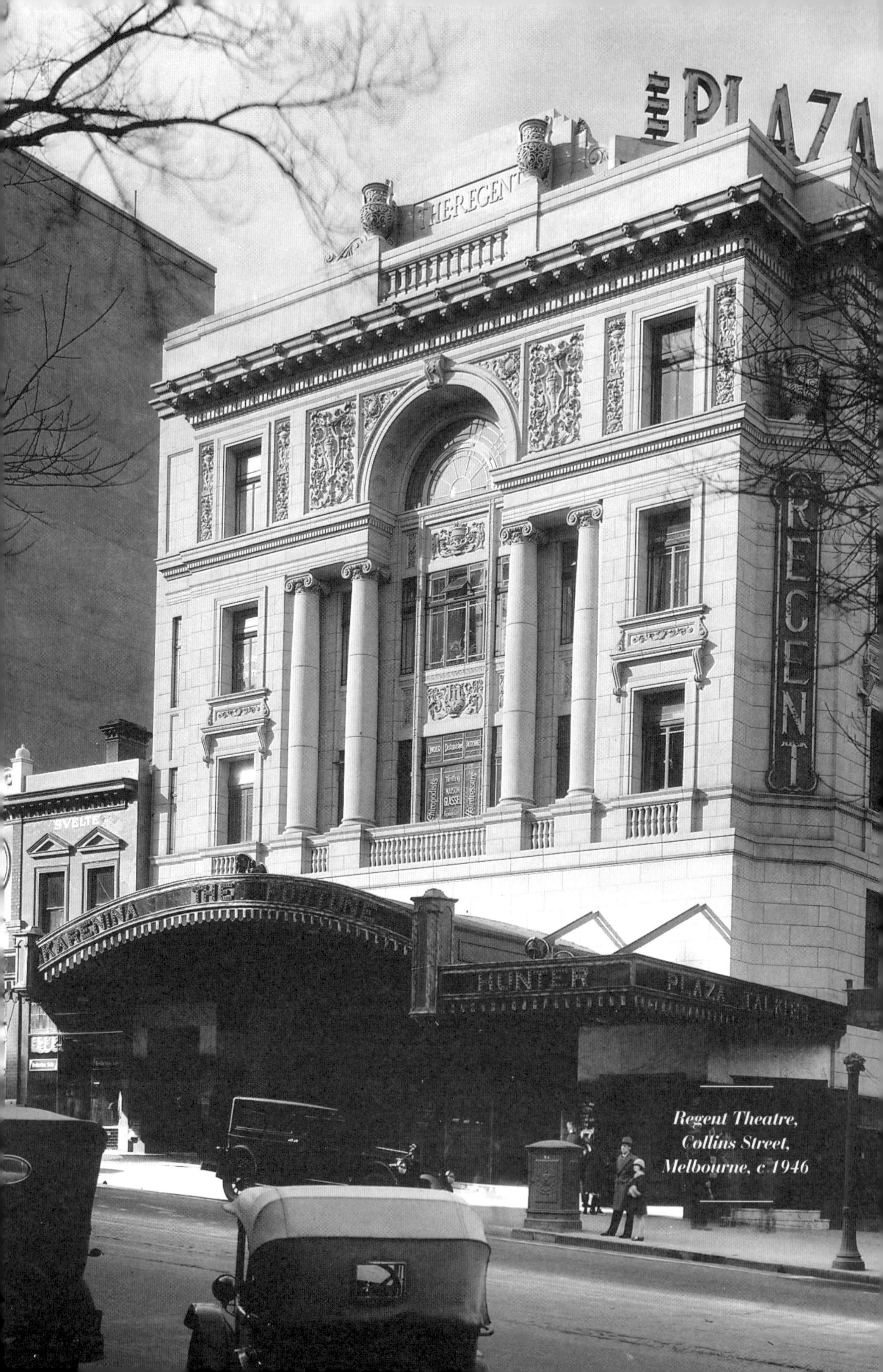

Regent Theatre, Collins Street, Melbourne, c 1946

– CHAPTER THIRTEEN –

Celluloid and Ether

'We know', said Hugh Ward in August 1921, 'eight styles of shows – namely drama, pantomime, musical comedy, straight comedy, farce, opera, vaudeville and comic opera such as Gilbert & Sullivan plays. The only form of entertainment we have not yet run is a circus; and that we shall do one of these days when we find one big enough. The Williamson firm can do all this as it controls theatres all over Australia.'[1]

Ward was then in London searching for shows and talking up the Firm. But thanks largely to the efforts of chairman of directors George Tallis, the Firm's portfolio in the early twenties expanded even further. Having acquired the concert business of J&N Tait, Williamson's in 1924 added the Tivoli vaudeville circuit to its live entertainment list. By the mid-1920s, the Firm had increased its management across Australia and New Zealand to the equivalent of fourteen live theatres full-time, and up to thirty additional theatres part-time.

The Firm's thrust into vaudeville, however, had not been as smooth as Tallis would have liked. He had negotiated with Hugh McIntosh to take over the Tivoli circuit at what he considered a reasonable price, but it was thumbs down in the boardroom. The deal had been lost. It seems that, as a consequence, McIntosh had sold his business in 1921 to Harry Musgrove. Some time afterwards, George wrote to the Taits, 'As you know, this [rejection by the board] cost us dear later on.'

Harry Musgrove did not last long. Mistakes and bad luck brought out his accountant's red ink, and the Firm, which for years had been trying to gain control of some of the Tivoli houses, was at last rewarded for its persistence. In 1924 it took over Musgrove Theatres – Harry Rickards' old Tivoli circuit – and enjoyed five years of profitable management.

Meanwhile, George Tallis was quietly ensuring that Williamson's would meet, and enjoy, the challenges issued by the newer medium of cinema. By the start of the twenties, the industry was huge. It was estimated that in Australia, with a population of five million, there were then seventy million visits to the cinema annually. This compared with eleven million visits to live theatres, ten million to concerts and six million to other types of entertainment. Writer Spartacus Smith justly remarked: 'It is a pleasure-loving community that lives in this part of the world!'[2]

Earlier we told how George threw a lifeline to JCW Ltd in 1916. He developed JC Williamson Films Ltd with his own money, installed Frank Thring as manager, and established a source of films and a string of theatres in which to screen them.

Soon, a second company followed, Electric Theatres Pty Ltd, which operated in Sydney under the same management. This successful beginning blossomed into an enormous business for the Firm. Tallis expanded into New Zealand in 1923 by setting up the JC Williamson New Zealand Picture Corporation Ltd, for many years managed by Beaumont Smith and John Mason. Tallis then in 1926 supervised the merger of JC Williamson Films with Hoyts Pictures Ltd on a fifty–fifty basis. Hoyts Theatres resulted and, under Tallis's chairmanship, the new company became one of the two biggest moving picture outlets in Australia, with over seventy cinemas under its control.

The second of the local movie Goliaths was Union Theatres. Competition between it and Hoyts was cut-throat. Which one would rise to supremacy, or which would provide the juiciest takeover target for marauding American companies like Fox, Paramount and Metro?

Before 1920, the Firm had established a direct 17.5 per cent interest in Union Theatres by merging Electric Theatres with it. Moreover, there were additional cross-investments, so Williamson's had all bases covered. JCW Ltd even had its own representative on the Union Theatres board. So, by the time these enormous corporate manoeuvres had been stitched up, the Firm controlled, or had an interest in, over a hundred cinemas across Australia. George claimed that this was more than any other Australian company.

It is interesting to note that the 'Picture Palaces', the collective brain-child of the two film giants Hoyts and Union, were foreshadowed as early as 1919. An article in the *Theatre Magazine* in 1920 described a proposal to erect two enormous 'entertainment centres', one in Sydney and the other in Melbourne. The plans were formulated by the directors of Union Theatres and JC Williamson Films. Much was made by the writer of the executive expertise that such a project required:

Never before in the history of the picture business has such an ideal working combination been placed under one head . . . With such men as George Tallis, WA Gibson, Edwin Geach, Stuart F Doyle and FW Thring to direct the policy of the big concern, little doubt can be left in the observer's mind of the result of the undertaking.[3]

Although it was eight years before these ideas became reality, George Tallis and Frank Thring were steering the picture palace movement for Hoyts from the start. Thring helped organise the construction of the theatres, and as chairman of directors of the various companies Tallis provided leadership and the necessary financial structure. The partnership between the two friends had flourished.

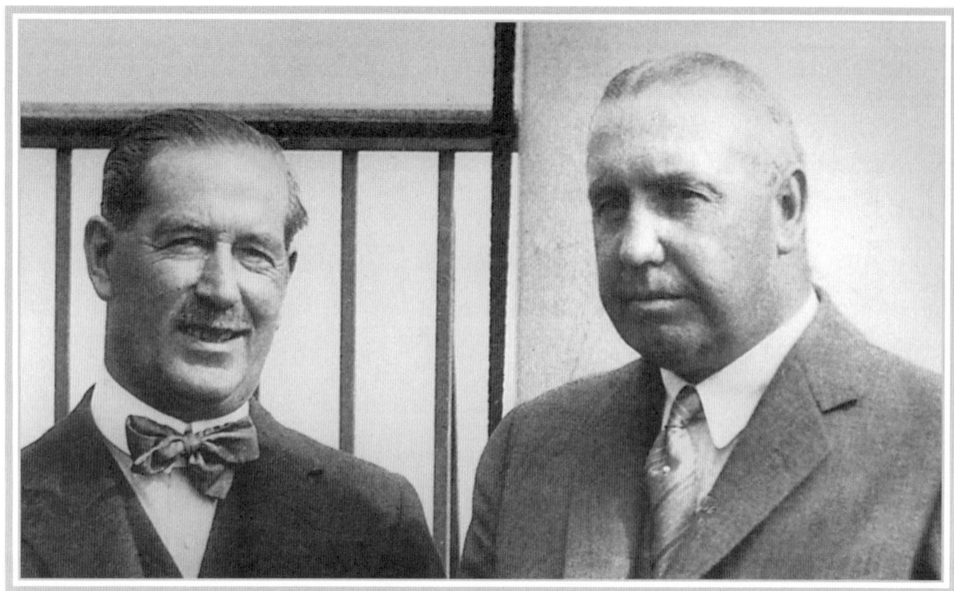

George Tallis and Frank Thring – the Hoyts–Regent chain partnership

Even before the picture palaces appeared, the facilities for showing films improved as the industry developed. Patrons gradually learnt to expect more comfort than that provided by old halls and unbooked theatres. The public was tired of the fleapits. As competition grew between the large distributors, especially Hoyts Pictures and Union Theatres, their concern for audiences became overwhelming, and by the late 1920s they were building movie houses to more than rival the best of the live theatres.

Hoyts set up its Regent chain of lavish cinemas.[4] The picture palace in Collins Street, Melbourne, was designed by Cedric Ballantyne and was constructed in the French Renaissance style, with liberal use of marble and imported furniture. The main auditorium featured an enormous central dome elaborately decorated and surrounded by eleven smaller domes, all fitted with magnificent chandeliers. The theatre's capacity was 3250 people, who enjoyed the strains of a full orchestra that disappeared gracefully into the floor on the pit-lift as the curtain rose. Robust musical support was supplied by a massive

Wurlitzer organ. Other five-star Regents were in South Yarra, Sydney, Brisbane and Adelaide.

Union Theatres countered by introducing even more innovative designs, with managing director Stuart Doyle at the wheel. The State Theatre, Sydney, was one of the most luxurious picture palaces that Australia has seen. It was completed in 1928, and was restored in 1981.

An example of the 'atmospheric' cinemas is Union Theatre's Capitol Theatre, also in Sydney. It has a roofed auditorium with an imitation blue sky and moving clouds. Its sister theatre in Melbourne was the State. With seating for 3370, it was the biggest in Australia.

These enormous picture palaces were fitted with orchestra pits, and they were able to handle vaudeville shows as well. This ability to

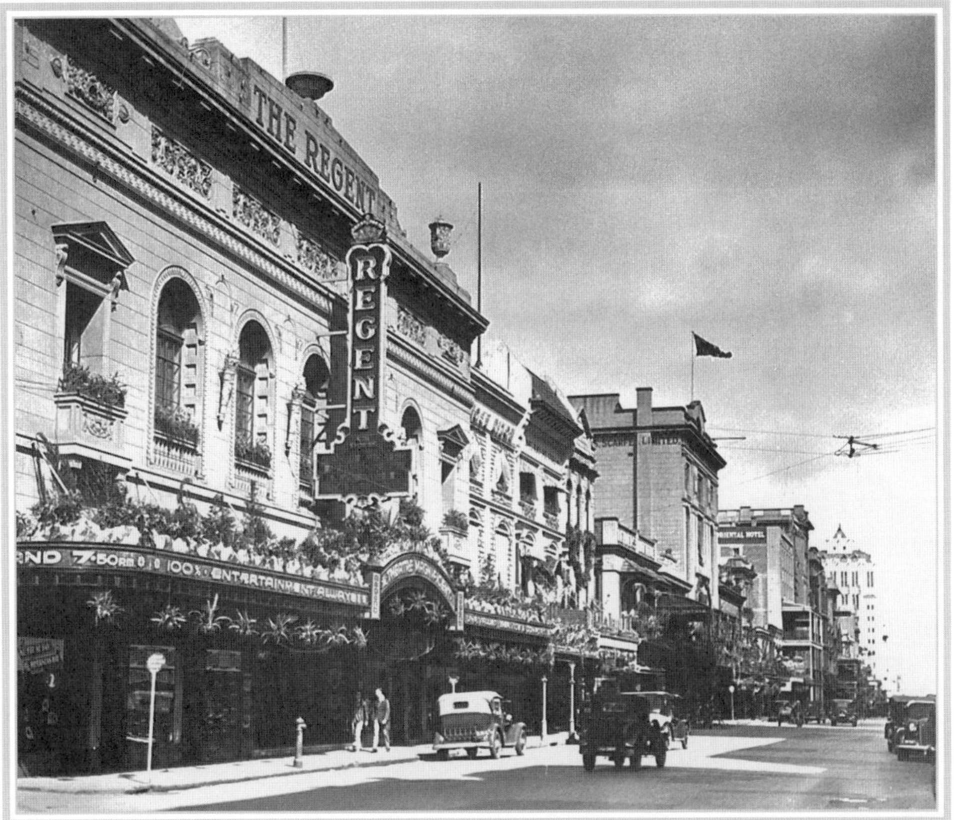

Regent Theatre, Adelaide, 1936

The Regent
Sir GEO. TALLIS
F. W. THRING, Esq.
G. F. GRIFFITH, Esq.
Realisation
TO five men the Regent Theatre represents the realisation of dreams.
Years ago they saw in motion pictures a potent force trammelled by disrespect; for motion pictures lay in bondage to blind minds. Few shared their vision, until the great chain of Hoyts Theatres Ltd. stretched throughout Australia.
There is now a Regent Theatre in Melbourne, Sydney, Adelaide, Perth, and Wellington, Auckland, and Dunedin (N.Z.). Soon there will be one in Brisbane; but, besides these splendid metropolitan cinemas, Hoyts Theatres Ltd. directly control over one hundred others in Australia and New Zealand.
JOHN TAIT, Esq.
F. CHALLINGSWORTH, Esq.
The Directors of Hoyts Theatres Ltd. are Sir George Tallis (Chairman), G. F. Griffith, Esq., F. W. Thring, Esq., John Tait, Esq., and F. Challingsworth, Esq.
Their faith is in Australia, in Australian skill and craftsmanship, to which the Regent Theatre stands as a tribute.

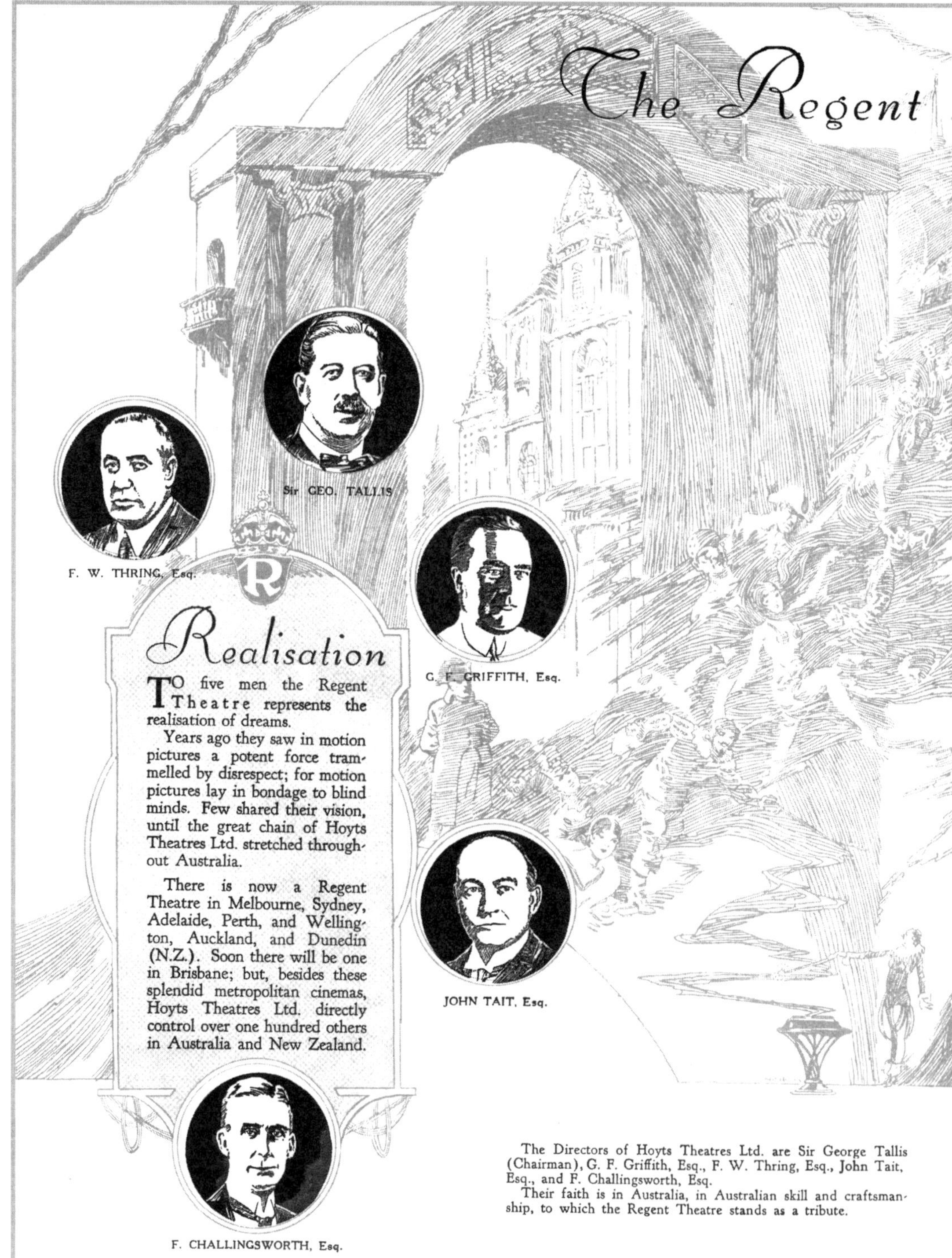

From original Regent souvenir program

provide auxiliary entertainment for enhancing the silent films fell into disuse when the talkies appeared late in the 1920s.

The talkies started to make an impact in the United States in 1927 and the following year the pressure was on the Australian film industry to screen the new sensation. Overnight the silent films died and the talkies were in. This required some gearing up on the part of the local film companies, who realised immediately that the old adage 'first up best dressed' applied.

In 1928, Tallis was overseas. He had been looking into the latest equipment for screening the talkies and reported his findings in a letter to his board:

> Broadway Melody *is miles ahead of any of the other talkies. It is so very far in advance that one can now see what an absolute menace the talkies are going to be to the legitimate theatres before very long. The feeling in New York is that before three or four years are over most of the legitimate houses will be devoted to talkies and I am inclined to agree with this. Therefore I think we are on the right track in wiring up the two Royals and eventually we will have to equip all our houses. I came over on the same boat as Warner [the American film producer] and had a long chat with him. He tells me positively that within three months the Western Electric will have complete equipment that can be bought for $6000.*
>
> *The thing is: Can we wait until this is on the market?*

As for Hoyts, work started immediately. Sound equipment was installed in all of the chain's cinemas. This cost so much that there was some delay in shareholders' dividends, but for a very short while Hoyts was first.

The Firm is remembered for its virtual monopoly of the live entertainment industry in Australia in the 1920s, but its massive influence in the developing cinema business is less often considered. It really did not matter who won the battles, or who won the war – Hoyts or Union – because either way the Firm was well and truly covered. Clearly, this was Tallis's financial architecture.

He went to the movies occasionally to see the latest block-buster, or to assess some particularly praiseworthy piece of acting, but his experience with live theatre was his yardstick. The films he saw did not so much impress him as concern him with their curiosity value for the public. Although he disliked the endless stream of poor quality films, he knew that they would attract some section of the public. Above all, whatever George thought of the product, he never underrated its danger to the live theatre industry.

The success Tallis had in putting together a huge safety net to insure the Firm against loss of its audiences to films rests largely on his choice of a partner, Frank Thring. Both men had vision, and both worked enormously hard to grasp an opportunity which, with nurturing, developed into a massive business investment. There were no crippling arguments, and the pair worked as friends to map out a dream. It was in such collaborative ventures that George was at his best. He saw what had to be done, financially and artistically. He steered the partnership into corporate structures to deliver simultaneously an exciting investment, and insulation for JCW Ltd from lethal opposition. That Thring and Tallis achieved this without falling out flies in the face of the old adage that the best way to lose friends is to do business with them.

During the 1920s Tallis also introduced the Firm to the rapidly developing business of radio.

The Italian physicist Marconi had created history in 1901 by sending the letter 'S' in Morse Code across the Atlantic, thereby heralding the new era of wireless telegraphy and telephony. Just four years later, the enterprising Marconi company built the first two-way radio telegraph station in Australia. It transmitted between Queenscliff, near Port Phillip Heads in Victoria, and Devonport on the north coast of Tasmania. The Australian government heard the till ringing, and gave the Postmaster-General control over the developing wireless transmission industry throughout Australia, encouraging bureaucratic interference from the start.

Wireless telegraphy developed quickly. Around 1910, the main operators were Italian and German companies, Marconi and Telefunken, who tendered to build large towers for an Australasian and Pacific Islands telegraph service. However, a brash new local syndicate of investors called Australasian Wireless Ltd walked off with handsome contracts. George Tallis, always interested in new media, was a minor shareholder, and when the company went public and became the Australasian Wireless Company Ltd, George found himself on the board.

In late 1912, Marconi and the Australasian Wireless Company Ltd merged. The result was Amalgamated Wireless (Australasia) Ltd, AWA. This company became the major driving force in the technical development of commercial wireless across Australia for the next twenty years.[5]

The first regular broadcasting stations began operation in America and England in 1920. The English opened with a program featuring Dame Nellie Melba, perhaps stirring Australian entrepreneurs to enter the field. In July 1923 one of the early radio licences went to 2FC in Sydney. The ownership syndicate of this station consisted of Farmer and Company, a Sydney retail store; John Fairfax Ltd, publisher of the *Sydney Morning Herald* and *Evening News*; Dalgety Ltd, stock and station agents; and JCW Ltd and J&N Tait. George Tallis was a member of the board.

2FC's first public broadcast took place on 5 December 1923 but the 'official' opening was delayed until 10 January 1924. The highlight of this was a direct broadcast from Her Majesty's Theatre Sydney of Gladys Moncrieff and Williamson's Royal Comic Opera Company in *A Southern Maid*.[6] Also in January 1924, AWA conducted a demonstration involving excerpts from the JCW Ltd musical comedy *Sally*. The studio was the AWA offices in Collins Street, Melbourne,

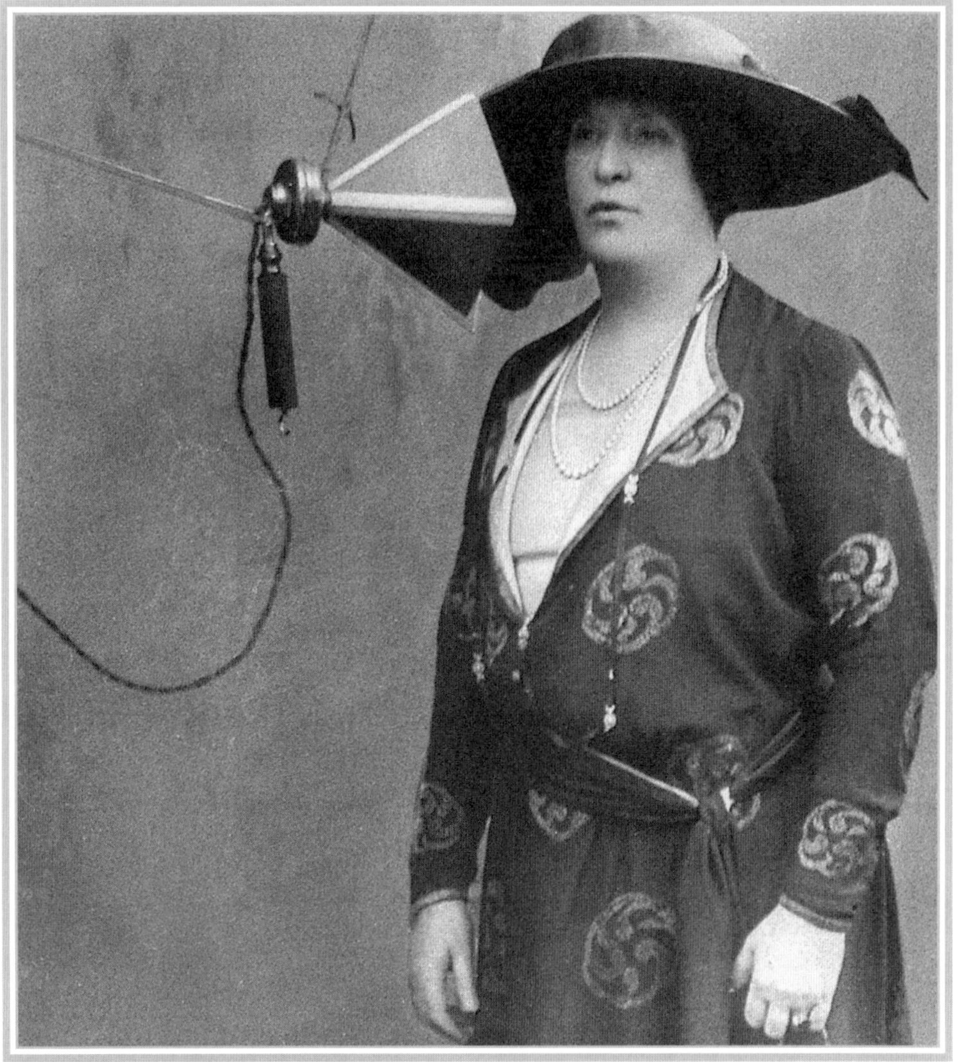

Dame Nellie Melba introducing broadcasting in London, 1920

and the broadcast transmitted clearly all the way to Flinders and King Island in the Bass Strait. These early broadcasts stunned listeners, who left doors and windows open to let in the magic.

AWA was to establish many firsts. It was the first, in 1924, to broadcast from Australia to England; the first – 1927 – to use beam radio between the two countries; and the first – 1930 – to set up an international radio-telephone service. No wonder the company became a monopoly!

In mid-1924 the government muddied the water by introducing two grades of broadcasting licences, A-class and B-class, each issued for a period of five years. A-class stations attracted licence fee revenue and, in return, they were expected to cater for country listeners with chains of relay stations. Advertising was the bread and butter of the B-class stations. By 1927, in addition to eight A-class stations, there were twelve B-class stations across Australia.

The two A-class stations in Melbourne were 3AR and 3LO. The licence for 3LO, the stronger of the two stations, went to the Broadcasting Company of Australia. 3LO made its first broadcast on 13 October 1924.

A formidable syndicate assembled by George Tallis had formed the Broadcasting Company of Australia. Forty per cent of the company was owned by JCW Ltd and J&N Tait, and forty per cent by Farmer and Co., proprietors of Sydney's 2FC. The Melbourne Herald and Weekly Times Ltd, publishers of the *Herald* and the *Sun News-Pictorial,* and the Melbourne retailer Buckley and Nunn Ltd held the remaining twenty per cent.

The board consisted of members from each group in the syndicate, all well known to George Tallis. He and John Tait acted for the JCW Ltd and J&N Tait interests, company executive George Wright represented Farmers Ltd, Theodore Fink and Keith Murdoch stood in for the board of the Herald and Weekly Times, and company executive Felix Lloyd was the Buckley and Nunn representative. Because of his long experience with wireless, Tallis was made the chairman of directors.

Station 3LO was built by AWA, and an AWA employee TW (Bill) Bearup became the studio manager. The transmitter was located at Braybrook, about ten miles from Melbourne, and the studio was in four rooms in the Cambridge Building, 139 Collins Street, later moving to nearby Kurrajong House, a building belonging to Tallis and the Taits.

The managing director of the station was Major WT (Wally)

Conder. Wally had extensive experience in leadership, discipline and motivation gained in the army during the First World War, and subsequently as Inspector General of Prisons. Every now and then a company needs an army presence, and a military mind.

How did Conder enter the Williamson orbit? It was very simple. Wally and George Tallis were fellow members of the Athenaeum Club in Collins Street, Melbourne. The Firm had been looking for someone to investigate box-office receipts, which had been unexpectedly low. Wally's background recommended itself for this problem, and a friendly chat and a drink settled the matter. Wally's bullet head, athletic build and blunt manner put in an appearance at the theatres, and takings mysteriously showed an abrupt improvement. Conder then moved on to the less physical task of managing director of 3LO, but everyone knew that he was on call.

On opening night, 13 October 1924, 3LO offered Melba singing Mimi in the Melba–Williamson's production of *La Bohème*, transmitted from His Majesty's Theatre, Melbourne. Although the transmission itself was only fair, not a wireless, nor even a spare valve, was available anywhere. The event was so successful that Melba's agents forbade her to sing for wireless broadcasters again. Radio reached too many non-paying customers – it was exploitation!

In 1925 the Firm broadcast the musical *Sally* in its entirety on 3LO, taking pride in the all-Australian production. This embellished the AWA experiment of the previous year. At the same time it was a significant pointer to the future when much of the station's success would flow from its close association with the theatre, vaudeville and the concert circuits controlled by JCW Ltd.

One of the early entertainments of 3LO was the Buckley and Nunn Studio Orchestra, a five-piece ensemble consisting of a violin, viola, cello, piano and trumpet. Bill Bearup had the whole orchestra play first. Then he brought in a soprano. There followed a violin solo; then a piano solo; then another soprano; finally a trumpet solo. 'By which time,' he said, 'you were half way there.' The Buckley and Nunn tea rooms provided refreshments, and in return for publicity Allan's Music Store lent the instruments, music and records.

Williamson's provided artists who had rates for wireless appearances written into their contracts. They also supplied some of the music used as accompaniment to silent films, as well as the music from their shows. Less frequently the Firm attempted live broadcasts directly from theatres. Wally Conder convinced Allan's to sponsor concert parties, and, on his suggestion, they ran a radio song contest.

Station 3LO flourished. It could draw on George Tallis's abilities to develop the necessary corporate structure, Farmer and Co.'s experiences with radio 2FC, Keith Murdoch's newspapers for publicity and JCW Ltd and J&N Tait to guide the broadcasting of concerts and shows. Coupled with the management team of Conder and Bearup, it was not surprising that 3LO dominated broadcasting in Victoria from 1924 to 1929. The programming set a benchmark for the industry, and 3LO became the most popular station in Australia.

In his book *The Music Sellers,* Peter Game writes about the 3LO investment. Within five years the Broadcasting Company of Australia had an annual income of £50,000, made from a mere £6250 initial investment. He concludes that 'it was one of the most sensational success stories of the century.'[7]

In line with the federal government's demand that A-class stations share and widely broadcast good quality programs, in 1928 Tallis merged the Broadcasting Company of Australia with Associated Radio, which controlled station 3AR. The new entity was called the Dominion Broadcasting Company Ltd. Naturally Tallis was the chairman of directors of the board. *Smith's Weekly* succinctly summed up the situation:

Station 3LO, from tiny beginnings, has grown like the bean stalk in the fairy tale. It has linked interests with 2FC (Sydney), it controls the Tasmanian service, it has latterly acquired control of the Perth broadcasting service, and it has been in treaty with the Adelaide company, 5CL. The amalgamated scheme with 3AR Melbourne means that the broadcasting service will be in combination, and the Brisbane station will also come into line in arrangement of programmes and other essentials.[8]

Late in the decade, Victorians held over fifty per cent of all listener licences in Australia, and the number of licences was still growing. Eight in every hundred Victorians had a valid listener licence, a world-beating figure by twenty-five per cent. Putting it another way, one in every two or three houses in Melbourne had a licensed receiver, and this penetration came about in five years or less. After due consideration, *Wireless Weekly* concluded that:

There can be only one reason for this extraordinary position in Victoria, and that is the excellence of the services of 3LO, which have dominated the airwaves since the commencement of broadcasting in Australia . . . It is the result of vision and enterprise on the part of the directors of that station in supplying at all times the best and the most comprehensive services possible.

Similar success flowed to the other stations associated with 3LO. When the world-wide reputation of the station's short-wave broadcasts, operating on a wave-length of 31.55 metres, is added to the list, the total service assumes phenomenal proportions.

As early as 1929, *Wireless Weekly* indicated that 3LO may have already sown the seeds of 'Radio Australia' programs. The article reported that the station's regular Monday morning short-wave broadcasts, from five to six o'clock Melbourne time, were heard loud and clear world-wide. Even the long-wave broadcasts were received in far-away Alaska. The report continued:

At a jungle mission outpost at Tanganyika, Australian listeners gather to hear the special Government news bulletin issued from Canberra exclusively for broadcasting by 3LO – the importance of the world broadcasting being thereby officially recognised.

The Prince of Siam was an enthusiastic listener to 3LO, and he thought it an important medium for bringing about a better international understanding. Reports came in from California, from the deserts of Asia and Africa, Northern Scandinavia, the Holy Land at Jerusalem, and also from Damascus and Baghdad. 'In America 3LO is regarded as one of the foremost short-wave services in the world,' the article concluded.[9]

But what of the country listener? According to the *Wireless Weekly*:

3LO applied to the Commonwealth Government for the necessary permits to erect four relay stations of the same power as the main station at Braybrook . . . Had 3LO been granted the permits, these relay stations would have been operating as early as 1927, and a chain system similar to that of the BBC would have been established.[10]

Was this not the sort of leadership that the government had been seeking? Yet there were cries of monopoly; the same cries JC Williamson himself had heard when he formed his Triumvirate management team more than forty years earlier. Lucky Williamson! He had not been plagued by major government interference.

By 1925, the Firm had been so successful with its multi-media activities that George announced that the Firm now had 'wonderful additional assets' in the form of wireless, pictures and vaudeville. To celebrate, and to bring his friend Arthur Allen up to date, George sent him 'a beautiful new wireless instrument – six valves, loop aerial. It is what they call a Super Heterodyne set and with an aerial you can easily get Melbourne and other places'.[11] Now, in Sydney, even Arthur could experience the wonders of 3LO.

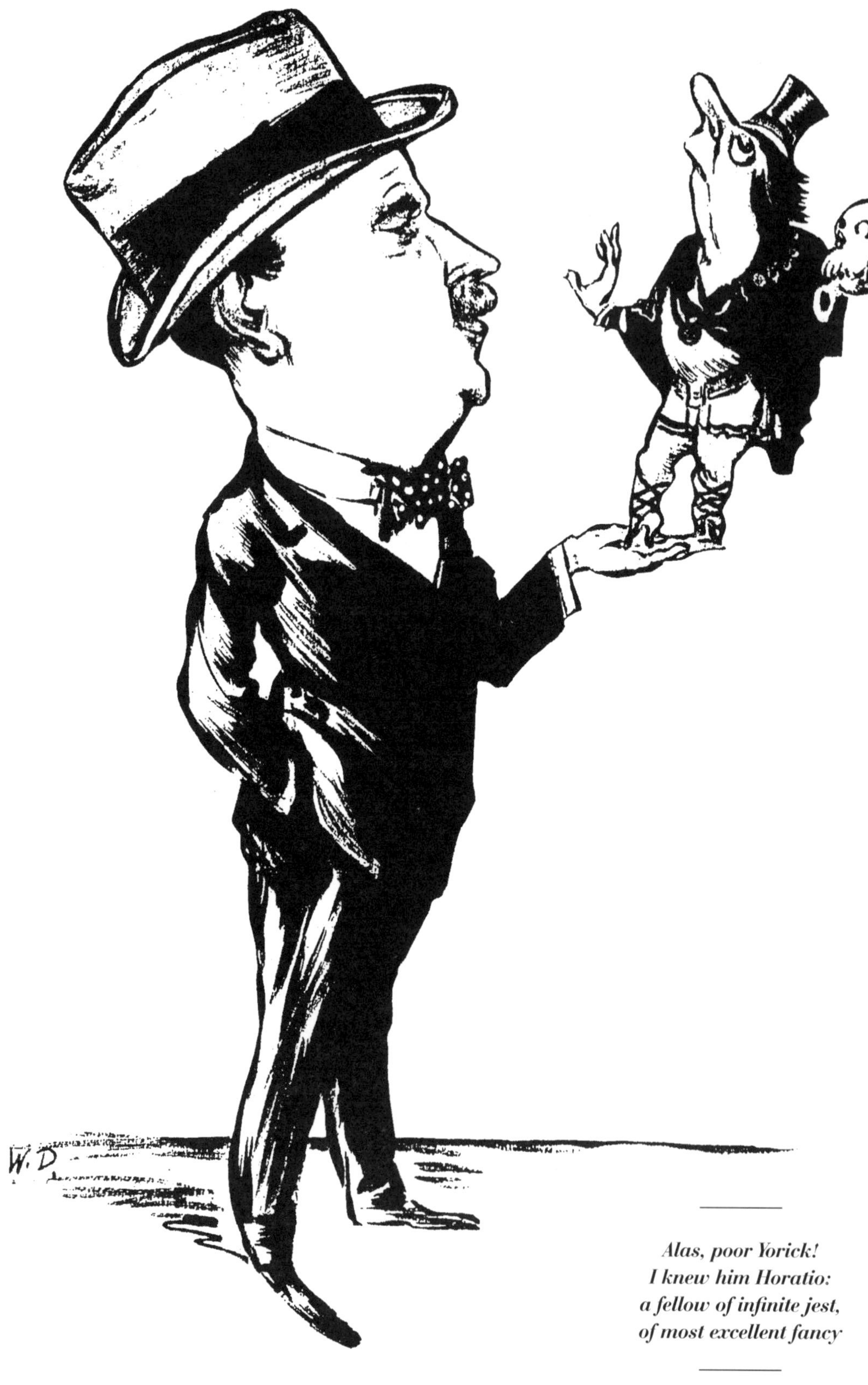

Alas, poor Yorick!
I knew him Horatio:
a fellow of infinite jest,
of most excellent fancy

CHAPTER FOURTEEN

Old Lightnin'

In 1921, the year after the amalgamation with J&N Tait, George spent three months in Sydney. Head office was there, and the new management was looking for fresh initiatives. The bigger team had not led to a more relaxed working life for him. In fact business was hectic because ambition was generating from another quarter.

It was during the negotiations for the lost McIntosh vaudeville deal that George noticed how slow the Tait brothers were to reach an agreement among themselves, and that this was delaying their decisions. A niggling worry developed, although Tallis, characteristically, reasoned that it was a problem easily fixed with a friendly chat, so he pushed it aside.

In spite of great tidings from the accountants, the London end of the business had been unstable. Nevin Tait felt uncomfortable about the arrangements. In fact, he had emphasised some years before the merger that J&N Tait was a privately owned concern with no liabilities, and there was no board of directors or group of shareholders hampering family decisions, or those of its bankers. Nevin was not convinced that amalgamation was a good idea.

But John, Frank and Ted were seduced by the immediate advantages of joining with the Williamson company, and the Taits' business model was turned on its head. Before the end of the decade, they may have looked back wistfully at Nevin's view, and on the good old days, unencumbered by boards and hostile shareholders. Although adopting Nevin's cautious attitude might have meant missing some of the rewards of the 1920s boom years, it may have allowed the brothers to sail through the turbulent years of the 1930s like a cork on a wild sea.

More immediately, though, Nevin anticipated problems to do with the doubling-up of responsibilities, and indeed he was right. Perhaps the main issue to bother him crystallised as early as 1921, when he found himself in America at the same time as Hugh Ward. Both were conducting business for the Firm; Ward as a managing director of JCW Ltd and Nevin as a managing director of J&N Tait. Nevin felt compromised, and he complained to his brothers that he should also be a managing director of JCW Ltd. He could not command the respect of the English or the American agents otherwise.

Nevin had been a casualty of the negotiations. There were already two members of the Tait family on the company's board, and that remained the agreed representation for some years. Moreover, although the Taits wanted Pat Malone, the Firm's long term representative, off the payroll to allow Nevin to have sole responsibility for the London office, Tallis renewed Malone's contract. George's reason gave food for thought, and a sense of *déjà vu*.

Hugh Ward was about to leave JCW Ltd to join the Fuller Brothers, and this new team looked set to organise some real competition. If Malone did not work for the Firm, he would work for Ward. In this event, a string of valuable shows that Williamson's could ill afford to lose would no longer be available to them. When told that Nevin could certainly hold his own against Ward in London, George must have felt giddy. Was there to be yet another Tait–Ward shoot-out, Nevin playing the role of Ted, and London replacing New York?

It was becoming clearer by the day that there would always be difficulties somewhere in the organisation. The Firm had grown so big that it was impossible to keep every department running smoothly, every director happy and every sphere of the operation performing at peak efficiency. There was bound to be big trouble sooner or later.

Ted Tait was looking into the very soul of JCW Ltd when he observed before amalgamation that it was a machine carrying enormous overhead expenses, principally for men with little interest in the company. The exception, Ted had written, was Tallis, 'the only brain in the concern'. Although overstated, his criticisms had some basis in fact.

In the early 1920s, George saw a great deal of Arthur Allen, the Firm's Sydney solicitor. Allen, born in 1862, was the grandson of George Wigram Allen, founder of the oldest legal firm in Australia, Allen, Allen and Hemsley, which has its offices in Sydney. As was expected of him, Arthur joined the family company. He became its driving force, and dealt with two of the big accounts, the Australian Gas Light Company and JCW Ltd. In her book, *The Allens Affair,* Valerie Lawson states that Arthur showed a great affinity for business, promoting the wellbeing of his company, and his own family, with many shrewd real estate transactions.

Allen had been associated with the Firm for years, first as JC Williamson's personal solicitor, and in 1913 he, Tallis and Williamson had worked feverishly together for some months on company business and finalising Williamson's personal affairs. It was natural that Allen and Tallis would get together during George's business trips to Sydney and review the old days.

Allen was a very keen theatre-goer. He enjoyed talking shows and productions with Tallis, and lunching or dining with him at whatever restaurant was the talk of the town. Tallis was usually in Sydney for meetings of the JCW Ltd board. Allen also attended these meetings as a director of the company, and issues raised there were the subject of informal debate by himself and Tallis long after the lights had gone out in the boardroom.

Arthur was the great 'facilitator' of the Firm. He knew more about the Sydney senior staff, and the goings on, than anybody else, and whenever George Tallis came to town it was Arthur he turned to for a briefing. Constantly keeping in contact with so many people would have wearied even a young, fit man, and Arthur Allen was a chronic asthmatic for most of his adult life. Many nights were a battle with breathlessness and insomnia. During his hours of wakefulness he would talk into a dictaphone, giving his two secretaries a flying start when they arrived for work the next morning. In part, the dictations were for his meticulously kept personal and business diaries. These documents, held at Sydney's Mitchell Library, are a fascinating window on life at the top of the social and legal worlds during the early part of the century.

Late in 1921 Tallis broke the news to Allen that he was planning to visit Europe and America. At the same time he also articulated his concerns about leaving the management of JCW Ltd for such a long period. Already there were signs of disharmony.

The two hot-heads, Ted Tait and Hugh Ward, had never managed to heal the enormous rift that pre-amalgamation competition between J&N Tait and the Firm had generated. Possibly neither man tried very hard, even though they worked out of the same office in Sydney. They had quite different agendas, and, in any case, it was becoming evident to Hugh Ward that his own future lay away from that of the Firm.

To cap matters, Clyde Meynell, usually the quiet man of the company, had a clash with *Smith's Weekly*. To his intense disgust the paper had published an article inferring that the only theatre manager in the Firm worth reporting was – Hugh Ward.

Meynell had long taken exception to Ward's strong penchant for personal publicity and at least once previously, in 1914, he had drawn Tallis's attention to the dangers inherent in it. At that time his hackles had been raised by some articles published in London as a result of a Ward visit to that city, and he wrote to George:

I must say that I take great exception to them. You know I am not a person who is bursting for publicity, but these interviews are likely to give a most erroneous impression in England. It would appear that he is sole Director in this business in Mr Williamson's place. People who have been associated in business with us for some years will naturally say, 'What has become of Tallis and Meynell, have they been pushed out or are they broke, taken to drink or in a lunatic asylum that no mention is made of them at all?'

With such disputes raging, it is little wonder that Arthur Allen noted 'Tallis is full of worries' as a result of a big JCW Ltd meeting in 1921. Much of it revolved around the Ted–Hugh and the Meynell–*Smith's Weekly* issues, and it was all extraordinarily difficult, Allen wrote, 'because there was so much jealousy and difference of opinion with respect to the production of plays and casts ...'

Eighteen months into the amalgamation George was getting a small preview of what the ride would be like. For the moment, though, it was time for 1921 to close and for him to exit overseas.

By March 1922, official news of Hugh Ward's resignation as a managing director of JCW Ltd reached the press. *Theatre Magazine* announced that month:

It had to come! Hugh J Ward announces his withdrawal from the firm of JC Williamson Ltd because of an 'over-abundance of directors, many without theatrical skill ...' [1]

Simultaneously, one bone of contention and a very experienced showman had left the Firm to join forces with the Fuller Brothers. The Taits were pleased, but the side was the weaker for Ward's going. Large theatrical companies benefit from the propaganda antics of an extrovert who knows what he is doing and, whatever the costs of his self-promotion and prickly personality, Ward had certainly kept the Firm in the public eye. In the years ahead, Tallis may well have felt the loss of an actor–manager who truly understood theatre and its people.

Also in March, George and Millie left for London, and they were to be away until December. It was a long time for the Firm to be without its captain and, by August, Meynell was expressing concern about the length of Tallis's absence. How the Firm would cope was creating some nervousness. George and his vast experience had been around the place for so long without a break that he was taken for granted. When things went wrong managers had instinctively called for him. Now, while he was away, there was no one to fill the gap. Tallis was not only missed, he was needed.

Late in 1923, because of the new administration at Williamson's, Clyde Meynell announced that he wished to retire and sell his shares. It is not clear who bought them, but since Arthur Allen was 'trying to help', they may have come under his control. In any event, Meynell sailed for England in March 1924 to start a new life and, from the point of view of Australian theatre, he disappeared.

Thus, within four years of the amalgamation, there was a theatrical vacuum on the JCW Ltd board as the old team of Tallis, Ward and Meynell broke up. Although the Taits had little time for either Ward or Meynell, the company had lost an enormous amount of theatrical expertise with their departure, and the incoming team could not hope to redress this deficiency in the short term. Of the four brothers, only Ted was properly trained as a theatre manager.

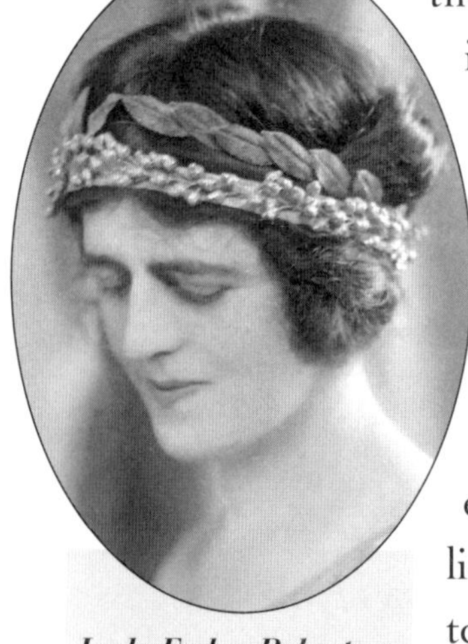

Lady Forbes Robertson

In any case, the new system was about to be tested. In 1922 George was in England assembling, as the London *Evening News* put it, 'probably the biggest series of theatrical engagements entered into by one organisation'. The article, published on 11 July, said that Tallis intended to 'carry off to the Antipodes' the three complete companies, with scenery and properties, of Oscar Asche, Lady Forbes-

Robertson, and the husband and wife team Dion Boucicault–Irene Vanbrugh. The collective repertoire was well over a dozen plays. George was quoted:

These three companies will include at least 40 principals. It is the biggest undertaking that I have arranged. Incidentally, we have bought outright Mr Asche's entire Shakespearian outfit of scenery and properties . . . Mr Asche is taking his six greyhounds; it was only on this condition that he consented to go. I had to cable to the Commonwealth Government for special permission to allow them in the country.

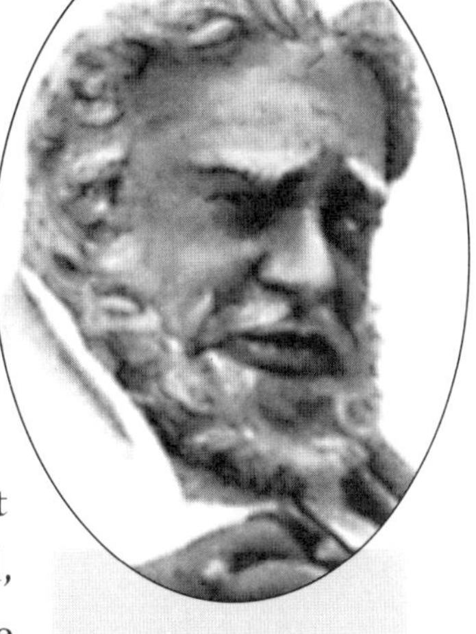
Oscar Asche

Oscar Asche gave the new Williamson administration some practice in handling fractious theatrical celebrities. He stayed in Australia until mid-1924, and by that time some unpleasant disagreements had arisen between himself and the Firm. Asche had made £16,000 on his tour, while the host company had lost heavily. In spite of this, it was public knowledge that the actor, disgruntled, intended to discuss his grievances with the audience on the night of his last appearance. While the orchestra played the national anthem, he stood before the curtain, and the orchestra continued to play—and play. Asche, an immense man, boomed at the audience; it whistled and cheered back. At last the leading lady, Doris Campion, stepped across the footlights and onto the piano, disarmed the conductor, and the orchestra died. Asche, with all impediments out of the way, then had the crowd at his mercy.

This incident was widely reported, locally and internationally, especially Asche's comment in the *Sunday News* on 15 June 1924 that:

I am astounded that the National Anthem was used to gag me. I have not heard before of its being played in the dark. It did not give me opportunity of saying 'goodbye' to my public.

Whatever the merits of the Oscar Asche case, the debacle was a poor advertisement for a mature theatre company like JCW Ltd. But an internal matter was of greater concern to Tallis. There was a growing tendency for the Taits to stall board decisions until family unity on issues had been reached, and an emerging pressure to stack the board with Tait directors.

In 1923 Ted wrote to George:

I see no reason why you should not arrange with John and Frank to purchase Meynell's shares and give the Directorate to John, Nevin or Frank. It seems a great pity that we do carry such a load of Directors and wish we could drop AW Allen who has never been very useful to us.

Of the 'old brigade' that would have left Tallis, Theodore Fink and Fred Smith on the board. Surely George must have wondered where he now was on the gold-watch list.

Claude Kingston, who at the invitation of John Tait worked for the Firm as a manager of celebrities from 1921, dedicated a page in his book *It Don't Seem a Day Too Much* to words that were extravagant in both their praise and blame of George Tallis. He wrote:

The Taits were all able men, each in his own way and particularly in the celebrity concert field. But none of the Taits was Tallis's peer as a live theatre entrepreneur.

I remember him for his mellow wisdom, his attentive way of listening to opinions different from his own, his faultless manners. I have never known another man who was, quite unstudiedly, as courteous as Tallis, not only to his social superiors and equals but also to his lowliest subordinates.

Then came the sting:

It is true that he had one dire weakness: this was an unconquerable propensity to run away from trouble, which inevitably led on to worse trouble in the end. If he had taken a stronger stand with the Taits when they first came into The

Firm, strains and conflicts which developed over the years would have died stillborn and never asserted themselves. Once the early tussles were over, life would have been more comfortable for him and for all concerned, but he could not nerve himself to face the immediate unpleasantness.[2]

What are we to make of Kingston's criticism? Tallis sometimes doubtless did procrastinate, and slip around confrontation in pursuit of his own goal, or the goal that he thought would best serve the interests of his firm. While he would later complain about the indecisiveness of the Tait-laden JCW board, George himself could be elusive in his business dealings, preferring to stall until the first move came from the other side. Nevertheless, the Kingston assessment requires some comment.

Before the amalgamation, the Taits had expressed surprise that Tallis was not governing director of the Firm as Williamson had been, with rights to set policy and to veto resolutions made by the board. As chairman of directors, Tallis had no such powers. If he had wished to inherit the Williamson governing directorship, the time to negotiate it would probably have been when he held most of the shares, before the Clarke–Meynell amalgamation. With that opportunity gone, he could have made the governing directorship a condition of the Williamson–Tait amalgamation, since the Taits had previously mentioned it as a possibility. We can only conclude, therefore, that George did not want special advantages in the boardroom, and that he wished to lead by consensus, fixing the occasional problem, as we have seen, with a friendly chat. But, when the predictable happened, and the Taits asserted themselves *en bloc,* there was no legislated way they could be contained.

Kingston claims that George had 'an unconquerable propensity to run away from trouble'. Had this been true, he would never have survived as a theatre manager where real trouble came by the barrow-load. Nor would he have confronted the 'troubles' brought on by cinema and radio so squarely, investing his own time and money. Kingston, it would seem, underestimated Tait determination, and overestimated Tallis's powers to control it.

In summary, perhaps the situation was this. In the same way that Tallis around 1900 – and certainly after the establishment of the Williamson, Tallis and Ramaciotti partnership – had lifted the burden of administration from JC Williamson's shoulders and allowed him to travel and pursue big prizes for the Firm, George hoped that with the Tait amalgamation the injection of managerial skills would free him from his day-to-day routine. The main difference, however, was that while George had been a loyal lieutenant to Williamson, the Taits worked to a different plan. They, and in particular Ted, wanted the company, and George's job.

HIS MAJESTY'S THEATRE
Melbourne
DIRECTION . . . . J.C. WILLIAMSON LTD
FAREWELL
OF
DAME NELLIE MELBA
MONDAY, OCTOBER 13TH 1924
ACT III LA BOHÈME
rall
a Tempo
Addio, senza rancor
Nellie Melba
THE PROCEEDS WILL BE GIVEN TO THE
LIMBLESS AND TUBERCULAR SOLDIERS APPEAL

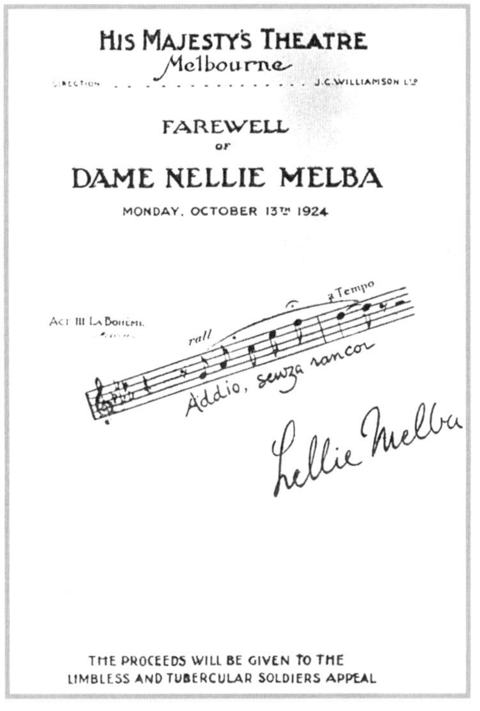

In 1924 Nellie Melba and JCW Ltd combined in a highly successful operatic venture. Toti Dal Monte was a new star for the season, fresh from successes in Milan and Paris, and wherever she went in Australia the press pestered her for interviews and photographs. Melba sang as Marguerite in Gounod's *Faust*, Mimi in Puccini's *La Bohème* and Desdemona in Verdi's *Othello*. However, the tour was tarnished by Melba's poor health and illness amongst the cast, leading to several last-minute cancellations. It was during this tour that Melba sang in the special gala benefit of *La Bohème* for the opening of radio station 3LO on 13 October 1924. The broadcast was heard by 150,000 eager listeners, who thought it was Melba's Australian swan-song.

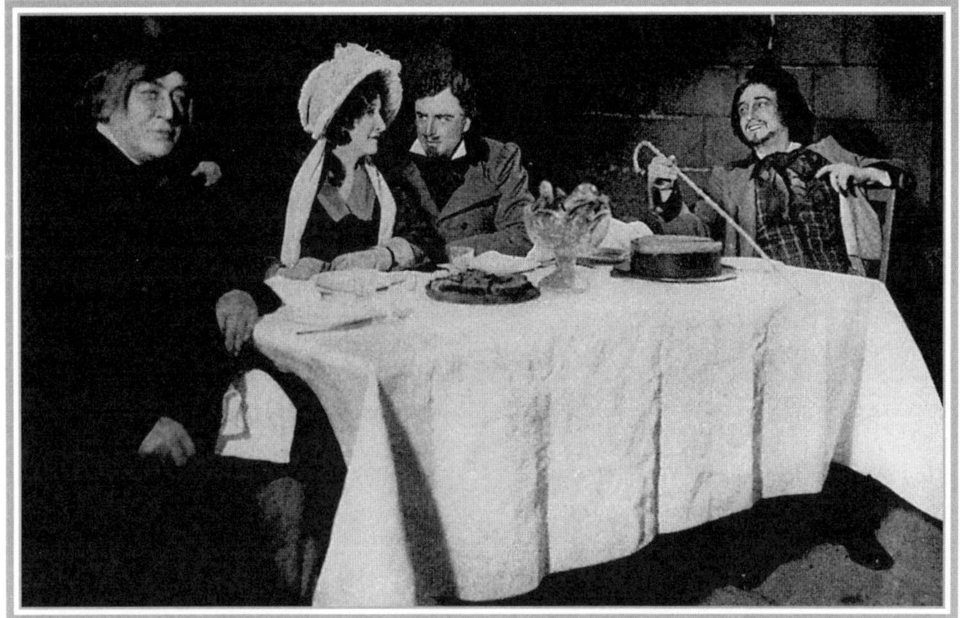

Dame Nellie Melba in La Bohème, *1924*

There were glowing reports following the Melba tour, and the takings reflected the artistic success of the performances. For once, the season had been an exception to the rule that grand opera spells financial ruin to managements.[3]

After the opening of the season the *Evening Herald* wrote on 31 March 1924:

Now that the opera début has passed off with such success, Sir George Tallis can lean back in his office chair with a sigh of thankfulness. Had it not been his personal ambition to revive grand opera in Australia on a scale greater than before, many years might have passed before Australians had a chance to hear the world's best music presented by distinguished artists. I am told that in the face of great opposition from many quarters, opposition dictated only by the prodigious cost, Sir George fought his great plan through.

But more theatrical fuel was necessary to stoke up the next year's offerings. In July 1924 George, accompanied by Millie, left for America, where he spent two months searching for shows. With

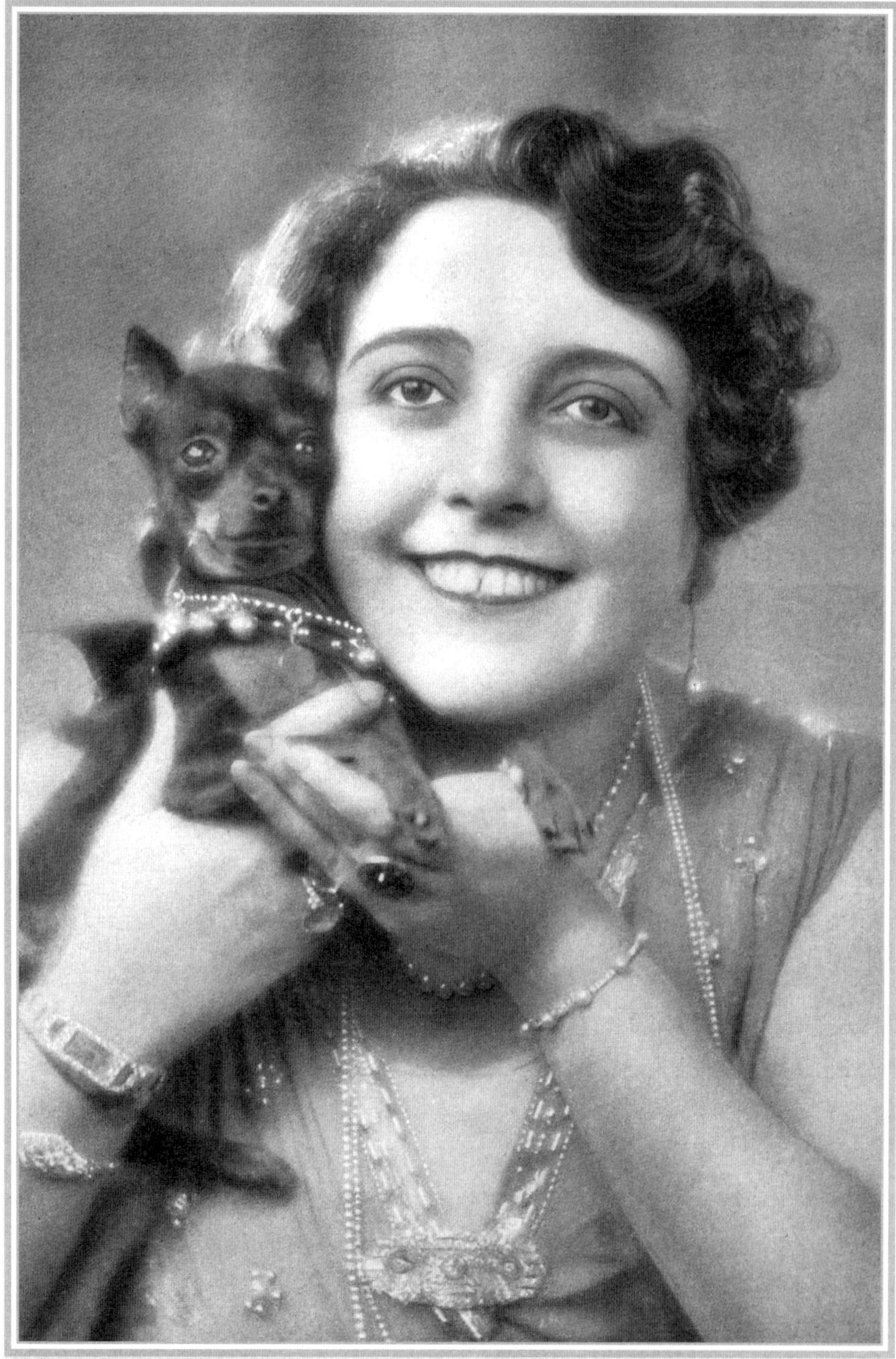

Toti Dal Monte, star of the 1924 and 1928 opera seasons

them was their second son, Pat, who had recently finished an outstanding schoolboy sports career. They motored across the United States west to east, and met up with their oldest son, Mick, in New York. Mick was studying engineering at Harvard University. There was a great reunion, and a list of likely productions to see, but Pat became continually frustrated when, just as the performances became absorbing, there was a tap on his shoulder. George had already made his assessment, and they were off to the next theatre.

The nicknames Pat and Mick had become so entrenched that very few people knew the men's given names, Jeffery and George. Strangers thought that Pat was older than Mick, because that is the natural order; so the confusion was absolute. The young men and their father were great friends, and George always enjoyed travelling with them, either together or separately.

Late September of the same year found George sailing for London, where his quest for more theatre fare continued. While in America, he had experienced great difficulty locating available shows. When he did find them, the prices were higher than he expected. There were faint memories among the agents of the good old days before the 1920s, when JCW Ltd and J&N Tait competed for popular pieces. They still rubbed their hands together whenever they saw an Australian theatre manager heading their way.

To counter this, George set up an international combination of managers, agents and playwrights to control, in part, the distribution of theatrical material on four continents: America, Europe, Australia and South Africa. While in New York in 1924 he obtained the English rights to the play *Lightnin'*, and the following year the London *Daily Sketch* wrote about this combination under the headline 'Old Lightnin' Strikes London':

One of the whirlwind forces of the world of entertainment is now in London. It is a new thing that while [Tallis] has been gathering up fresh spoils in America and here he should have been assisting in the formation of a great international organisation which aims at putting monkey glands, so to speak, into British theatrical enterprise.

Associated with JAE Malone in England, as he has been for some years, Sir George Tallis is co-operating also with AE Erlanger and CB Dillingham, the managers, and John Golden and Winchell Smith, the dramatists, whose names count for the best in America, for a big extension of British Empire–American entertainment exchange and development.

As a beginning … we have the coming of Lightnin'*. For three years the play has been touring the southern hemispheres. It was produced in New York as long ago as 1918 and has been one of the biggest dramatic successes there of modern times.*

'It couldn't come to London before,' Sir George Tallis told me, 'because of an understanding between Winchell Smith and joint author–actor Frank Bacon, that the actor should himself introduce it here in his original part, as soon as he could be spared from his native New York. Now, unhappily, he has died, and the embargo no longer exists.'

Winchell Smith is himself to superintend the production at the Shaftesbury [in January 1925], which will follow soon after the trial presentation at Eastbourne next Monday. To play Old Lightnin' is Horace Hodge, who has carried the part through South Africa.[4]

Lightnin', a comedy-drama, centred on a quaint old bedraggled fellow known as Lightnin' Bill. The plot has overtones of the old Williamson hit *Struck Oil,* in which JC Williamson had starred in the major role as the bumbling Dutch shoemaker John Stofel. *Lightnin'* survived because Horace Hodge blew life into old Bill, who came up with words of unexpected wisdom.[5]

George continued to say that:

We get plays and the big film dramas in Australia often much earlier than you in London. Where you have advantage, however, is in the abundance of acting talent and personality which enables a thin play to get across. With our much smaller population, repertory is inevitable and we require the very best in plays as well as first-class touring companies from England and America.

Tallis returned to Australia in March 1925, after his launch of *Lightnin'* at the Shaftesbury in London. Ted Tait had been holding the fort. By and large, matters were deemed by Ted to be 'very satisfactory' in 1924 and 1925. So satisfactory had business become, in fact, that the Firm moved into new Sydney offices. Most of the touring shows were doing well and, while George was away, Ted hurried up and down the eastern seaboard to keep an eye on the whole operation.

Whatever the situation at JCW Ltd concerning theatre management, the Firm had a bountiful supply of business expertise. George and the Taits conducted a great deal of the Firm's affairs together – a collaboration that spilled over to private Tallis–Tait investments in city real estate, and theatres. This activity kept everyone on the move by boat, train or car. The Melbourne directors headed for Sydney, and occasionally vice versa. The *ennui* of all the local commuting was relieved by overseas business trips. George was abroad with Frank Thring from March to December 1927, visiting America and England. He was back for the Firm's AGM, and the inevitable press interviews.

He observed that 1926 overseas had been prolific in musical comedies, and that his list contained five of the chief successes from the past and present London seasons. The most popular of these was *The Desert Song,* which had played for a year at Drury Lane. The others were *The Girl Friend, Hit the Deck, Princess Charming* and *The Vagabond King.* He continued:

Of course, our outstanding attraction for 1928 will be the grand opera company. At Florence, I met Mr Nevin Tait, who had already devoted upward of twelve months to the preliminaries of the scheme. He had then heard practically every voice of note in Europe, and had narrowed down the list . . . to the really great artists of the Continent.[6]

Together, Nevin and George had toured Europe for two months and made the final selections. This resulted in the 1928 Melba–Williamson Grand Opera Company, the most brilliant of its kind ever to visit Australia. Melba was paid a large fee for her professional input, and she did very well while the Firm lost money on the venture. The season generated a mixed reception, while the marriage of star singer Toti Dal Monte at St Mary's Cathedral, Sydney, was the social highlight of the tour.

Later, George was particularly annoyed by a criticism that the opera extravaganza was driven by profit motives rather than a desire to serve musical culture in Australia. He emphasised the £100,000 backing that the Firm had given the tour, and the enormous effort required to stage it. No governments, or other private backers had come up with money, and for the very good reason that 'it is an axiom all over the world that grand opera spells ruin'. Tallis then pointed out that opera in Europe and America was heavily subsidised by outside agencies, and in England Oscar Hammerstein and Thomas Beecham had gone to the edge of bankruptcy with their excursions into opera. He also pointed out:

I have personally been associated with every grand opera venture financed or undertaken by Williamson's since 1887 and apart from the 1924 season none has shown a profit except the Melba season in 1911 . . .

What Tallis did not explain, however, was that the 1911 Melba season had been in the black only because the singer had not charged for her time – the event celebrated her fiftieth birthday and Williamson's fifty years in show business. Had she charged, as she did in the 1928 season, even that earlier opera experience would have been a financial disaster.

In October 1927 – not 1922 as commonly believed – Hugh Ward's JCW Ltd shares were up for sale.[7] Ward had left the Firm in 1922 and was about to retire from show business altogether. Perhaps he was clearing the decks, but again Arthur Allen 'tried to help'. He mentioned the parcel to the Taits, but they considered them too expensive. Arthur did not, and quietly earmarked some 33,000 ordinary shares to join the growing pile that he already controlled.

But at the end of the year the Taits changed their minds. They had developed a definite interest in the shares, and they approached Arthur. To their surprise, he did not intend to sell on. This rejection of business opportunities on grounds of price, followed by afterthoughts and regrets, was a feature of some of the Tait dealings. It often cost them dearly, and it did in this case.

As required by the Firm's Articles of Association, the transfer of Ward's shares to Arthur Allen was raised at the board meeting of 31 December 1927, and it passed without objections. The item was well and truly overshadowed by a report of the glowing state of the Firm's finances.

That same evening Arthur Allen joined George Tallis and three of the Taits in a box at Her Majesty's Theatre, Sydney. The irony of the occasion passed unnoticed. No one could have foreseen that this innocuous share transaction would become one of the important events of the decade in Australian entertainment.

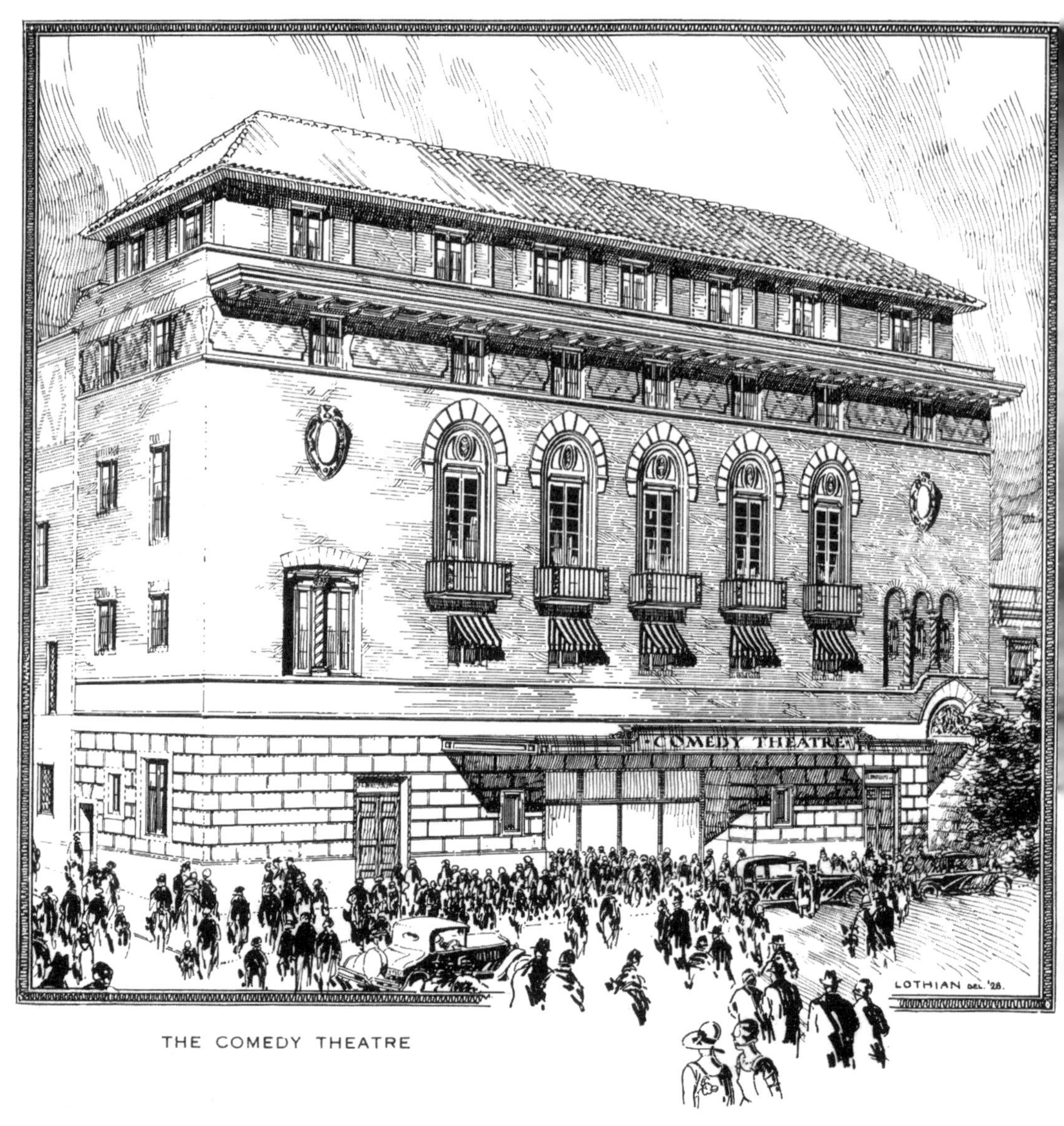

THE COMEDY THEATRE

Opened on Saturday Night, April 28, 1928

By

ANTHONY PRINSEP'S LONDON COMPANY

with

MARGARET BANNERMAN

in

"OUR BETTERS"

– CHAPTER FIFTEEN –

London Calling

As far back as 1910 JC Williamson and George Tallis had discussed the need in Melbourne for a small, intimate theatre. Harold Ashton wrote to Tallis presenting Williamson's idea to renovate the Princess Theatre into 'a first class, cosy and comfortable theatre for the playing of good comedies'.

By 1912, Williamson had changed his mind, and wrote to George at some length giving advice about the possibility of building a *new* theatre. He suggested that Tallis get all the:

details and particulars mapped out, and put on paper all ready to place before a meeting of the board as soon as we return to Australia. I don't know whether you intend putting up a theatre yourself, or to form a syndicate to build and let to the company, or for the company to build – I don't suppose it matters much how it is done so long as a really high class 'small theatre' is built at a reasonable expense.

But another dream was shelved with the passing of Williamson and the disruption of the First World War.

It was not until 1927 that JCW Ltd got around to building the Comedy Theatre, directly opposite His Majesty's Theatre on the south-east corner of Exhibition and Lonsdale Streets. The site was that of the prefabricated 'Iron Pot' theatre that George Coppin had ordered as a venue for the Irish Shakespearian actor Gustavus Vaughan Brooke way back in 1855. Now times were good, the idea had been on hold for over fifteen years, and there was a growing demand for 'intimate' theatres.

In his memoirs George showed his admiration for the refined fare presented by the Brough–Boucicault company in the 1890s, and in 1927 George was reported as saying that:

The [recent] success of the Boucicault productions had been a big factor in the decision. The welcome the public had accorded these plays indicated the demand which had arisen for plays of a similar type, and also for repertory plays, light comedies, and similar productions which required a small or intimate theatre. One of the objects of the new theatre was to house the Repertory Theatre organisation, which would play a season there of at least three months in every year.

The accommodation would be for nine hundred to a thousand persons, and only stalls and dress-circle would be provided. All the important details would be of the most up-to-date type, and special facilities for the rapid handling of scenery and quick changes would be installed.

Productions of a delicate light type, which were unsuitable for an ordinary theatre, would be staged at the new house. Sir George named the works of Barrie, Arnold Bennett, John Galsworthy, AA Milne, Bernard Shaw, Eugene O'Neill and Ibsen as suitable.[1]

The years had moved on. Some of the 'delicate light type' of productions would have been exactly the fare JC Williamson had so mistrusted – in 1890 he had wanted a company touring Ibsen's *A Doll's House* to change the ending so that the renegade heroine Nora would stay 'for the sake of the children'![2]

No expense had been spared in the construction of the new theatre. The foyer had an old Italian palazzo flavour, with its own gushing fountain, Spanish mirrors, fine tapestries and red upholstery to match the carpet. No cold air rushed out when the curtain was raised, by courtesy of a row of hot water radiators at the back of the stage. And was that a telephone for the convenience of the patrons to Melbourne's new playhouse?

The opening souvenir thundered:

It may be said without fear of contradiction that there is no theatre anywhere quite like the Comedy. In style, and the completeness of its atmosphere, it stands alone. Here we are in the stalls, and from any position, even at the extreme sides, a clear, unimpeded view of the stage is given.

Someone had heeded Williamson's views on theatre sighting, comfort and ventilation.

The theatre opened in April 1928 with Somerset Maugham's *Our Betters,* produced by Anthony Prinsep's London Company and with Margaret Bannerman in the lead role. According to the *Argus*:

The play is of the sex variety, but in the main the author's skilled treatment redeems the subject ... At the end of the play the forefront of the stage was a bank of flowers that brought the beauty of autumn into the theatre. Conspicuous among them was a bouquet of crimson roses flung from her box by Dame Nellie Melba, a gift gracefully acknowledged by Miss Bannerman in her speech when she referred to the presence in the audience of the world's greatest artist as one of the many things that made the occasion a memorable one for her.[3]

Maugham had written in the program:

I don't know if it is still the fashion to say that in order to see good acting you must go to France or Germany, but if it is it can only be because when you have once said a foolish thing it is easier to say it again than to say a sensible one. You will have to go far before you see better acting than that of Miss Margaret Bannerman.

Initially, there had been some consternation concerning Miss Bannerman (Mrs Margaret Holm-Sumner) and Mr Prinsep. Mrs

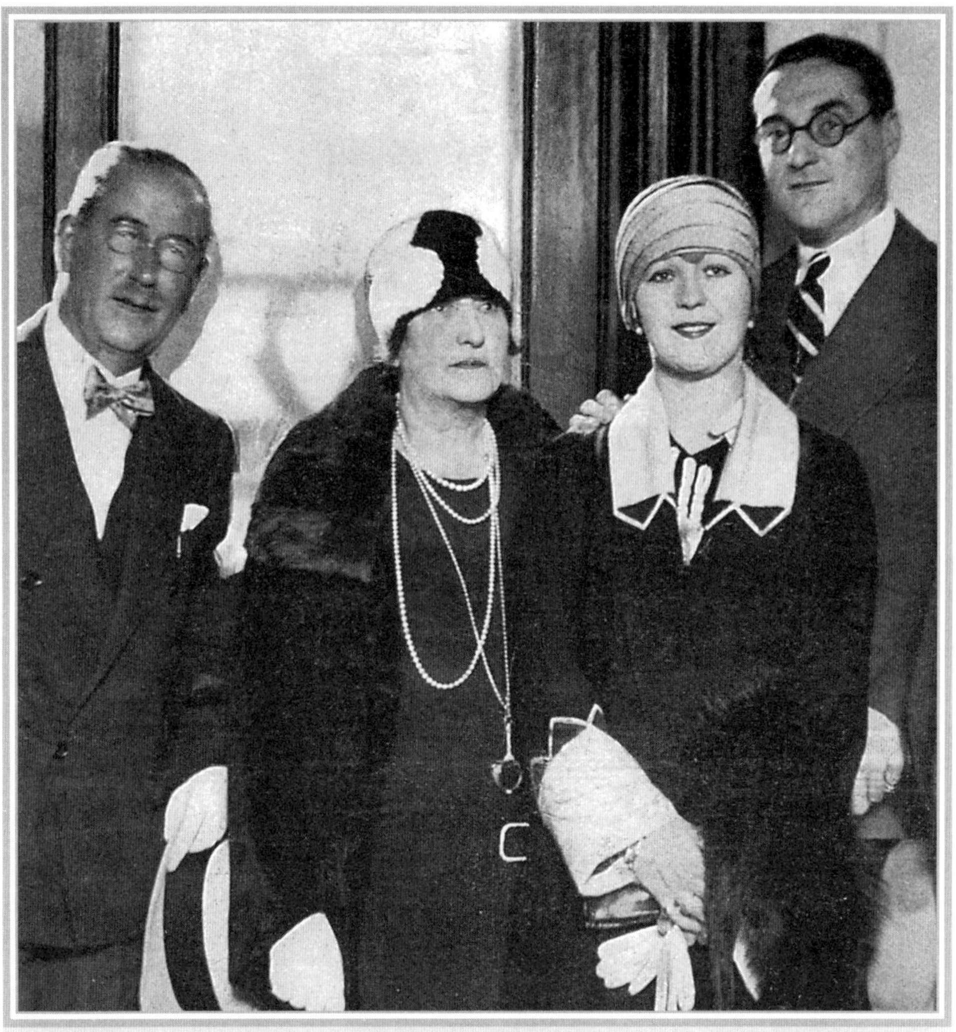

The wedding of Margaret Bannerman and Anthony Prinsep – Dame Nellie Melba and Sir George Tallis in attendance, 1928

Prinsep was about to be granted a divorce; Miss Bannerman had been cited. The problem was, should the sailing of the Prinsep company from London be delayed until after the scandal blew over? Of course not! There is nothing like a scandal to sell seats. The company left as scheduled, Miss Bannerman played, and the Bannerman–Prinsep wedding took place quietly in Melbourne during the tour. In attendance were Sir George Tallis and Dame Nellie Melba.

While George Tallis may be remembered as a businessman in the entertainment world – as one newspaper put it, he had a 'special gift, almost a genius, for finance'[4] – his affection for, and work to popularise, less commercial theatrical entertainment, including grand opera, should not be forgotten.

A comparison with the tired, old His Majesty's Theatre across the road was unfair, but George made it anyway. As a result, he moved from the weary office he had occupied for decades and crossed Exhibition Street. His morale lifted as he inspected the new accomodation with its lavish appointments. At last here was ambience appropriate for the head of the mighty Firm, and he settled in with pleasurable anticipation.

Tallis was now fifty-nine, but he could have seen no reason why his reign at JCW Ltd should not continue far into the future. He felt uneasy that the departures of Ward and Meynell had severed connections with the old days, and concerned about problems arising with the new senior management. But there is nothing like success to soothe transition and stem bickering.

Looking back, George would have acknowledged with pride that the years between 1920 and 1928 had been a period of vast expansion. During that time, the Firm's cinema and radio interests became highly developed and profitable. The Taits maintained the concert business, and Williamson's had branched into the vaudeville market. The Firm's investment in both legitimate and movie theatre buildings had increased sharply, and the number of productions had also risen. In Melbourne alone, immediately upon amalgamation an additional theatre, the King's, had come on stream. For a brief period late in the decade there were four main theatres in use there, the new Comedy Theatre, the Theatre Royal, His Majesty's Theatre and the King's Theatre. The Melbourne Tivoli Theatre was not simply under the control of the Firm, it was owned by a Tallis–Tait syndicate. In Sydney in 1926 five theatres were operating for Williamson's, and fifteen stage attractions were on show across Australia at the one time.

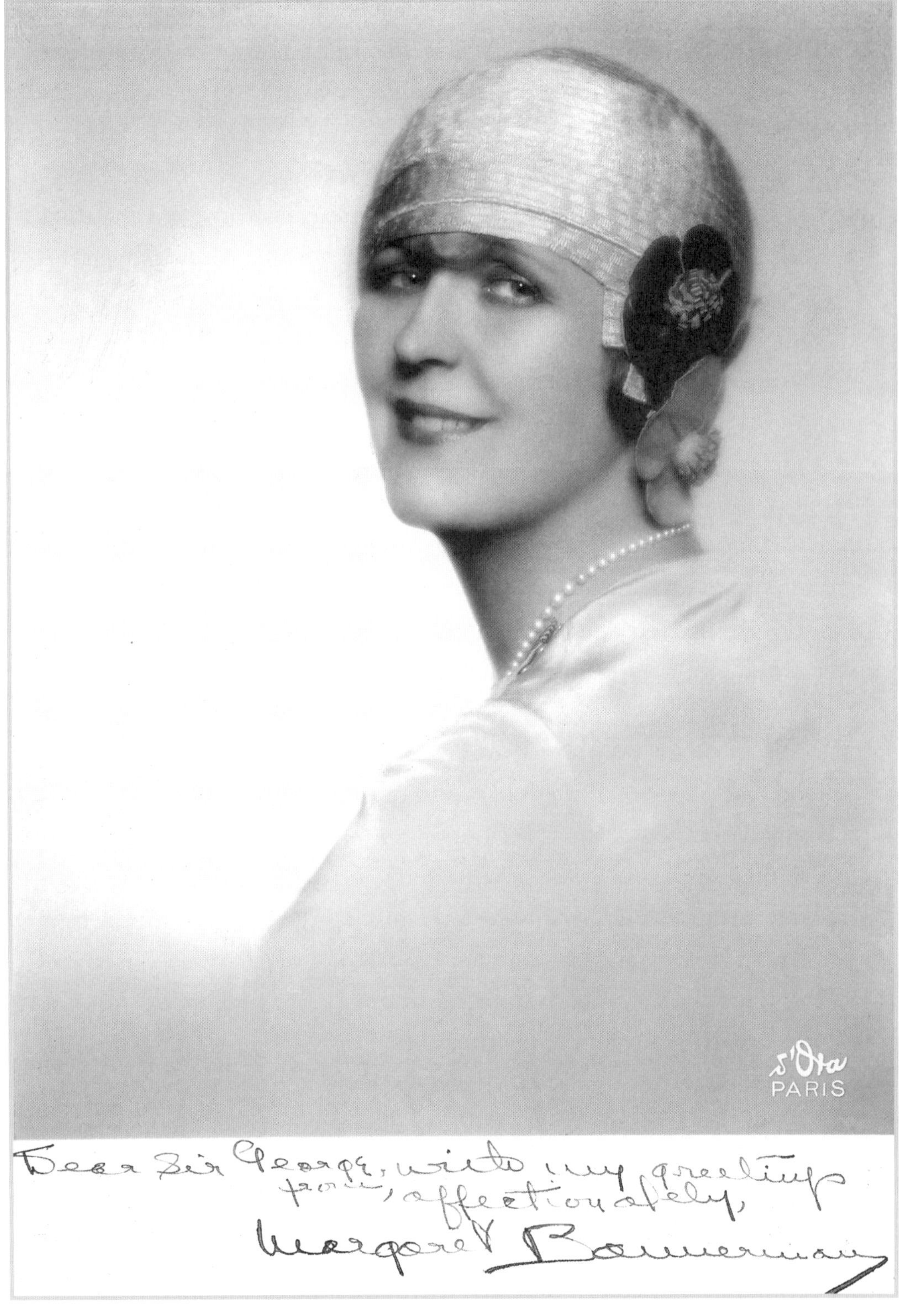
d'Ora
PARIS
Dear Sir George, with my greetings
affectionately,
Margaret Bannerman

In 1926 George was able to speak with pride to the Melbourne *Herald*:

JC Williamson Ltd is now by far the biggest theatrical organisation of its kind in the world. Certainly there is no combination in England which handles anything like the same number of attractions. In America there are two or three big theatrical firms controlling a number of theatres; but, on the whole, in comparison with the Australian firm, the number of productions which they launch during the year is quite limited.

The Williamson firm's interests are not confined to dramatic or musical productions. It is equally at home when presenting opera, pantomime, revue, musical comedy, drama or comedy. In addition, it controls the big Tivoli vaudeville circuit of Australia and New Zealand, while the picture end of its business is probably more extensive than that of any other individual firm in Australia, as directly and indirectly it is interested in or controls more than a hundred picture theatres, and in conjunction with Electric Theatres it is now erecting two large picture and vaudeville houses in Auckland and Wellington for the New Zealand circuit.[5]

At that stage George would not have realised that the Firm was in its golden years; at its very peak. Equally, he would not have dwelt on the fact that it was he who had led it there, to the dizzy heights of the largest entertainment company in the world.

After a delay of at least twelve years, the notion of opening permanently in London appeared again in the JCW Ltd boardroom in 1928. Like wine, it was as if new proposals gestated for long periods in the company's ideas bin. The Comedy Theatre in Melbourne had spent fifteen years maturing, and the London venture twelve. George noted that the Firm was well placed financially, and he proposed to extend its horizons yet again. The feasibility of this plan should be tested immediately. Echoes of Musgrove's ambition in the late 1890s?

Ted Tait had supported the idea when it had been raised some years earlier, but it was never going to be easy. Venture capital was essential, and the Taits were not keen to divert funds to underwrite a scheme of such uncertainty. Perhaps the clinching argument was provided by Tallis. He pointed out that if the Firm owned a theatre in London and produced its own shows, 'it would make the expensive London office self-supporting and profit-making'. This idea appealed to John Tait, and the board nodded agreement.

George sailed for America on 4 October 1928. Ted Tait was also scheduled to go, but he became ill and had to remain in Sydney. Tallis moved on to England some weeks later having, among other attractions, secured the rights to the two most popular Broadway musicals, *Show Boat* and *The New Moon*.

For the first test of the London theatre circuit Tallis selected an American play, *The Patsy,* described by one London newspaper as 'a sort of *Peg o' My Heart* plus wise-cracks', using JCW Ltd's George Parker as producer. The play had run in Melbourne for a season of three months in mid-1928, but before opening night at the Apollo Theatre on 19 December Tallis thought it seemed to lack sparkle. He wondered if it would do for London after all. Fortunately, the next day the London newspapers approved the play. One critic wrote:

Sir George Tallis's ventures on the London boards have been few, but that his shrewd judgment in Australian theatrical matters holds equally good here seems almost proved by the first night of The Patsy *at the Apollo Theatre last night.* High Jinks *and* Lightnin' *he had previously presented to London, but now the new vehicle looks like a winner from the start.*

Indirectly last night's ovation was Sir George's triumph, but public acclamation went to [the unknown American actress] Helen Ford, who caused the simple Londoner to sob all over his boiled shirt and cheer madly at the curtain call.[6]

The London *Times* went further:

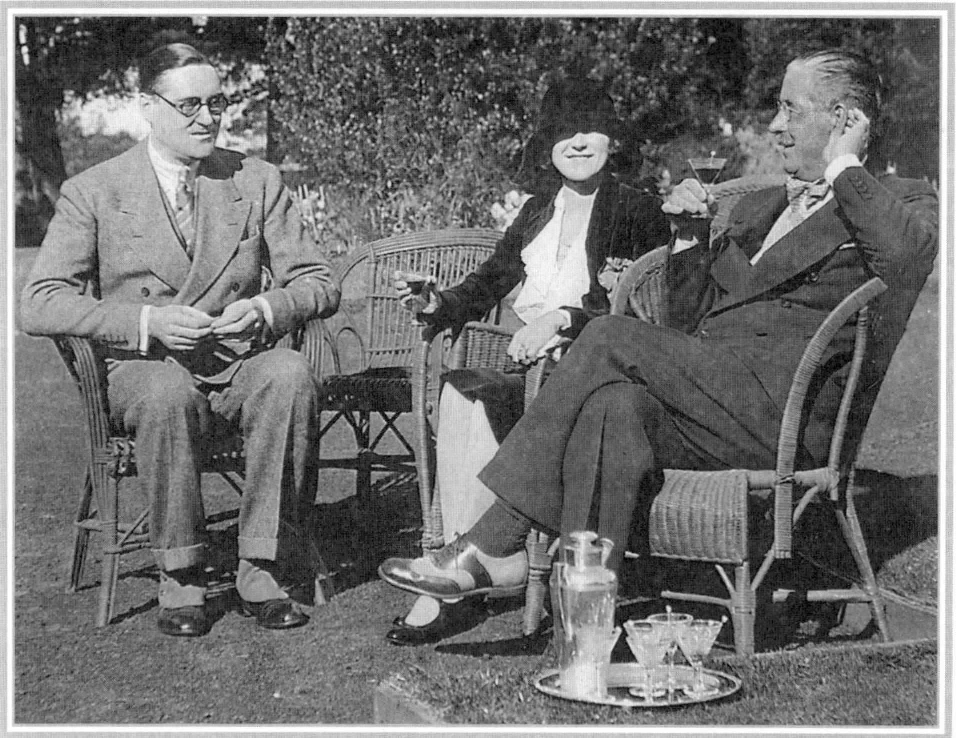

George enjoying cocktails with Margaret Bannerman and Anthony Prinsep at Grosvenor

The curtain went up five times to cheers at the end of the first act; six times to louder cheers at the end of the second; and nine times to still louder cheers at the end of the third. It could have gone on for at least another nine so far as the delighted audience were concerned. This time it was not mere hysterics. It was a genuine welcome to a charming young actress in a charming play.[7]

While in New York, George had heard about a new musical comedy, *Mr Cinders,* that was showing promise in England. He had contacted the JCW Ltd London representatives, who found that *Cinders* was doing very well in the provinces with Julian Wylie as producer. For what Tallis considered a good price, the management of the *Cinders* company offered JCW Ltd a half interest in the show, including a royalty in the profits of the provincial tour. This offer was referred back to the Taits in Australia for a decision. There were delays, and a lost opportunity.

When George finally reached London, *Mr Cinders* was still being tried out. He boarded a train for Glasgow on 24 December, and viewed the production with the Scottish test audience. Greatly impressed, he bought the show, and *Mr Cinders* headed for the Adelphi Theatre in London. However, because *Cinders* had been doing brisk business, the terms were now much steeper than previously. By letter he sharply pointed out to Ted that 'through lack of a quick decision I had to pay through the nose for the London season'.

Mr Cinders nevertheless was critical to Tallis's strategy. A big musical was needed to get the Williamson name on the high road in London, and *Cinders* seemed just the show to do it.

George personally supervised the production in an attempt to give London his best shot. He found a wonderful supporting cast for the stars Bobby Howes and Binnie Hale, but he had difficulty in locating female support singers and dancers among the local talent.

In his book *The Foot Lights Flickered,* distinguished theatre historian W MacQueen-Pope devoted several paragraphs to *Mr Cinders* – an honour that was not given to all musical plays:

There was another great musical play in 1929, and a homemade one too. That was Mr Cinders. *It had a book by Clifford Grey and Greatrex Newman, with music by Vivian Ellis and Richard Myers. It was produced by Julian Wylie ... he engaged and teamed up with Binnie Hale and Bobby Howes. He considered them an ideal stage team and he was right ... The great Australian firm of Williamson's saw the show and liked it; they were invading London and here was a fine card to play. Wylie [sold] them an option ...*

AE Malone produced Mr Cinders, *with many alterations, for the Adelphi where it opened on 11th February, 1929. It was one of the coldest nights for many years and some of that frigidity got into the audience and into the critics. Yet the merits of the show were fully apparent. Binnie Hale and Bobby Howes were ideal; the story was good, a variant on the never failing Cinderella theme;*

the music was delightful, and one of Vivien Ellis's best numbers 'Spread a Little Happiness' has become a classic. Yet, somehow the show hung fire ... The Williamson firm decided that some magic had gone from the show. They [called] back Julian Wylie to put it back into its original form. Wylie went back, restored his magic touch, ... and Mr Cinders *soared to success and, what is more, finished [a] run of 528 performances ... It was one of the romances of the 1920s.*[8]

The casual observer could be excused for thinking that George Tallis was on a roll. London theatre critics were hard to please and, by all accounts, in a difficult and unpredictable market George had achieved two popular successes in as many months. If JCW Ltd was to remain in London on a long-term basis, it was the start it needed. Unfortunately, there was more to the story, much more.

Pat Malone's sudden death on 4 February 1929, exactly a week before *Mr Cinders* opening night, threw Tallis's program into a spin. To top this, an influenza epidemic hit not only George, the casts of *The Patsy* and *Mr Cinders,* but London audiences as well. However, the *coup de grace* to this latest attempt by the Firm to enter the London theatre circuit was the advent of the 'talkies'. Londoners were closely considering their options to live-theatre entertainment. For London, all these forces combined to turn 1929 into the worst year for theatre in living memory.

George wrote to the Tait brothers and complained:

The flu is playing the deuce with The Patsy *business. In fact, all the commercial world at present is suffering. The tragic loss of Pat Malone ... has made everything very worrying ... We sadly miss [our own] producers like Highland, Burcher and Minnie Everett. They would be a godsend.*

If *The Patsy* opened with a roar, it ended in a whimper. The play outstayed its welcome. The American theme, combined with the other factors making 1929 such a bad year, forced an early retirement from the Apollo. Banished to the provinces, it toured quite profitably, but the lost financial ground in London was not reclaimed.

Mr Cinders was a different matter. London agents chastised each other for having rejected the rights to the play, and George's confidence in it was vindicated. It was still playing long after he returned to Australia in mid-1929.

A later thrust at the London theatre market came with the play *Coquette*. George saw it in New York, thought it had potential and bought the rights. The play tested at Brighton before opening at the Apollo Theatre on 3 June 1929. It failed to draw big houses, and JCW Ltd's excursion into London's West End was terminated for all time.

Realistically, there had been only a slim chance of making a big financial success of the experiment. A great deal of local knowledge was needed to obtain the right shows at the right prices and to establish reasonable lease agreements with the managers of the West End theatres. The Firm had to become theatre-smart in London, and that particular piece of education would be costly. The right contacts would materialise slowly, and then only if the Firm could establish a respect for its professionalism and integrity in a city where it was hardly known. With Malone gone, it had been a battle all the way.

However, the more modest goal of making a splash had surely been achieved. London now knew that JCW Ltd had been in town, and that it meant business. One smash hit in the form of *Mr Cinders*, one well-received play, *The Patsy*, and one fizzer out of three was reasonable batting on a difficult pitch.

During this period managerial disputes beset the Firm. These were profound enough that, on their own, they would have thwarted any further attempts to expand to London. The talkies, influenza and other problems simply finished off a venture that was already doomed.

George's difficulties with the JCW Ltd board spilled over into his letters from London. Following the debacle in obtaining the rights to

Mr Cinders, he asked the Taits to make quick decisions, and to stick to them. He pointed out how difficult it was to do business with his hands tied.

As he became aware that the boardroom delays were persisting, Tallis wrote to Ted more desperately:

You brothers will definitely and positively *have to make up your minds whether we want to come here permanently. Up to date there has been a great deal of indefiniteness and indecision on this point, and I think you ought to let me have your views fully and positively as soon as you get this letter.*

Later:

It does seem a pity though to give up now having cleared the decks, as it were, and an enormous amount has been learned during the last six months, both as far as London and the provinces are concerned. I am sure that this office would gradually become an important factor in the amusement world in England.

The idea of building a Williamson theatre in Leicester Square was another plan that George found attractive. The site in question, and one which John Tait had inspected during his last visit to London, became vacant. George sent a cable to John putting the proposition of constructing a comfortable, up-to-date theatre to seat about 1500 people – another Comedy Theatre perhaps. The property market was looking good, so the proposal warranted serious consideration.

It was a big request, and George knew the answer long before he received the return cable. 'After deliberation board considers ...' The cable provoked a very enlightening response from Tallis, in which frustration built up over decades spilt over:

Of course I anticipated your reply about the theatre site. That is the traditional policy of our firm, and naturally I agree that we must walk warily and with discretion, but at the same time it is well worth recollecting that this particular

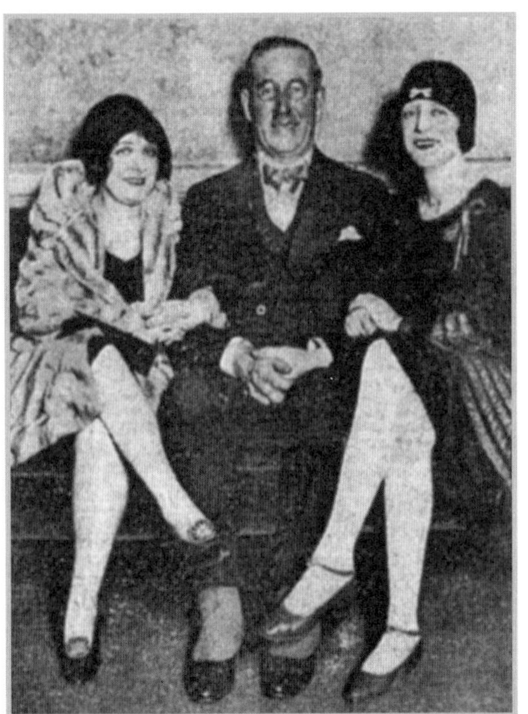

Sir George Tallis, London's latest theatre magnate, with his two leading ladies, Binnie Hale (right) and Helen Ford, who are the stars in "Mr. Cinders" and "The Patsy" respectively.

non-speculative policy has perhaps lost us a great number of opportunities in the past. It was this policy that turned down the Criterion in Sydney when it was offered to us at 60,000 pounds. It was the same influence, with Ward dominating at the time, that tried to squelch the picture deal. If I had not taken the responsibility of the finance during the war period, JCW Ltd would have no interest in pictures at this moment.

Likewise the arrangements I made with McIntosh originally to take over the Tivoli at six per cent with nothing down were turned down by the Board and, as you know, this cost us dear later on. A couple of years ago the London Victoria Station picture scheme was also rejected and events have now shown that this would have been a great move for us. The Americans are willing to pay almost anything for theatres in which to show their films. If we do turn the London proposition down now in some form or another, in all probability in four or five years time we may be forced to take it under much more onerous terms.

The letter shows Tallis's difficulties in having his ideas accepted, and it confirms that a number of good opportunities were lost. Even back in the early days Williamson, known for his caution, eventually discovered that Tallis's advice was worth taking.

The mail had not all been one way. If success stems bickering, lack of it does just the reverse. During this period, Tallis received a string of letters from Ted Tait meting out blame for London losses and poor results in Australia, where theatre attendances were also down.

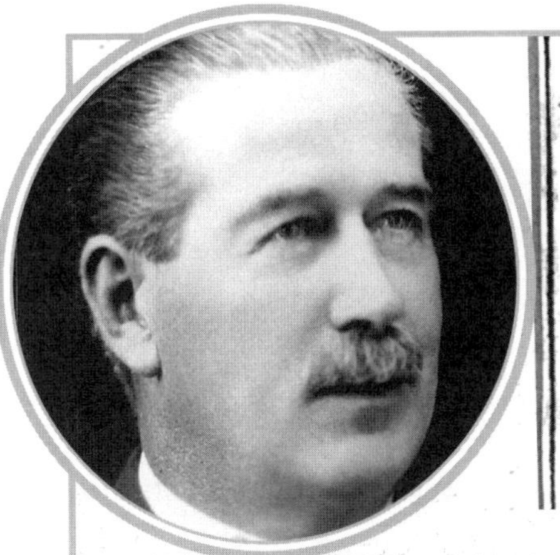

THE BEST MUSICAL SHOW FOR YEARS.

"MR. CINDERS" JUSTIFIES BRITISH PLAYS.

SPARKLING COMEDY.

TALLIS PLAY SUCCEEDS IN LONDON

"The Patsy" Well Received

(By Our Special Correspondent)

Daily Telegraph.
24. 12. 28.

ADELPHI THEATRE UNDER NEW MANAGEMENT.

Late on Saturday evening negotiations were brought to a point by which the Adelphi, following close upon the departure of Cicely Courtneidge and Jack Hulbert, will pass into the hands of Sir George Tallis, the leading spirit in the long-established firm of J. C.

PUBLIC STILL FLOCKING

THEATRE NEWS OF THE DAY.

"Back to Variety."

Concerning Cochran's New Revue—and a Noel Coward Opera : : : Sir George Tallis's Plans in London.

BY—
PHILIP PAGE.

Daily News.
21. 12. 28.

"MR. CINDERS."

LONDON STAGE CHANGES.

A NEW AUSTRALIAN ENTERPRISE.

A New London Management.

Once again, this week, "The Patsy" looked gloomy at the last rehearsal. Sir George Tallis was wondering if it would do for London. When the curtain fell on the first night at the Apollo, he knew he had such a success —Miss Ford had twenty curtain calls— that it strengthened his desire to become permanently a London producing manager.

I expect he will be buying "Mr. Cinders" before long, and that he will find it that London home which, in his opinion, it deserves so much that he considers it the best musical play he has seen for years.

Even *Mr Cinders* was caned, although the show still had months to run in London, and its initial poor profits were largely due to indecision at the Australian end.

As part of his analysis, Ted constructed a 'Year of Disgrace' list for 1929, and this contained all the London shows, and three of the local productions, including *Show Boat*. This was a musical play with the credentials of greatness: lyrics by Oscar Hammerstein II and PG Wodehouse, and music by Jerome Kern. It had been an enormous hit in America, but made heavy weather of the Australian season.

As profits were squeezed by a downturn in the industry, Ted's analyses may have simply reflected difficult times. Many more 'disgraceful' years lay ahead. Nevertheless he made much of his list, until he, too, was to become part of it after a failed attempt to gate-crash Broadway.

In September 1929, a few months after George had arrived home from his London trip, Ted sailed for America. He was met in New York by Nevin Tait, and they agreed that it was time to test American luck. The vehicle was the play *Jew Suss,* which was working well in London. A joint American–Australian production ensued.

The play opened brilliantly in Newark, which is close to New York in location and name. This greatly encouraged the syndicate. However, *Jew Suss* failed when it moved to the Erlanger Theatre in New York, and it failed again in Philadelphia some weeks later. It was officially declared deceased and, due to some strange customs regulations, the 'running gear' was unsaleable. Everything was burnt, and when the smoke cleared there were losses to explain. On this occasion George was the observer, and half a world away at that – not in America as reported by Viola Tait in *A Family of Brothers*.

It had been a very demanding few years for the management of the Firm. Everybody had worked hard to stage great theatrical events, but ultimately it was the sheer size of the business that caused stress, and frayed tempers. After nine years, disharmony was palpable on the Firm's board, which now consisted of Chairman of Directors George Tallis; Managing Directors Ted and Frank Tait; and Directors John Tait, Arthur Allen and Theodore Fink. This was in line with the history of the company. None of the Williamson partnerships had lasted for more than nine years, and the directorate since incorporation in 1910 had been bristling with personal conflict. It was all part and parcel of the impatience and ambition that inevitably come with the top theatre jobs.

When George returned to Australia in July 1929, the memories of the London venture were still fresh. The operation had been necessary, if only to test the feasibility of a long-mooted expansion. By theatrical standards it had been successful; it was just unfortunate that the patient had died.

Yet the fiasco had uncovered more worries. Apart from disagreements to be expected in the running of a giant business, flaws in the JCW Ltd management, which had been evident in a small way years earlier, were now flourishing. Indecisions and bloc voting were rendering the board itself almost non-functional, and it was now absurd to entertain any further ideas of new projects until these managerial problems had been fixed. George recognised that something most *definitely and positively* would have to be done.

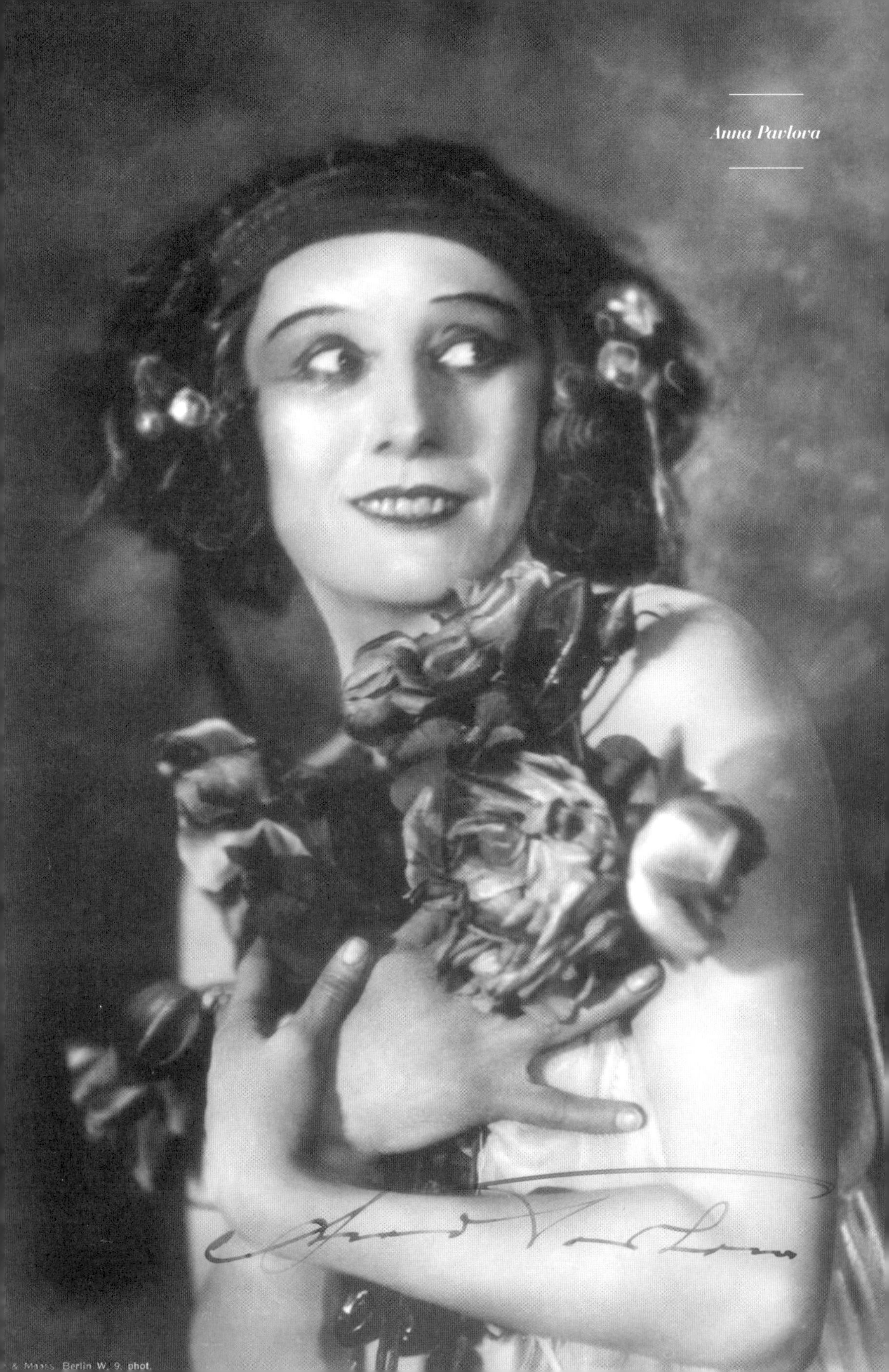

Anna Pavlova

CHAPTER SIXTEEN

Not So Firm

The radio telephone service between England and Australia first opened for business in late 1929, not quite in time to ease communication problems that developed during George Tallis's long overseas trip in 1928. Contacts needed restoring, and his return to Australia could not be delayed indefinitely. When he arrived in Fremantle on the *Narkunda* in late July 1929, he gave press interviews.[1]

In summary George said that he did not think the talkies would harm the legitimate stage. He reasoned that talking pictures were booming at the expense of theatre business because of the many artists they had absorbed from dramatic and musical circles. In the end, he mused, these people would return disillusioned and with new ideas. He felt sure that in this way the talkies would actually assist the theatre. The human appeal of the stage could not be equalled by anything else, he said, although many people in London were pessimistic about the future. Ruefully he reported that it had been a bad season in London – the worst for theatre in the last forty years. One pleasing factor he found was that the vacuum created by the exodus of live theatre artists to film production was being filled. The old musical comedy authors were gone, and there was now room for new theatre writers. He concluded that a transition period had been reached, and something novel in plays could be expected.

Tallis, as usual, took the train from Adelaide to Melbourne, where he was met by Ted Tait with sober tidings, and problems galore. The JCW Ltd vaudeville circuit had folded as patrons flocked to cinemas for their laughs. At the same time, the Great Depression had begun to bite. This was also the year when the company's interest in radio was terminated with the expiry of all A-class licences. All live theatre attendances were down as talkies caught on, and there were specific complaints about the legitimate theatre itself. Generally, theatres had become old and tatty and they did not compare favourably with the plush comfort of the new picture palaces owned by Hoyts and Union Theatres. In addition, there were rumblings of discontent about the number of revivals JCW Ltd was staging, as well as fading production standards.

An article in *Smith's Weekly* in 1931 addressed the question of theatre comfort, pointing out that there was more to increasing theatre attendances than 'play construction'. The writer had abandoned the talkies for some 'flesh and blood' entertainment, but he greatly missed his cinema comforts. He noted that some cheaper theatre seats had an obstructed view of the stage, and that the shabby carpets, tired decor and listless ushers added to an impression of decay. He concluded: 'Would talkie-fans patronise these badly ventilated theatres, enduring extreme cold in winter and unbearable heat in summer? They would not!'[2]

It seems that Tallis and the Taits might have been too busy painting the big picture to notice that the frame was cracking. The result was that the Firm's theatrical producers, who had been run off their feet, were letting standards slip. The heavy use of theatres during the frantic days of the mid-twenties took its toll on the buildings themselves and they became dilapidated at the very worst time.

In 1929, other prime detractors from profits were the Victorian and New South Wales state taxes, which were crippling the theatre business – double taxation. The Commonwealth took its dues, and then the states put out their hand. Here was something else to use up nervous energy; one more force chipping away at the foundations of Williamson's. By mid-1930, Arthur Allen was moved to write in his diary: 'Business at the present moment is very bad. It is the same with pictures and everything else.' In November, George was visiting Sydney for the umpteenth time that year, and Arthur noted that 'he is very low and depressed about theatrical affairs.'[3]

A giant economic downturn was affecting the country. The American stock market crash of October 1929 sent shock waves around the world. It ushered in the Great Depression, which lasted in one form or another for a decade. In Australia the effect was immediate, and as the crisis deepened the Bank of England's Sir Otto Neimeyer was appointed a consultant to the Australian government. He told Australia that it needed to make sacrifices to cut foreign debt and that 'there was not enough pessimism in the country'. It would have been better, he said, if 'Don Bradman and Co. had lost the last Test cricket match [against England]'.

Don Bradman was a record-breaking member of the 1930 Australian Test side that toured England. He left a reputation behind for all to consider – Sir Otto was certainly giving it some thought. But despite the Bradman euphoria, long-term interest rates halved, industrial activity faltered, stock market values fell up to fifty per cent and businesses closed. Unemployment exceeded twenty-five per cent of the work-force, and population growth slowed. Forty-five years on from George Tallis's arrival, the streets were no longer paved with gold.

Hordes of men roamed from town to town seeking work, living on rabbit stew and scrounged vegetables. At night, they formed make-shift camps, where they exchanged campfire yarns before moving on. No way could they afford a theatre or cinema ticket.

For others without work, there were large public demonstrations. The crowds were demanding an increase in the 'susso', the sustenance

To dear Mr & Mrs Tallis
with my love
Dorothy Brunton

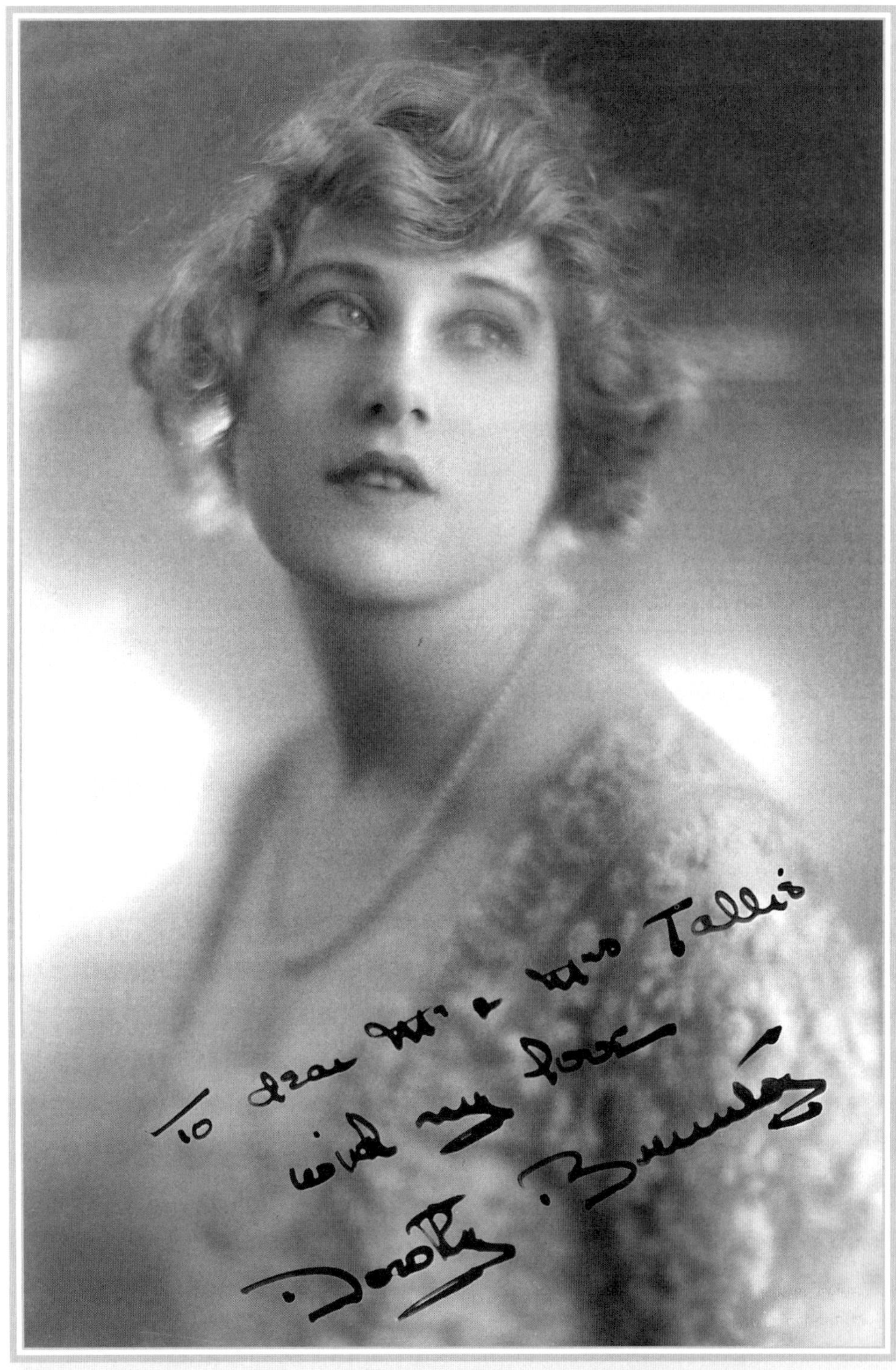

Dorothy Brunton – musical comedy star of the 1920s and 1930s

allowance for the unemployed. Nothing had been effective. Despite subsidised bread, soup kitchens and food depots, there was rising malnutrition in the community.

People grasped for inspiration, and along with Bradman the Depression era brought with it other heroes. The names of Australians Charles Kingsford Smith and Charles Ulm – the first to fly from America to Australia – and Bert Hinkler – the first to fly solo England to Australia – were on everyone's lips, and there were gala theatrical performances in their honour. These exploits heralded serious commercial aviation.

There were many sad occasions. Dame Nellie Melba died in Sydney on 23 February 1931 aged sixty-nine. A funeral train moved her from Sydney to Melbourne, and thousands of mourners at crowded country stations along the route paid homage to the great star. In June, Nellie Stewart died at the age of seventy-two. Affectionately known as 'Sweet Nell', she was one of Australia's most popular stage stars. This was not a good time to be losing theatre favourites.

Stresses of the depression were felt by George's daughter, Biddy, who wrote late in her life:

On my return to Australia in 1931 I became more interested than ever in the theatre and stage. My first opportunity came with the musical Florodora, *starring Dorothy Brunton. Some friends and I took part in the chorus. This was during the depression years, when we were lucky to have three people as audience. We were paid two pounds ten shillings per week, and the catchy number 'Tell me Pretty Maiden' was our specialty. Mother sat well forward in our theatre box proudly while Father sat well back and without comment.*

When I started to rehearse with Leo Franklyn in The Merry Widow, *I inadvertently took somebody else's place. Members of the cast showed their disapproval by spiking my make-up with powdered glass. I did not realise that I was keeping someone else out of a job in those difficult times. When news of this reached my father, he firmly put his foot down and ended [my] theatrical career forever.*

George was somewhat over-protective of his children, and dissuaded them from joining the theatre. In the 1930s this may have been due to his assessment that the trade would be down, and possibly out, for a long period into the future, and that the young would have better lives elsewhere. Or it may simply have been a result of his own career which, stripped of its glitter, had entailed long hours and little family life.

Tallis saw a lot of Arthur Allen during these turbulent days. Millie was in London with the two unmarried children and George spent weeks at a time in Sydney on business. In his diary Allen portrayed a friendship that whiled away weekends and evenings with luncheons, dinners, theatre visits and motoring trips. George was 'delighted' with everything. He particularly enjoyed some very happy hours with the artist and *bon vivant* Norman Lindsay, and was impressed by his art and conversation.

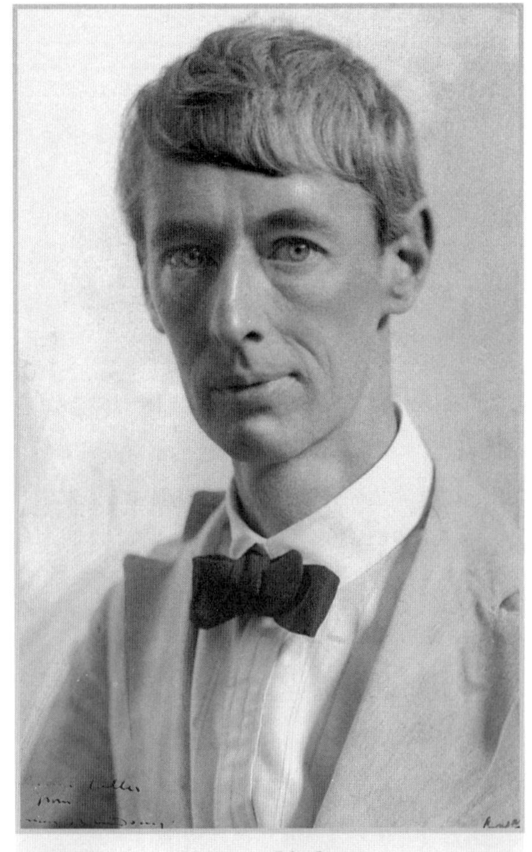

Norman Lindsay

But George and Arthur knew that they were sheltering in the eye of the hurricane.

If the depression affected the whole of Australia's economic and social structure, it devastated the live theatre industry. In 1929 there were ten live theatres operating in Sydney. By 1930, there were only three. For Melbourne, eight theatres also became three. This was not a uniquely Australian experience. It was the same on Broadway, where the demand for theatres peaked in 1928, never to be equalled in later years.

Representing JCW Ltd, George Tallis announced stringencies: activities were to be halved, the Melbourne Theatre Royal was to be sold and the refurbishing of Melbourne's His Majesty's Theatre, owned by the Firm and badly damaged by fire in 1929, was postponed indefinitely.

What ignoble changes were afoot! The old Melbourne Royal became a drapery store in 1933, and Her Majesty's Theatre Sydney vanished in the same year. Demolished, its site was absorbed by the Woolworths chain. The Sydney Criterion lasted until 1935 when a performance of *The Patsy* closed its doors for the last time. Half the site became an expansion of a roadway, and the other half the Criterion Hotel. The Theatre Royal remained the only JCW Ltd theatre in Sydney; it was still owned by the Ramaciotti family.

The King's Theatre, Melbourne, jolted along until 1941, when its lease terminated. A refurbished His Majesty's in Melbourne eventually reopened in July 1934, and Melbourne's Comedy Theatre remained part of the JCW Ltd theatre portfolio long into the evening of the company's history.

Asked about the depression and its effect on his company, George told the Melbourne *Age* in 1931:

It is true that, like all amusement organisations throughout the world, we have suffered severely during the past two years, and in the very lean period we have been passing through recently, our very strength proved to be our weakness. Instead of running fourteen or fifteen companies throughout Australia and New Zealand, as in the past, today we have been required to restrict our operation to three or four organisations at the most. Thus we are obliged to keep more than half of our theatres closed in the various states with disastrous financial results. But I have been through financial depressions and lean periods before, and we have always survived them, as we shall survive the present one. I think the theatres were, if anything, more severely hit in the boom smash of the nineties than at present.[4]

As a concession to morale, George failed to elaborate that in the 1890s there were fewer conflicting dynamics working to change the very concept of entertainment. In 1931, live theatre was competing not only with the Great Depression, but with the talkies and radio as well. There was even news of a brand new medium, television, which the *Washington Evening News* had reported as early as 1925:

By 1935, or perhaps sooner, any public spectacle will be visible to persons without leaving home, as a result of the recent success in radio vision experiments. Broadcasting motion pictures will be the next outstanding advance of wireless communication.[5]

Tallis encouraged the Firm to cut its losses and wind back activities to market demand. Nevertheless, faced with empty theatres – leased and owned – a large staff, and hungry shareholders, the spectre of liquidation was ever-present.

To further reduce costs, the Firm relied on revivals of old plays, and it all but eliminated imports. In time the company developed its main live theatre business around musical comedies, because that was what the people wanted. JC Williamson would surely have applauded that.

The troubles at the Firm raged on well into the future. Should the remaining Williamson theatres be converted to cinemas as a result of the downturn in the popularity of stage productions? This vexed question was just one of many examined by the board. The cost alone of converting theatres to a class of cinema that would compare favourably with the plush picture palaces was enough to scuttle the idea as a general solution. Practically none of the Williamson theatres was sufficiently modern to be a serious candidate. In particular Her Majesty's, the Williamson flagship in Sydney, had a style of architecture and decor that would be intolerable to cinema goers. The forest of structural posts blocked views of a central screen, and refurbishment was out of the question.

And there were other immediate financial headaches besetting the Firm: live theatre overhead expenses that JCW Ltd could not avoid. The company would have to honour outstanding contracts with star actors. This meant negotiating releases from existing arrangements, or else a blind adherence to old schedules in the hope that Lady Luck was looking.

Also on the books was the cost of owning expensive options and performing rights to theatrical pieces. This was a legacy of the company's policy. The Firm invested heavily in rights to 'stage futures' on a regular basis, and it had an agent in each of London and New York keeping its portfolio of shows on-hand up-to-date.

The depression played no favourites. It took its toll on the movie industry as it did on every business. Among movie fans, some did not even have money for food, and their Saturday night at the local cinema went on hold. Belt-tightening was everywhere. Yet these problems did not prevent the giant American company Fox Film Corporation from expanding its interests in Australia. Fox had control of 1100 cinemas in America and 350 in England, and it made a play for Hoyts Theatres Ltd. The upshot of this was that, in 1930, the syndicate headed by Tallis sold most of its 'second-class' shares to Fox. The other investors sold Fox their entire holding.

The total made a tidy sum, between 1.3 and 1.4 million shares, thus putting Fox in control of the Hoyts company. This was a good move for Tallis and partners. By retaining only their 'first-class' preference shares, they greatly reduced their risk profile in the company at a very volatile period.

This step marked the end of the Tallis–Thring partnership. Frank

Thring took a greater interest in film production until he died in 1936 at the age of fifty-three. He left a wife, a daughter by his first marriage and a son, Frank Thring, by his second marriage. His daughter married theatrical entrepreneur Tom Holt, and one of Holt's sons by the previous marriage, Harold, became Prime Minister of Australia. Frank Thring junior achieved world fame as an actor.

If Tallis and his partners cut their losses with cinema investments, radio was a different story. The board of the Dominion Broadcasting Company Ltd (chairman George Tallis), controller of 3LO, 3AR and other stations across the country, had tried to satisfy government demands for leadership in the developing wireless industry, but their efforts were ignored. As A-class licences expired, they were not renewed when pressure built within the Postmaster-General's Department, under the leadership of HP Brown, to nationalise all the A-class stations. Not everyone agreed with this idea, and one country listener voiced the concerns of many:

The wireless is a great asset to country listeners, but I doubt if the licences of many would be renewed if a professor of music was directing the broadcast . . . We people do not like so called classical music, as we are not trained for it. How many are?[6]

But the necessary bill passed in parliament in May 1932, sealing forever the fate of the A-class radio stations. Ownership of them passed to the Australian Broadcasting Commission, the ABC, which was to be governed by five commissioners. The prime brief of the new commission was to provide 'adequate and comprehensive' programs, and to foster local talent. It had some broad powers of autonomy, although the Postmaster-General had the ultimate power of censorship.

There was great speculation about who the first five commissioners would be. More than 150 people expressed interest in the position of chairman, including the writer AB (Banjo) Paterson. Two days before the official announcement, the press listed George Tallis as among the five most likely to be approached.[7] The aim of the Ministry was 'to combine literary, artistic, and business interests so that all sections of the community may be represented'.

The public received the final appointees with scepticism. Not a showman was among them, and the political inclinations of the group were the subject of debate. Tallis may well have provided some earthy balance from his unrivalled experience in entertaining the people with theatre, film and radio. He had grass-roots business experience where it mattered. He was also popular, apolitical and unavailable.

Tallis was actually in England while all this was going on, and he remained there for eighteen months. He had retired late in 1931. To break forty-five years of continuous theatre, film and radio involvement, his best trick was to vanish, and he did!

Under Tallis's chairmanship, the Dominion Broadcasting Company had established the most successful broadcasting system in Australia, and had set standards for those who followed. The early story of 3LO, 3AR *et al* is similar to the story of JC Williamson's development of his enormous theatre company. Williamson had based his reputation on quality, as had the Dominion group, and it proved to be a magic formula.

Furthermore, it seems that the Prime Minister, Stanley Bruce, had agreed in private discussions to reward the Broadcasting Company of Australia by renewing its A-class licences for a further period of five years. When the government later refused outright to honour the promise as the licences fell due in 1928–1929, a claim of £60,000 was lodged against it. This move produced only a small *ex gratia* settlement.

HP Brown was a 'bowler-hatted engineer'[8] whose background had been with the British Post Office. It was said that he knew better than anybody else how things went 'at home', and therefore his agenda was to steer the government towards an Australian version of the British Broadcasting Corporation. This was despite opposing messages from the Australian Prime Minister. The political climate of the day successfully stifled private enterprise in broadcasting and the survival prospects of the Dominion Broadcasting Company can be summarised by a popular play on the name of one of its partners, the Buckley and Nunn department store:

They had not even Buckley's chance,
No chance whatever! Nunn.

Bill Bearup, the 3LO program manager, recalled that Tallis had once said about radio: 'We came into this thing not because we wanted to, but because we were afraid not to be in it.'[9] What Irish nonsense! In spite of the disappointments, there was no way in the world George would have missed all that fun.

In 1926 George Tallis could boast to the newspapers:

Unlike other managements in England and America, the firm of JC Williamson Ltd is practically self-contained in all departments. Thus the entire productions are prepared from beginning to end in their own workrooms. It maintains a big staff of scenic artists, both in Sydney and Melbourne, and its wardrobe and property departments are the most extensive in the world.[10]

By 1930 such sentiments were reason for lament. 'Our very strength proved to be our weakness,' George said to the Melbourne *Age* in 1931. Indeed.

In its core live theatre business, the Firm was carefully 'vertically integrated'. It owned theatres outright and in partnership, and it held leases on the rest of its theatres. By means of a clutch of departments, the company took care of all the needs of even the biggest theatrical productions including scenery, lighting, costuming, directing, and producing. Managing directors made regular overseas trips to snare the best plays and musicals on the international markets, and to attract specialist touring companies for the Williamson circuit. A whole department arranged the touring schedules, and extended seasons to country centres and New Zealand. In short, apart from the writing and composing of the productions – and it sometimes did that as well – the Firm handled shows 'from cradle to grave' as it conducted its massive theatrical enterprise.

This great concern was designed to withstand moderate economic downturns. In the 1929 depression, however, all the negatives came at once. A total collapse in world economies synchronised with a swing away from live theatre to talkies. At the same time, patrons noticed just how drab and uncomfortable the live theatres themselves had become. To add to the woes, during the previous decade expansion had been a principal boardroom theme, a dangerous initiative given the impending crash. As a result the Firm's young vaudeville venture failed and the company was wrong-footed when it attempted to extend its activities to London. Last, and certainly not least, the Australian government knocked out one of the main JCW Ltd props by failing to renew its A-class broadcasting licences. Add some squabbling in the boardroom, and no wonder the company reeled and bit the dust.

All the positive strength translated into inflexibility, even inertia. When demand for live theatre evaporated, the Firm had a circuit of houses it could not fill, lease or sell. There was overstaffing, and expensive new plays were gathering cobwebs. The old adage of 'the bigger they are the harder they fall' certainly applied to JCW Ltd.

The original JC Williamson model of the complete theatre company providing total and continuous entertainment was now a dinosaur; a relic of a past age, standing before a Jurassic wilderness of sparse and mutated theatre opportunity. There were no quick fixes. The party was over.

George starting to feel his age

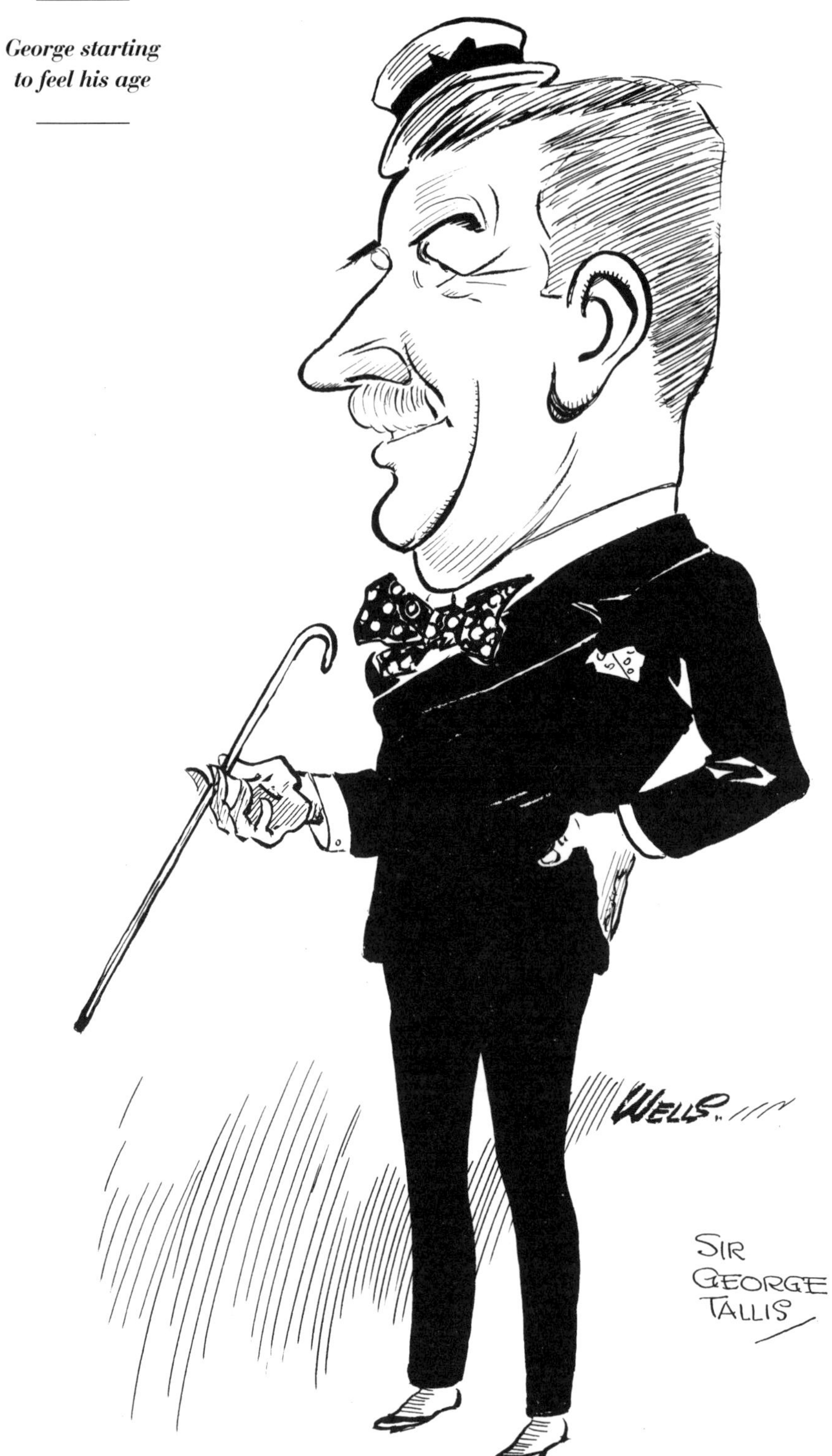

CHAPTER SEVENTEEN

Too Many Cooks

When you are approaching sixty-two and feel eighty-two, it is time to consider your options. In 1931 George Tallis's doctor considered them for him, and told him to take a long rest. Was it time to exit?

No matter what was to happen to the Firm in the future, the golden days of live theatre were obviously gone. George knew that competition from other media would supersede stage shows. Films and radio, once vital supports to the Firm's finances, were now largely in the hands of specialists. The pioneering days of these two media were also past.

The problems with the JCW Ltd board remained. These could no longer be overcome with friendly chats. Tallis realised that he had been overseas for nearly a quarter of the previous twelve years. During his absences Ted Tait had become used to assuming control of the company. At press interviews Ted already described himself as the 'Chief' of the Firm.[1] Perhaps George had flashbacks to 1912 when Hugh Ward did the same to JC Williamson.

Pondering his possible retirement and one last attempt to rationalise the board he set out his thoughts in a letter to Arthur Allen in August 1931:

So far as I am concerned, if I do continue with the company, I certainly would do so only under one condition and that is that the Managing Directors should be limited to two instead of four as at present. The old axiom that 'too many cooks spoil the broth' still holds good, and it is practically impossible under the present conditions to arrive at any definite decision on a point of policy or otherwise.

Important matters requiring immediate decision are referred over to Ted, back again to Frank, then John – each has different ideas, and the original idea is torn to pieces and lost in the process. In the meantime, the business of the Firm is suffering.

Where an immediate decision is required it is often difficult enough to get unanimity from two individuals; but it is almost impossible to get it from four, all pulling in different directions.

George had put it in a nutshell. He delivered his ultimatum to the Taits and this time received an immediate response. It was, predictably, negative. Tallis relinquished his position as chairman of directors, and retired as a managing director on 13 November that year, forty-five years after he had joined the Firm in 1886. The resignation immediately reduced the number of managing directors from four to three, and removed George from managerial decisions affecting the future of the company. In that sense, he and all the shareholders were in the hands of the Taits, although at no stage did the Taits ever control the company financially in their own right: George Tallis and Arthur Allen each led a syndicate owning about 100,000 shares, giving the two groups a combined fifty-three per cent holding in JCW Ltd. This situation dated back to 1927, when the Taits turned down the Hugh Ward parcel of shares, allowing Allen to buy them instead.

On 13 November 1931, most newspapers carried articles saying that: 'Sir George, acting on the urgent advice of his doctor, has announced his retirement as chairman of directors of JC Williamson Ltd after forty-five years with the Firm'. At that time, Tallis wrote an interesting article for the Melbourne *Herald* in which he reflected on theatre's changing fortunes:

Forty-five years represents a long association with the theatre; and now, when I am about to sever my connection with the Directorate of 'The Firm,' I look back and there comes before my mind a varied pageant of theatrical folk, scenes and times.

There have been years of change and progress, and today life's passing show, now under the shadow of crisis, finds reflection in the theatre. Present difficulties are calling for a new era on both sides of the footlights; but, just as there is a way out of the depression for the people, so there is one for the stage.

Apart from the natural consequences of the depression, the theatre has been recently up against two obstacles. First, there has been the dearth of good plays. That may seem surprising, but when you look into it it does really seem that the brains of the world's playwrights have dried up! Unquestionably, we are in the creative doldrums at present.

The coming of the talkies, with new standards of luxury for cinema palaces, was the second challenge. They were novel, and they housed themselves in new buildings that made lavish attractions. Most of our playhouses have been built for years.

As for the charm of the new talkie entertainment, I believe that the films are now undermining the once formidable position they held. The system of 'blind booking', by which exhibitors [Hoyts and Union Theatres] must contract to take the whole of a producing corporation's [Paramount, Fox and Metro] output, irrespective of quality, is a bad principle for any business.

If we had worked on those lines, 'The Firm' would have been out of business 20 years ago. Actually, I think the cinema is helping a reaction of public taste towards the stage. You cannot, I feel sure, kill the flesh and blood theatre. There will always be a place in the hearts of the people for the living stage.

And the return of the theatre? There is a clue to that, by the way, in a most successful recent film. When I saw Viennese Nights *I was convinced that the secret of its popularity lay in the fact that Rhomberg had written three or four truly delightful melodies for the film, and to the appeal of these the public instantly responded.*

That is the type of musical play we want again from our lyricists for the legitimate stage. Their advent will do more to revive the theatre than all the nostrums put together. They used to supply the need, and will do so again.

All the same, the stage has its lessons to learn; it is coming back, in a chastened way,. to the conditions of 25 years ago – and that is exactly what Australia in general must do. The theatre will move with the times, and we shall have tuneful music in our musical shows, and still the glamour, and the glorious, irreplaceable charm of a living art. And no doubt there will still be endless funds of theatre stories for my successors to tell!

As you can imagine, a great store of memories remains from these forty-five years of my work with J.C. Williamson Ltd. Strenuous work it was; but I don't think I would have chosen otherwise – although my first intention, when I came to Australia as a youth from Ireland, was to be a journalist. I had some training in that career in the Old Country. Fate put me in touch with J.C. Williamson when I arrived here, and, well – here I am!

Forty-five years makes a canvas crowded with memories of men, women and events, and of a public taste in entertainment which, after all, has changed but little. Perhaps Australian audiences have been spoilt in late years, and it is now a little more difficult to tickle their theatrical palate. They haven't had the task of the manager who goes overseas and sits through, perhaps, a hundred plays before he selects three or four to bring back with him.

I have had twelve months directing London theatres, and I can say unhesitatingly that our Australian stage staff (mechanists, property men, electricians, etc.) are immeasurably superior in every way to the best staff in any London theatre. I have often been amazed at the uncanny resourcefulness of our property men especially. There seems to be nothing that they cannot do or make.

Our Australian chorus and ballet are also far ahead of the best English chorus that I have ever seen. They are more virile, more intelligent, better dancers, and, needless to say, they have much better voices.

On the business side of a long association with the theatre, the manager must look back with regret to the possibilities of other days. About this time of year he thinks of pantomimes. Our biggest pantomime production, and the greatest money-making success, was the Mother Goose *show that we put on at the Princess about 30 years ago.*

It was a splendid show. The book, scenery, costumes, 'props', rehearsal fees, and the hundred and one expenses that must be paid out before the curtain rises, cost us £2000. Fifteen years later the same preliminary charges had risen to £15,000. The result of these rises was that the Firm had to curtail its pantomime activities.

The cost of all other productions rose in approximately the same ratio. Before the curtain goes up on the first scene of a comic opera nowadays the producing firm has expended anything from £7000 to £15,000. Costumes comprise the main item. They may be worth £5000 or £6000. Nowadays about 95 per cent of the dresses are made in Australia, but in the old days nearly all were imported from London and Berlin. Then there are publicity, rehearsals, theatre charges, printing, lighting, scene painting, labour – a host of activities set in motion and paid for before the fateful first night.

Competition used to be keen in securing the Australian production rights of notable overseas successes. We have had to pay as much as 11 and 12 per cent on the gross takings for some shows. We had one great advantage, from the start, in having the sole rights of the Gilbert and Sullivan operas, but there was some keen bidding in the theatrical market.

A new company is now being formed to play Autumn Crocus, The Barretts of Wimpole Street, *and* Mariegold *for production early in the New Year. Then there will be a fine musical piece,* Waltzes From Vienna, *which is now playing to big houses at the London Alhambra. We hope to follow these with other musical attractions from America. In addition there will be a season of grand opera, return of the Gilbert and Sullivan Company, and the production of* Blue Roses, *which will bring back our Australian favourites, Madge Elliott and Cyril Ritchard. The theatre, you see, is still very much alive. Recovery from the 'dark patch' which at present holds so many playwrights and lyricists will give a great impetus to brighter days in the Green Room.*[2]

On 4 January 1932, the board finally ratified some significant changes to accommodate George's retirement. He was stepping down as chairman of directors, and Charles Alfred Wenman, one of the Williamson producers, was to replace him as an ordinary director. Should Wenman ever retire, George could appoint another director, or rejoin the board himself as a director. As usual, for all this to take place it was mandatory that Tallis hold at least 15,000 ordinary shares. The other ordinary directors were Arthur Allen, Fred Smith and Sir Robert Wallace Best, who had replaced Theodore Fink. The three Tait brothers, Ted, Frank and John, were the managing directors of the new board.

A few days later George ran into his friend Judge Jo Wasley, who asked, 'Why are you retiring? A youngster like you needs a job. You'll miss all that theatre razzmatazz. What on earth are you going to do?'

George answered that he intended to do some travelling, a reply that annoyed the judge.

'We've had months upon months of delays in our golf, and the excuse you have given me is that you were either in London, or in New York or somewhere in between. Doesn't that count as travelling?'

George explained that he wanted to see Europe properly. 'England has one culture and America another, and the two blend. In Europe it is totally different; there you find dozens of completely different nations living side by side, and I want to see that for myself.'

There were times when Wasley found George difficult to fathom. From a standing start, Tallis had built castles; yet still he was restless. His *wanderlust* had already taken him around the globe many times. Was this appetite for travel just a part, and now a residue, of his theatre life, or was it a more fundamental need? Chillingly the answer dawned on Wasley. George was without a country. He had become a man of the world, and now it had claimed him. Because he was wise, Wasley asked no further questions.

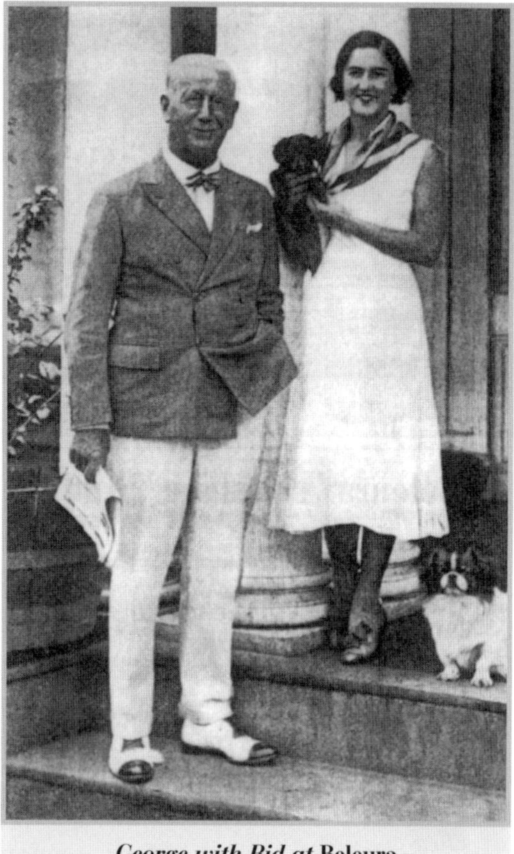

George with Bid at Beleura

In 1931 the Tallises moved from Melbourne. *Grosvenor,* the grand family home that stored so many artefacts and memories of better times, was closed. George and Millie leased it as a function centre, and its great ballroom started to pay its way. Its owner disappeared from the Melbourne business scene, and became hard to contact. Arthur Allen noted in his diary that 'it is very difficult to get him to take an interest in things now that he is retired'. In fact, George was at Mornington, farming.

At an earlier time, under the headline 'May cow him yet' one paper had reported:

Of all the men in Melbourne, well-groomed George Tallis looks about the least likely to spend time going round shows in order to prod bovine creatures of more than the usual ponderosity.

Yet it is one of his diversions, and at the Dandenong show yesterday, Tallis added a long list of successes as a breeder of Ayrshires by winning six of the prizes. He carried off a champion award for Ayrshire cow, champion for bull, and four firsts.

Presently, when he finds himself once again surrounded by stormy Italian prima donnas and tenors who want to slay the villainous baritones in real

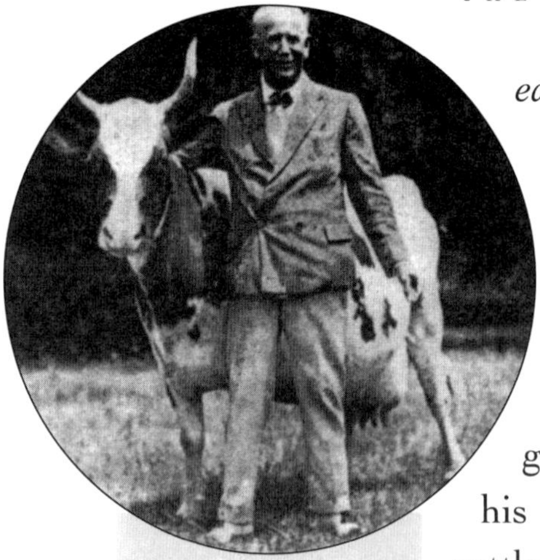

George with Beltana of Olive Dale

earnest, Tallis will no doubt wish that he could inoculate them with the 'germ of placidity' which is in the natural order of things among all decently raised Ayrshire milkers.

Somehow, George's prize bull, Starlight, missed his dose of the placidity germ. He disgraced the breed by lining up all his handlers and trying to fasten them to the cattle yards with his massive horns. His behaviour was no better in the paddock, where he built up impressive speed as he rushed to assist any moving target over the fence. Champion or not, when one day Starlight headed off to some unknown address in a butcher's truck, not a tear was shed by onlookers.

Close to the milking sheds and yards on the farm was George's orchard. He grew some of the finest apples on the Mornington Peninsula, and plenty of them. The orchard included seventy acres of trees bearing four main varieties of apple, which ripened in turn, allowing the pickers to keep pace with the maturing crops. George boxed and sent his best apples to his friends. Those who scored a box knew they had made the short list.

Add to George's dairy and orchard interests two thousand acres of grazing sheep and cattle and the breadth of his farming emerges. Nonetheless, it seems that he tired of his rural pursuits rather quickly, since he left for England late in April 1932. Tallis was as free as a bird – for six months. Then, in October, Arthur Allen cabled him about necessary adjustments to the JCW Ltd board. There were rumblings of disquiet among the Firm's preference shareholders, who were not receiving regular dividends. Some morale-boosting was needed. A surprise rabbit, perhaps? George came under increasing pressure to rejoin the board as the conjurer.

Board meetings of the time concentrated (again) on merger possibilities, and adjustments to managing director salaries. They were heavy weather. The ordinary directors resisted the rises claimed by the Taits, and insisted that any long-term agreements sought by the managing directors would cloud merger negotiations. The Taits argued that they did most of the work ... and so on *ad infinitum*.

As news of the boardroom roughhouses filtered through, George resolved to remain out of sight. He made good his promise to travel, and visited England, France, Holland, Belgium, Germany, Austria, Italy, the Scandinavian countries, Poland and Hungary. He was playing golf at the famous Gleneagles course in Scotland when he received the tragic news that Millie had died suddenly, at Mornington, on 9 August 1933. He returned on the first available ship, but it was not until 23 October that he disembarked at Port Melbourne. It was a foul day of extremes. Victoria turned on a blistering northerly wind, and the temperature was some sort of record for October.

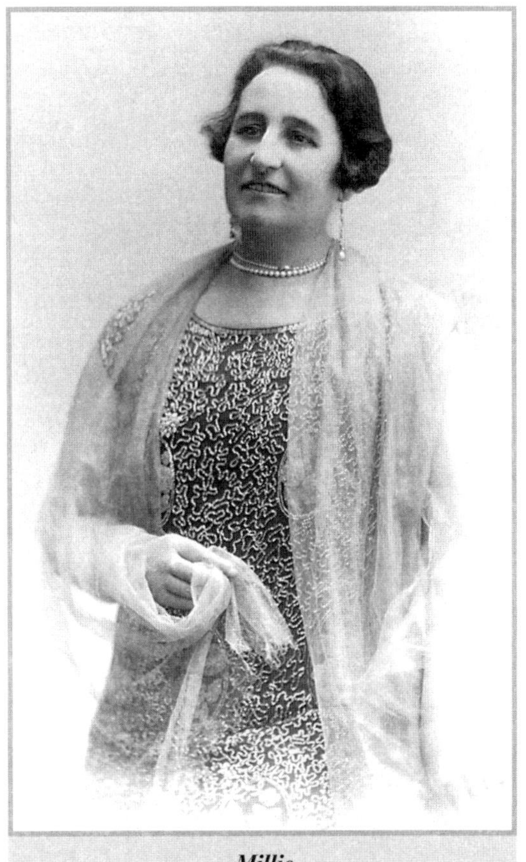

Millie

George was met by his family; at last they could mourn together their tremendous loss. Millie had cared for the children and managed the homes while George was absent, and she had been the central figure in the family. Now she was gone, and they were devastated.

The obituaries emphasised Millie's charming personality, which served her well in so many charitable works. She was a leading figure in the Blind Institute, the

Queen Victoria Hospital, the Ambulance Guild, the Anzac Club and many other organisations. She inaugurated the Grosvenor Auxiliary of St Vincent's Hospital. For 'Unselfish Service and Assistance Rendered' she received many citations, perhaps the most satisfying being the one of Honorary Life Governor of St Vincent's Hospital.

Millie was never happier than when she was entertaining her large circle of friends, or making visiting theatrical artists feel welcome. She was renowned for her wonderful parties, which were planned down to the last detail. She had led a full and happy life, and shared her husband's love of golf. They were members of Riversdale Golf Club, and in 1927 she had been elected the first Associate President of the Victoria Golf Club.

As he left the ship, George wearily faced the usual press interviews, but he had less to say about the theatre, preferring to remind the public of his retirement from active management. Then he slipped from view to rejoin his Ayrshires and apples.

About this time, vigilant Mornington residents would have seen truckloads of quality loam heading towards the Tallis house, *Beleura*. What was going on? The local sandy soil was certainly impoverished, but surely this was over-doing it!

The main action was at the front of the house. Trees were coming down, and a knot of sweaty, ill-tempered workmen removed the last traces of the residual stumps. An area the size of a tennis court was being prepared. Restraining boards appeared, levels were taken, and the men started to spread the tons of fresh loam. The final surface was smoothed and checked repeatedly for humps and dents.

'Perfect, mate. What in the hell are you going to do with it now?'

George, who had been taking a keen interest in the work, looked at the spokesman. 'Grow some grass,' he responded.

This irritated the man on the shovel, who was used to more direct conversations. 'Then bloody what?'

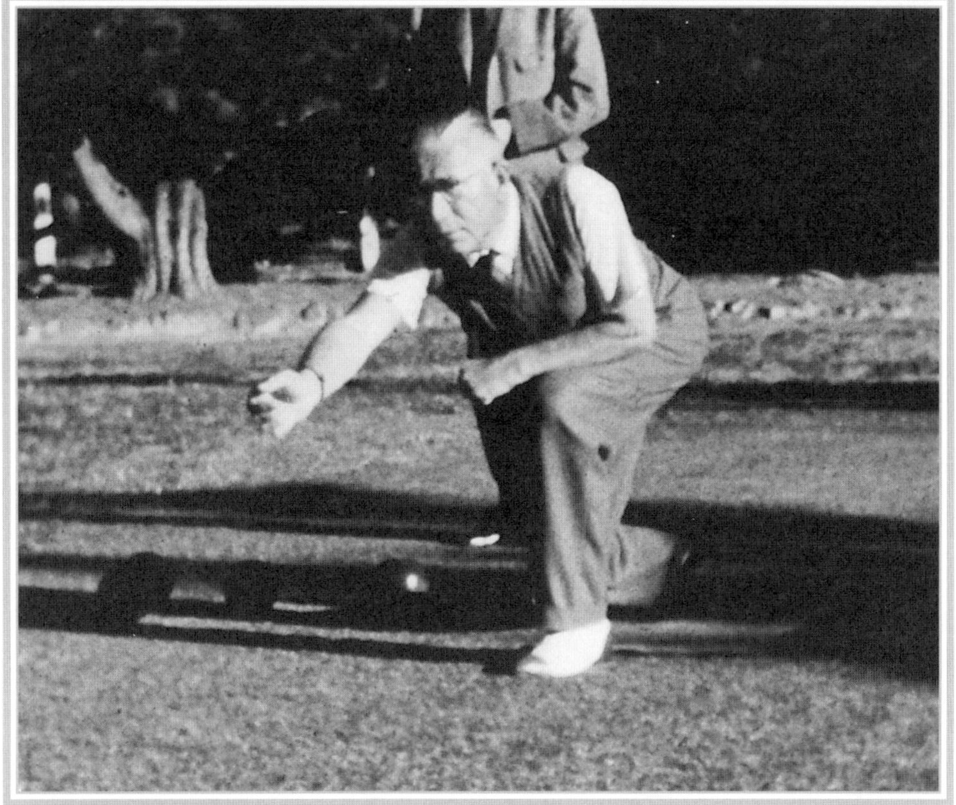

Bowling at Beleura

'Then,' said George, fixing his gaze on the man, 'we bloody well play bowls.'

To show his appreciation of a job well done, George ordered a keg of beer for the men. And that was how the inaugural party of the Beleura Bowling Club took place long before the grass arrived.

There they were, four old men dressed in white: white shoes, white trousers, white shirt, and any old blazer. They stood before the brand-new bowling green, each with a brand-new set of bowls. Judge Wasley told George to 'send down' the jack and to fire the first shot. A cheer for George. His bowl went six feet past the jack. Wasley was six feet short. Fred Smith was sixteen feet wide due to a misconception about the bias, and Fred Krcrouse was on the jack.

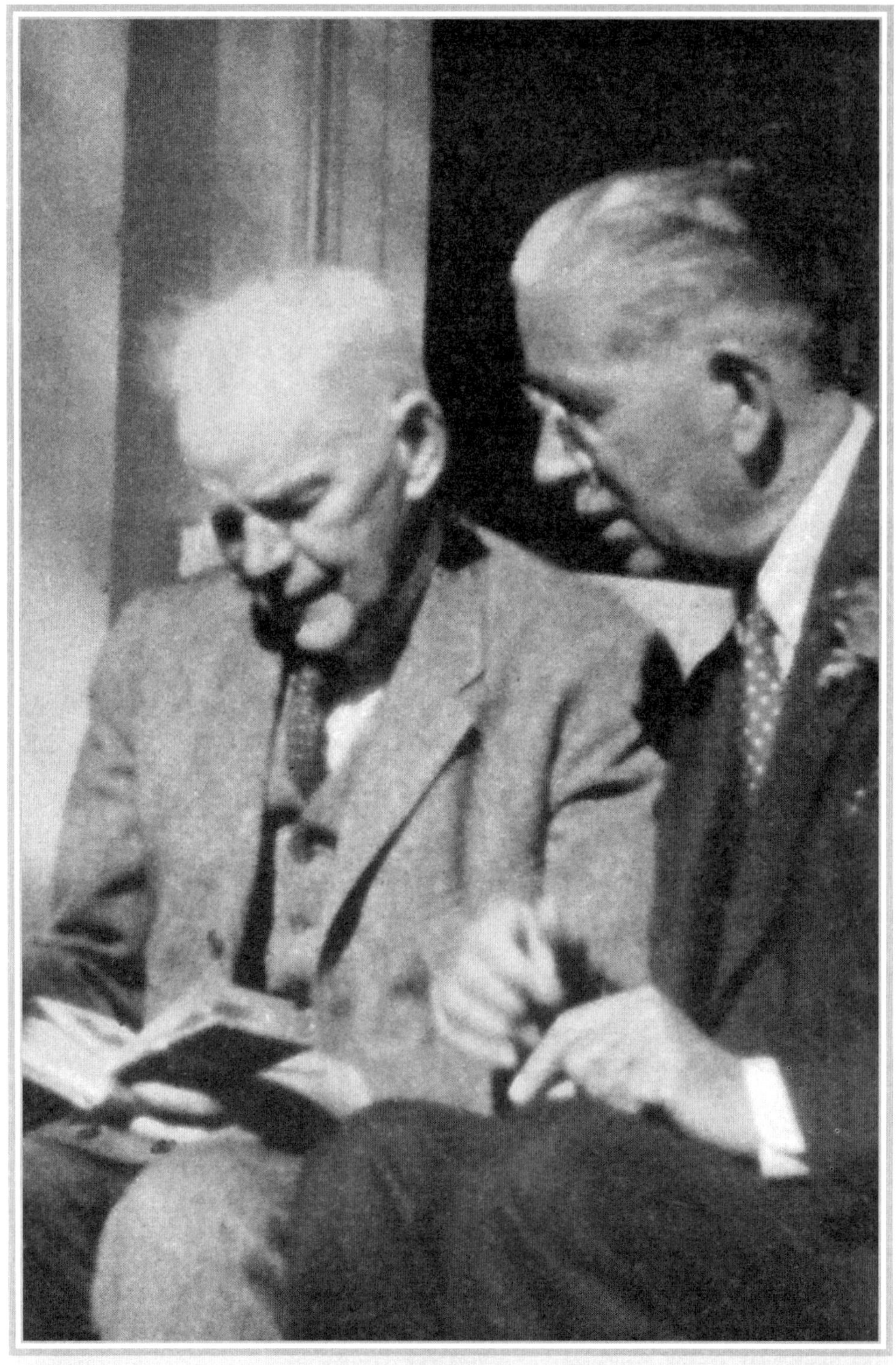

George with Judge Wasley

Krcrouse was the family solicitor, and he lived conveniently close to *Beleura*. He had married an actress well known to George and Millie, and was a lively source of theatre gossip. Smith was a JCW Ltd director and the company accountant. He often came down from Sydney on business. His health was bad, but he still had a competitive streak.

Wasley was the odd man out. He probed the others for theatre information, and somehow developed a source of his own. Krcrouse was the danger man on the new green, but when the cards came out in the evenings, or when rain ruined 'the track', Wasley was the one to beat. He picked up a pack of cards and had them dealt, and his hand sorted, while the others were still adjusting the score from the previous play. He memorised the cards, and at the end of the session could repeat every move.

One day Wasley said, 'I don't know why you don't play better bridge, George. You don't seem to try.'

'I keep forgetting the cards,' George mumbled, but Wasley would not let go.

'No you don't. You have one of the sharpest minds I have ever struck, and certainly the best memory. I think you just don't have the killer instinct.'

Bowling became an important part of George's life. The Beleura Bowling Club built up its membership, and hectic tournaments ensued. Good fellowship, friendly bowling, afternoon tea, dinner, bridge and reminiscences formed an agenda that suited the four crusty old professionals, who confronted their afflictions with humour and derived solace from the past.

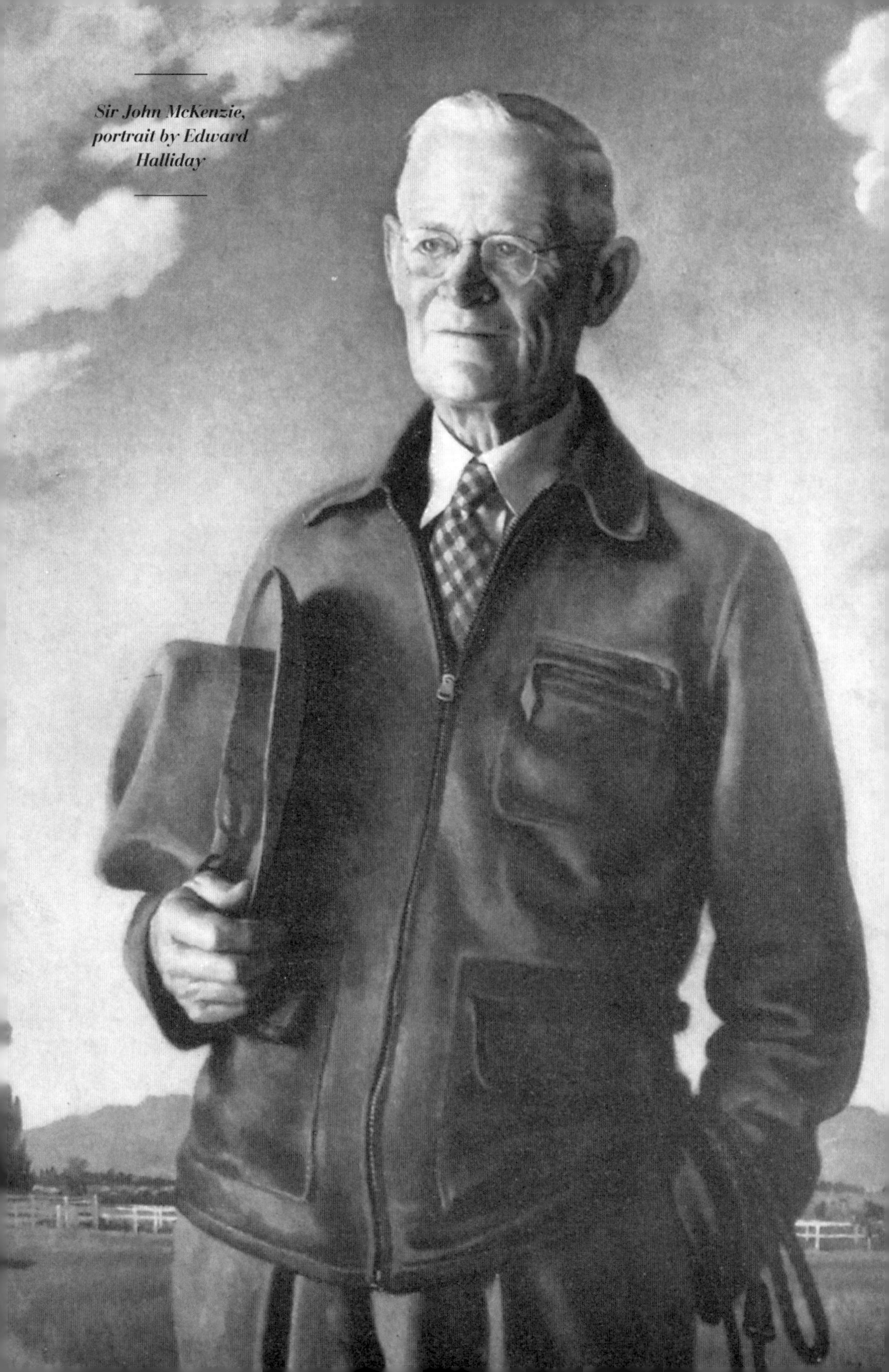

Sir John McKenzie, portrait by Edward Halliday

CHAPTER EIGHTEEN

Rangatira

Tallis was under increasing pressure from all sides to rejoin the JCW Ltd board. Charles Wenman, who had been keeping George's old seat occupied, stepped down in late December 1934, and George was slotted in as an ordinary director. He found very little change. Over the next month, Fred Smith and Sir Robert Anderson, a new director, created crises and threatened to resign. Only the persuasive powers of Arthur Allen coaxed them back from the brink. It was business as usual.

George's plans to rejoin the boardroom did not alter his travel arrangements. He was in England and Europe from June to December 1934, and part of the trip he shared with his two unmarried children Bid and Jack to celebrate his sixty-fifth birthday. There was a sudden split in the itinerary at Cannes when George elected to travel to Toulon by bus over a spectacular, but dangerous road known as the Grande Corniche. The other two voted for safety, and took the train. This was a decision of some merit, for the bus was wide open to the balmy breezes and spectacular vistas – canvas awnings were the only shelter from the elements. Somewhere along the Grande Corniche the weather turned nasty. A brutal storm tore away the awnings and ripped into the passengers. 'Experience of a lifetime' crowed the advertisement, and George had no reason to dispute it.

When he rejoined his travelling companions, they quickly decided that a tactful silence was the best way to discuss with their dishevelled father the marvels of the Grande Corniche.

Early in 1936, Tallis sold *Grosvenor*. Leased out for the previous four years, its number had come up. Most of the contents went under the hammer. George was changing his life by cutting the ties with the past. As *Grosvenor* was dismantled, all traces of his most successful era faded.

The sale was followed by a trip to America, and in addition to the usual boardroom dramas, when he returned, he struck one of Ted Tait's bad patches. All the Williamson senior staff knew that Ted needed a long rest, and they pressed John Tait to discuss the matter with him. This John refused to do. Ted's declining health, accompanied by bouts of irrationality, became a worry to all around him, and a big problem for the future.

Early in 1937, Sydney dominated George's business life. Even he was bored with the endless Melbourne–Sydney trips. Partly to relieve some of the travelling, he bought a 2300-acre grazing property near Wagga Wagga, New South Wales. Known as *Braehour*, it was on the banks of the Murrumbidgee River. For George it was a 'halfway house'.

This was real farming: drought, floods, fires and pests. Tallis thought that the local mail train to Sydney might prove novel, but after one trip the novelty had worn thin. The drive was really not so bad after all. But people looking for him in those days were often out of luck. If he was not supervising his Mornington estate, he was somewhere in New South Wales.

By mid-1937, most of the Williamson board had joined the Firm's accountants in believing that the best way out of the financial mess was to sell or lease out their theatres. The numbers men conducted feasibility studies and, although conflicting figures cluttered the boardroom table, they all supported this view. Word got around the business world, and the sharks started to circle.

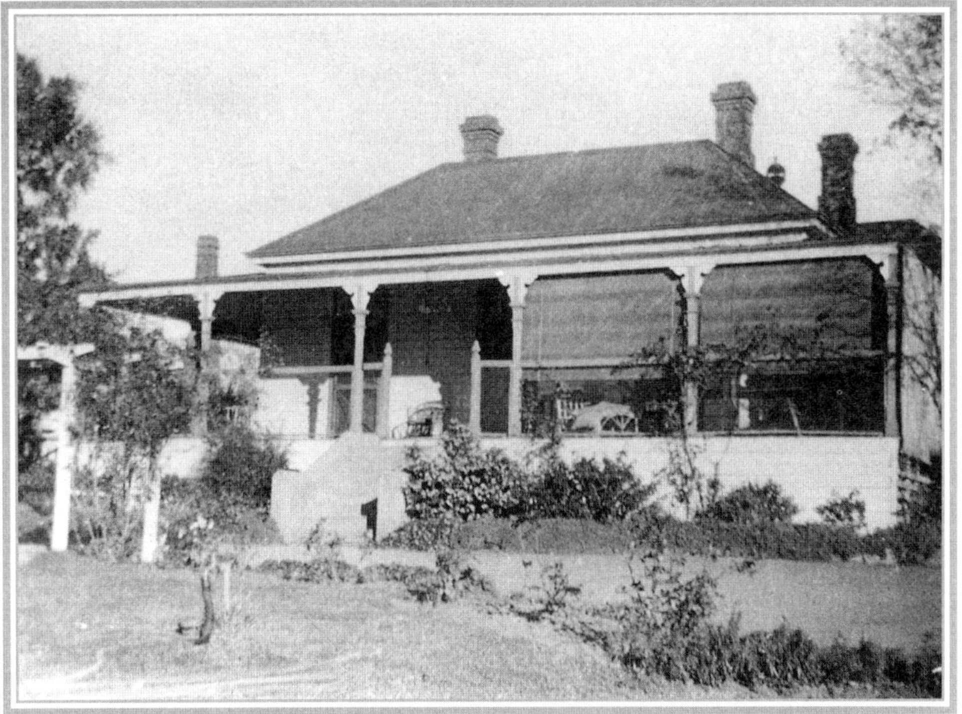

Braehour – *peaceful homestead on the banks of the Murrumbidgee River*

Ernest Rolls was a theatrical producer and entrepreneur who had experienced some mixed success. Originally Rolls Darewski, he was born in London and developed a flair for producing lavish revue-styled musical comedies. He was a showman, and he and his wife had presented successful productions for the Firm in the early thirties. His over-confidence and lavish staging, though, had often led to financial trouble. But in August 1937 he had a chat with Ted Tait in Sydney. Less than a few days later Ted headed for Melbourne to discuss with his brothers a preposterous nightmare. Rolls had mentioned something about gaining control of fifty per cent of the JCW Ltd ordinary shares. The idea was ridiculous! Wasn't it?

On 3 September, Rolls arrived in Arthur Allen's office and an impossible game started. The bookies would have had it at a hundred to one. Its details are complicated, but here we cling to the essentials required to give an official version of the affair.[1]

Arthur learnt about a syndicate consisting of Ernest Rolls and two newcomers, Eric Campbell and Hugh Chambers. They wanted a month's option to buy the controlling parcel of 200,000 ordinary shares held by George Tallis and himself at one pound per share. The syndicate's task was to locate a buyer. This was an interesting proposal to Arthur, as he and George wanted to retire and cash in their shares at a reasonable price. Moreover, a takeover might provide the necessary injection of capital and new blood the company needed so badly. The only problem was to find the right buyer, and a formula that would not jeopardise other directors or shareholders who were not part of the Tallis–Allen consortium.

On 15 September Allen wrote in his diary: 'Tallis is very keen to offer the shares to the Taits first.' He went on to write that a Mr Hill, from the Firm's accountants, Smith, Johnson and Co., had contacted the Taits and offered them the parcel at a pound a share. Arthur thought this a 'weak step' because he felt that, should the Taits take up the option, they probably would not proceed to purchase the shares, and in the process he and Tallis would lose valuable time and opportunity. Hill phoned later in the day to let Arthur know that John Tait was on his way to Sydney from Melbourne. Upon hearing this, George decided to wait until John's arrival 'as he wished to give the Taits the one chance of buying the shares'. But Tallis already knew what the response would be.

The following day, 16 September 1937, Arthur wrote in his diary that both John and Frank Tait were in Sydney. 'They said they would sell their own shares at 25/- but would not give GT or AWA more than 15/-.'

Clearly there had been a meeting between John, Frank and Ted, and they had decided not to treat the matter seriously. Nevertheless, Tallis and Allen reiterated their position and informed the brothers through Hill that there 'was nothing doing under one pound'. This provided a second opportunity for the Taits to take up the option, but they gave no response. Only then did the option go to Eric Campbell.

Tallis saw John and Frank Tait the following day, 17 September, when the two intimated that they did not believe that the Rolls–Campbell–Chambers syndicate was serious. On 21 September Eric Campbell gave the Taits a copy of the option signed by Tallis and Allen so that they could check that, as Allen wrote, 'we [Tallis and Allen] had tried to protect the other shareholders in every way'.

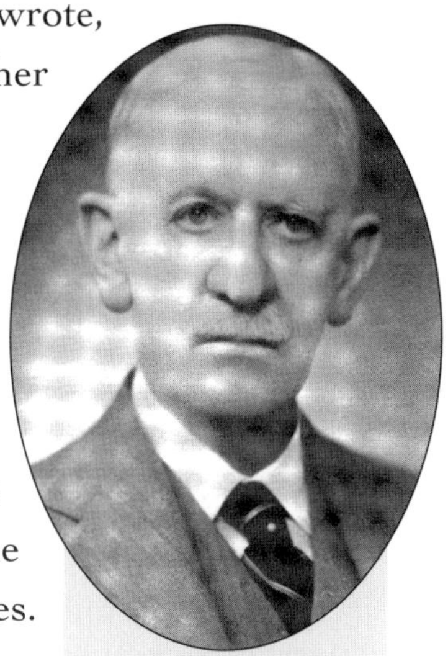

This version of the birth of the Tallis–Allen option, taken from the meticulously kept diary of the Firm's solicitor, can be compared with two other accounts: one by Viola Tait in *A Family of Brothers,* the other by Claude Kingston in *It Don't Seem a Day Too Much.* Both authors assert that the Taits were given no opportunity of taking up the option for the sale of the 200,000 Tallis–Allen shares. Kingston expands this issue in his book by developing a theatrical story, attributed to Ted Tait himself, that George had sold his shares as the final shot in a long-standing feud.

Arthur Allen

The real, and obvious, reason for the sale – Tallis and Allen wanted to retire – has already been given. However, as it turned out, not only was this the way forward for the intending retirees, but it seems that it was also the way forward for JCW Ltd and its managing directors.

The Firm had been staring an enormous shake-up in the face for over five years. The choices included liquidation, a complete takeover by another company, or a major sell-off of some of its asset portfolio, while keeping control of the production side of the business. A large injection of capital was needed, and at this stage, no progress towards a major rationalisation had been reached by the board. The company was coming under pressure from its shareholders who, starved of dividends, were demanding that something be done quickly.

With this background, what was the true attitude of the Taits to the Tallis–Allen option? Twice they were given 'first refusal', and the option was around for weeks afterwards looking for a buyer; plenty of time for second thoughts, and for forming their own syndicate if necessary. With the prospect of having to send good money after bad perhaps, after all, the brothers were happy to let others kick the Firm into gear. Or did the problem go deeper? In a later company internal memo, Arthur Allen wrote: 'Some days we are told that JH Tait is quite willing to sell his shares but that EJ Tait will not allow him to do so.'

Kenneth William Aspery was a Sydney solicitor, soon to become a senior partner in Baldick Aspery Co. Aspery had been supervising the deals of the Firm's New Zealand Picture Corporation Ltd, originally set up by George Tallis in 1923. Through his associations, Aspery heard of the Tallis–Allen option that the Rolls syndicate had been offering to the film giants Hoyts and Union Theatres in vain, and he thought he could sharpen the pace. In early November he took charge of the option. Exit Rolls, Campbell and Chambers.

Through the Aspery contacts, news of the Firm's plight hit the New Zealand grapevine, and came to the attention of expatriate Victorian, John McKenzie. McKenzie – later knighted – had started a chain of retail stores across New Zealand. He was a most successful businessman and also a great philanthropist. A linchpin of his charity work was his investment company, Rangatira, Maori for chief.

In 1937 Rangatira was in its infancy. It was managed by a group of clever business professionals, and they were seeking good investments. One of the directors, Ken Campbell, heard of the Allen and Tallis parcel of shares. Campbell was a particularly astute investor, with a background in real estate. Later he would earn the uniform respect of his Australian co-directors on the Firm's board.

The name of Williamson had lived on in New Zealand and ownership of the company could be good for Rangatira, if the price was right. Incidentally, it would also profit the Firm, as Sir Roy McKenzie,

Sir John McKenzie's son and for forty-nine years a director of Rangatira, much later pointed out in a letter to the authors:

As I recall, JCWs would have been forced into liquidation without the sale of these shares. It was quite a risky investment at the time, the value being in the property held.

Aspery produced £5000 to establish his *bona fides,* and he then raised with Tallis and Allen the main impediment to the sale of the shares. For the deal to proceed, Rangatira required that the Firm's business be split in two. One section would manage the theatres and other assets, and a second arm would take care of theatre productions. The prospective buyers were insisting that Tallis and Allen make a major financial commitment to the latter, in the order of a £15,000 share purchase each.

Details of the two new companies developed quickly. The asset management company retained the title JCW Ltd, and the new production company became Australian and New Zealand Theatres Ltd. After two shake-ups, and the retirement of Tallis and Allen, the final board structure of JCW Ltd was: Chairman of Directors John McKenzie; Managing Directors Ted Tait, John Tait and Frank Tait; Directors Robert Best, Ken Campbell, Harold Edwards and Alfred Duncan. The last three were Rangatira men.

On paper, the original board of Australian and New Zealand Theatres approved by Rangatira was a potent one. The chairman was Ken Aspery, and the managing directorship was Frank Tait, Stanley Crick and George Dean. George Tallis was included in the list of ordinary directors, along with Hugh Dennison and Arthur Allen. George and Arthur would have to put retirement on hold for the moment.

Ken Aspery was on his way to the New South Wales Bar and a position on the supreme court bench. Hugh Dennison had played a major role in the early development of radio in Australia. George had known him from the days of 1910, when the two were part of the pre-history of Amalgamated Wireless (Australasia) Ltd. Crick had been in the motion picture business for many years, and had become one of the most powerful movie moguls in the country. He had recently resigned a handful of directorships to prepare himself for the lord mayoralty of Sydney. Dean was also a film man, with plenty of experience. With the theatre know-how of George Tallis and Frank Tait also available, the future looked rosy for the production company.

All the wheeling and dealing finished on 3 June 1938. From start to finish it had taken more than nine months and it was only Aspery's rare powers of mediation that saw the deal complete. The Taits' agreement to the takeover arrangements was essential. Although there had been some tough negotiations, they kept their directorships and supported the managerial and financial shake-up that blew in with Rangatira.

All that remained of the old brigade on the board of JCW Ltd was Sir Robert Best, who was well into his eighties. The replacements, four hard-headed businessmen led by John McKenzie, injected a new air of discipline into the boardroom. It was certainly long overdue. For years the board had debated a much-needed reshaping of the company, but it was Rangatira that eventually made the Firm bite the bullet. And it was Rangatira that gave hope of a new era for the Firm, but not before some costly mistakes were made.

Australian and New Zealand Theatres took up leases of all the JCW Ltd theatres, and it rented from the asset management company all of the scenery, wardrobe and general 'running gear' at a total price of fifty to sixty thousand pounds per year. The managing directors announced 'big plans to bring to Australia world-famous plays, artists, concert and radio stars'—as if the firm had been out to lunch for the previous sixty years. Tallis and the Taits watched with hope, liberally tempered with misgivings.

In the wings waiting patiently for the smoke to clear was Ernest

Rolls. He and Charles Wenman were producers for the company, and Rolls went to New York and London to rustle up shows. On Crick's advice, Rolls had become a managing director and chief producer of Australian and New Zealand Theatres in mid-September 1938, largely on the strength of cables received about his performance in his home city of London.

This was all contrary to advice provided by George Tallis. He suggested that Rolls go to New York only, and that Wenman go to London. Alarmed at the expense of everything, Tallis asked that costs be reined in. Frank Tait was no fan of Rolls, and he added some warnings of his own. But Aspery, Crick and Dean rejected the advice. Before the end of the year, Tallis resigned from the board in disgust but retained his shares in the company. By January 1939 Rangatira was on the march. Harold Edwards and Ken Campbell, the New Zealand trouble-shooters, arrived in Sydney. They had heard some silly rumours about losses.

As it happened, the rumours turned out to be conservative. In the space of nine months the managing directors of the new production company had dispatched £60,000 of company funds, and no one was sure which way the money had gone. Somebody needed firing; so they fired Rolls, just as he was leaving. His lavish ways with productions, mixed with some bad luck, had got in the way of a shareholder's party again, and in April 1939 he suddenly remembered an urgent appointment in London.

Anger continued to spill over. Frank Tait came in for a caning from Aspery for not containing losses. Tallis was castigated by Harold Edwards for his lack of leadership and for his bad sportsmanship in resigning from the board. George pointed out that he was rising seventy and had been attempting to retire from everything for the past six years. In addition, he had tried to help by giving cost-saving advice, but had been ignored. Only then did Crick and Dean start to see where the blame really lay, and in August 1939 they resigned.

Rangatira listened to the message. Cinema and live theatre were inherently different. You could not expect movie men like Crick and Dean to understand the nuances of picking, casting, producing and touring plays and musicals successfully. Unfortunately, it was too late. Australian and New Zealand Theatres owed masses of back rent to JCW Ltd, and even attempts by Ted Tait to breathe life into the company were unsuccessful. With at least eighty per cent of the capital gone there was no way home.

But it was only the end of the beginning. As Australian and New Zealand Theatres disappeared and shareholders lost their investment, a new production company was incorporated. In 1943, JCW Theatres Ltd rose from the ashes of the disaster, and finally vindicated the 1938 structural reorganisation of the Firm. The old and the new management teams learnt to work in harmony, as Rangatira watched over the profits and avoided the mistakes of its first brush with live theatre.

George Tallis – no doubt relieved to get away – sailed for London on 19 June 1938 for what proved to be the last time. War clouds were gathering and, to his dismay, when visiting his family in Ireland he encountered anti-British slogans on the streets of Dublin. He met with his sisters Anne and Susan one Sunday, after they had returned from church. George attempted to talk the two into moving to England, but they would not listen. In later years he remembered their sombre, black dresses, their fervent discussions of the minister's sermon, and how deeply he felt the time-warp of all expatriates who return to conversations and attitudes that never change.

In October 1939 Tallis went to see Arthur Allen in Sydney. They discussed the old days and the endless saga of the Australian and New Zealand Theatres shares. Arthur was still on the board of the company, engaged in a futile battle for some return on his investment. He died, suddenly, on 2 October 1941. His long association with Tallis had been a happy one. The two men came together by

To Sir George Tallis
as a souvenir and with
my gratitude for his
and generous help to me in
my work in
W. de Basil
4.6.1940
Maurice Seymour

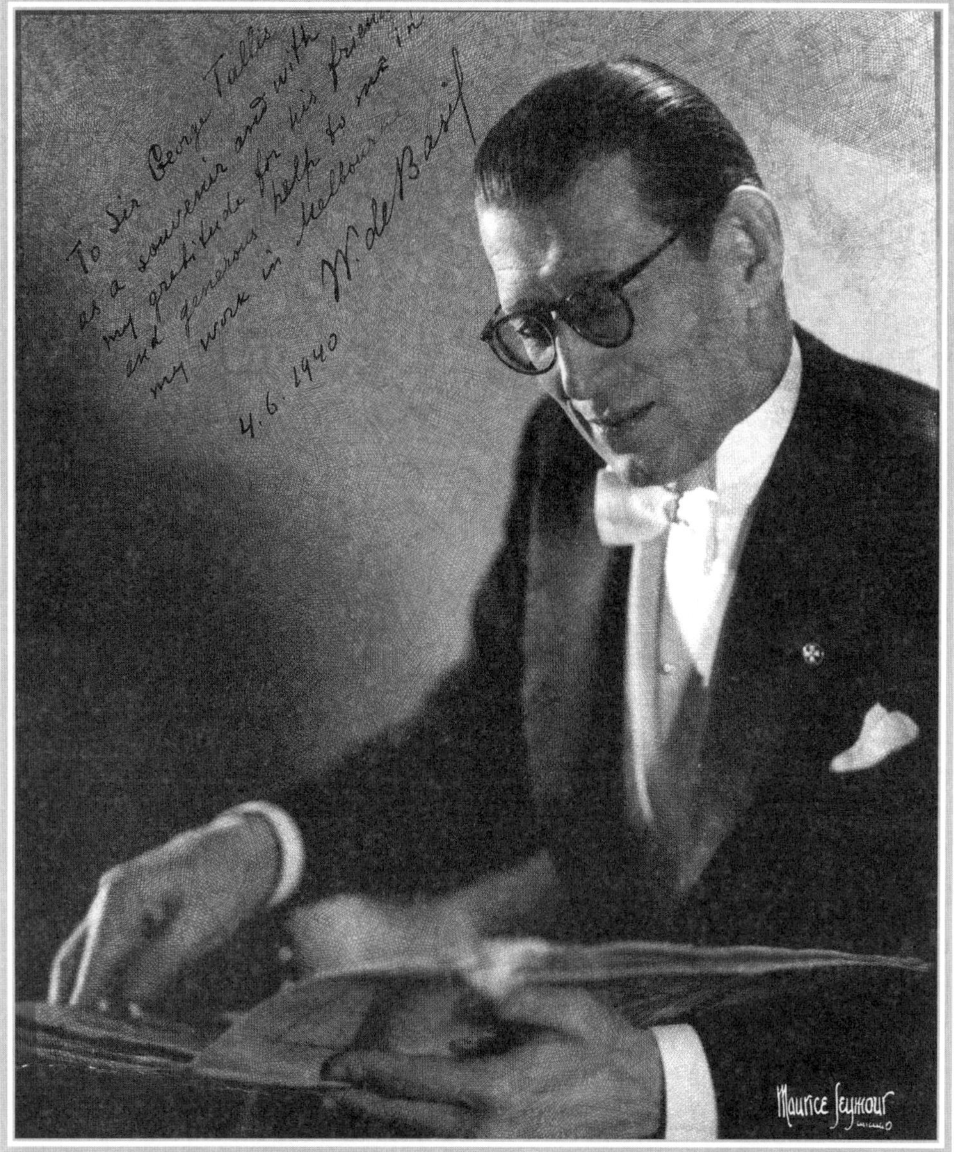

Colonel Wassilie de Basil, a great Russian ballet promoter

chance, and they had known each other from the Williamson days. During Tallis's frequent visits to Sydney, they mixed business with as much pleasure as they could muster. The Firm had monopolised them. Both reached for freedom. Arthur Allen never did quite achieve it, because the shambles that was Australian and New Zealand Theatres continued into the depths of 1941 and 1942.

Partners and Managing Directors 1886–1933

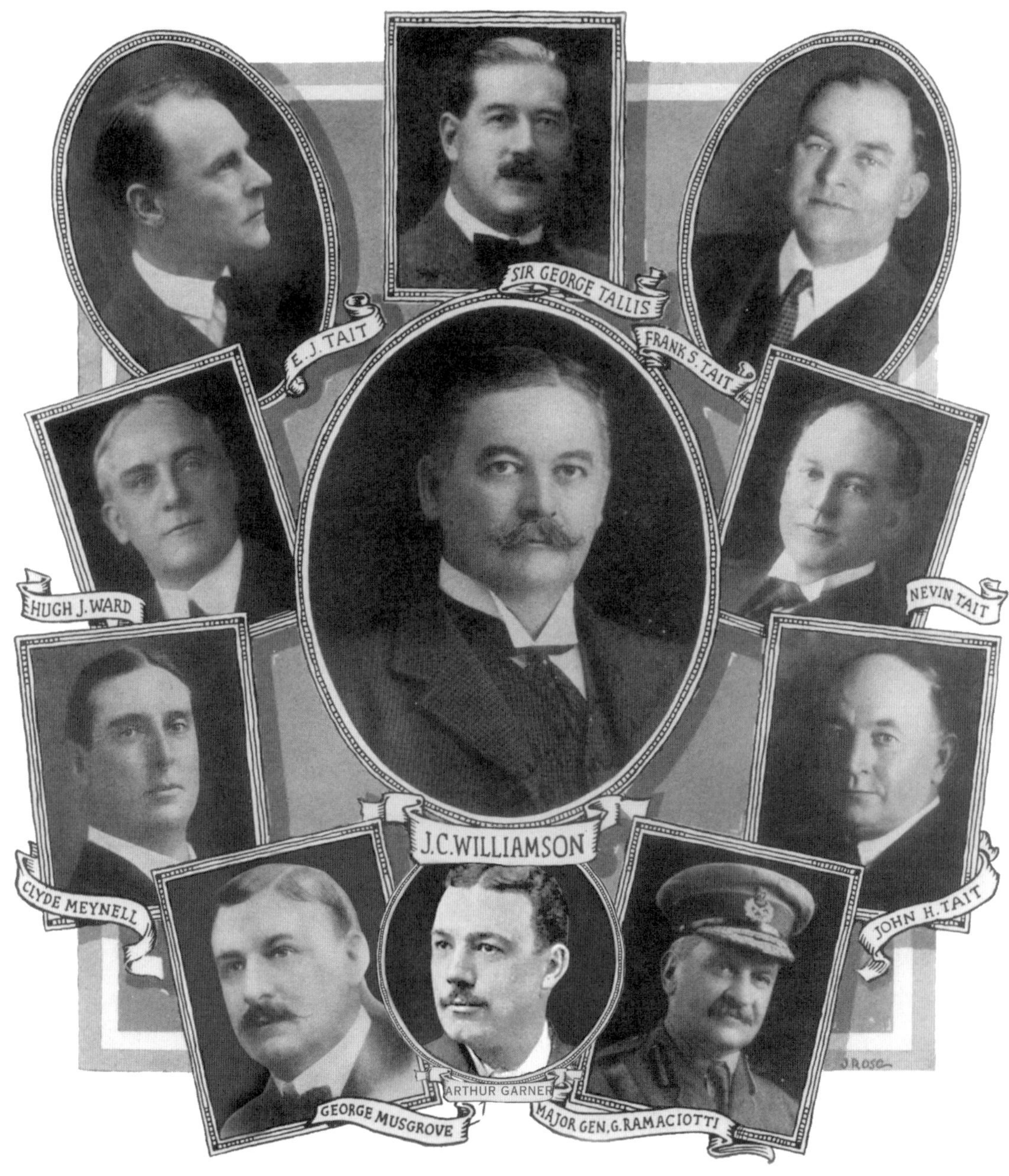

The depths of 1941! That was exactly ten years after George's retirement from 'active management' of the Firm. He had been involved with the Williamson theatrical concern, in one capacity or another, in every one of its partnerships and directorates from 1886 to 1938. This list does not include Tallis's chairman of directorships in the mid-to-late 1920s of Hoyts Theatres and the Broadcasting Company of Australia (3LO) – later to become the Dominion Broadcasting Company controlling 3LO, 3AR and other radio stations across Australia. He also held many other directorships during his life outside the entertainment industry. The list gives the partnership or directorate first, followed by Tallis's role. The dates are approximate.[2]

Partnerships

1886–1890 JC Williamson, A Garner and G Musgrove – the Triumvirate
G Tallis office junior

1890–1892 JC Williamson and A Garner
G Tallis treasurer Theatre Royal, Melbourne; junior on tour

1892–1900 JC Williamson and G Musgrove
G Tallis treasurer Princess Theatre; Williamson's secretary; business manager; manager in charge of touring

1900–1904 JC Williamson
G Tallis business manager, Melbourne and Sydney; manager in charge of touring; JC Williamson's right-hand man

1904–1910 JC Williamson, G Tallis and G Ramaciotti

JC Williamson Ltd

1910–1911 JC Williamson governing director; G Tallis and G Ramaciotti managing directors

1911–1913 JC Williamson governing director; G Tallis, HJ Ward and C Meynell managing directors
HJ Ward joins the Firm in 1911, followed by an amalgamation with the firm of Clarke–Meynell

1913–1920 G Tallis chairman of directors; HJ Ward and C Meynell managing directors
JC Williamson dies 6 July 1913

1920–1922 G Tallis chairman of directors; HJ Ward, C Meynell and EJ Tait managing directors; AW Allen, FJ Smith, T Fink and FS Tait directors
Amalgamation of JCW Ltd with J&N Tait in 1920

1922–1924 G Tallis chairman of directors; C Meynell and EJ Tait managing directors; AW Allen, FJ Smith, T Fink and FS Tait directors
HJ Ward resigns in 1922, and is not replaced

1924–1928 G Tallis chairman of directors; EJ Tait managing director; AW Allen, FJ Smith, T Fink and FS Tait directors
C Meynell resigns in 1924 and is not replaced

1928–1931 G Tallis chairman of directors; EJ Tait and FS Tait, managing directors; AW Allen, FJ Smith, T Fink and JH Tait directors

1931–1935 EJ Tait, FS Tait and JH Tait managing directors; AW Allen, FJ Smith, RW Best and CA Wenman directors
G Tallis resigns chairmanship 13 November 1931, retains access to an ordinary directorship through CA Wenman; T Fink resigns and is replaced by RW Best

1935–1938 EJ Tait, FS Tait and JH Tait, managing directors; G Tallis, AW Allen, FJ Smith, RM Anderson and RW Best directors
G Tallis rejoins board early in 1935. He and AW Allen sell their ordinary JCW Ltd shares to Rangatira in 1938 and resign

Australian and New Zealand Theatres Ltd

1938–1939 G Tallis director (with others)
Tallis resigns in 1939, and remains a shareholder until the company is reconstituted in 1942 becoming JCW Theatres Ltd

This was an enormous span of active involvement with the Firm, most of it at the top. George Tallis formed an administrative bridge between the days of Williamson and the depression years. During that period, he was the backbone of the company; he had seen it rise to the heights of the 1920s, and crash to the lows of the 1930s. Surely that was plenty, and more than enough, for one lifetime.

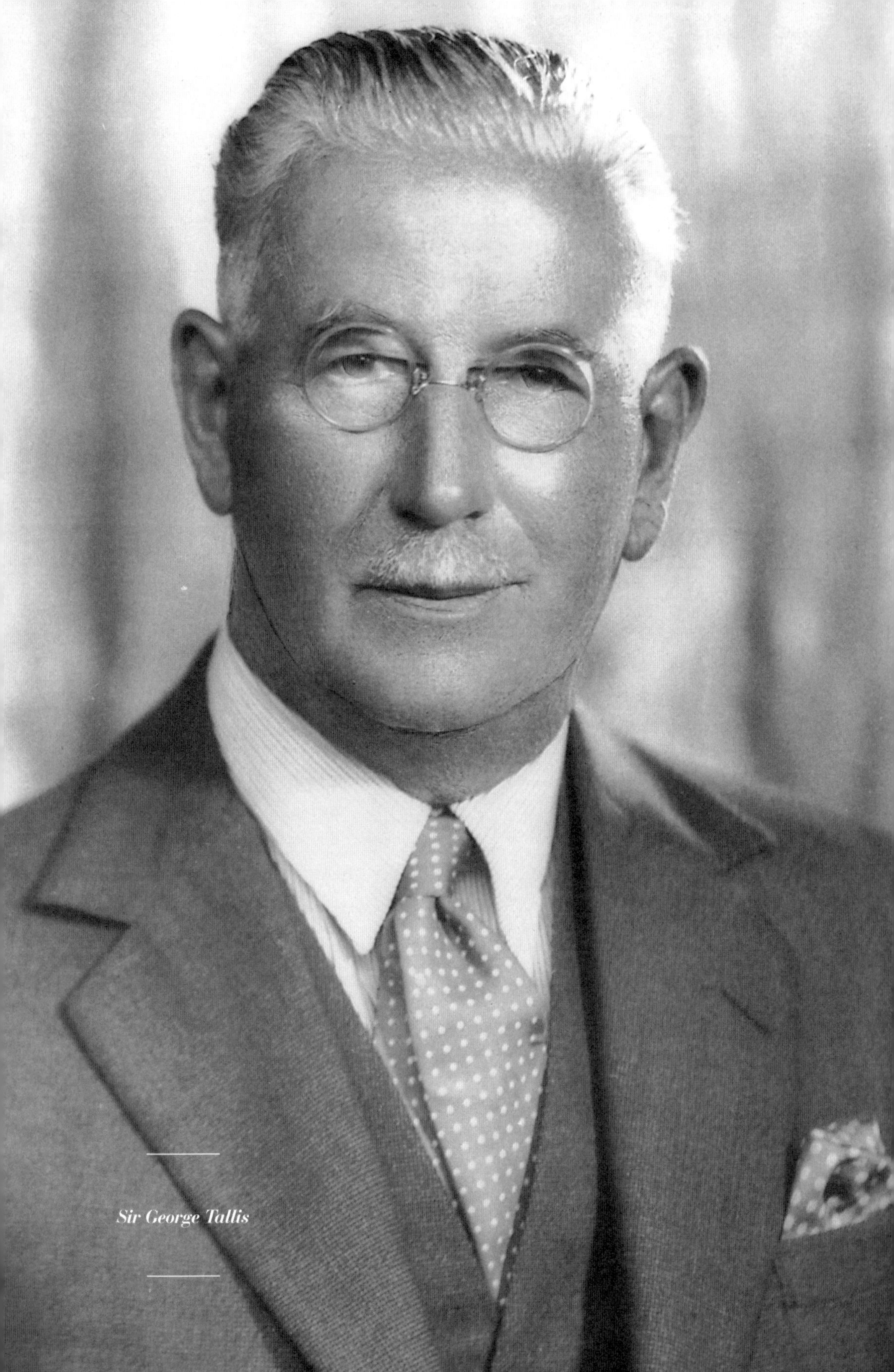
Sir George Tallis

CHAPTER NINETEEN

Rien ne va Plus

We do not know if that famous cry of the French casinos, warning players that there was no time left for further bets, ever roused Tallis, or whether he had a 'bob or two' on the horses. In business, he was a gambler, and the higher the risks the more he enjoyed his investing.

With serious projects he spent a long time gathering information, considering, and then waiting for the right time and place to make a move. With his own money George was a little more lenient. Investing was a social activity. If a proposal showed any merit at all, Tallis supported it to avoid letting the side down.

In 1930, for instance, George joined a group of Australian businessmen known as the Broom Syndicate.[1] With the help of two small European republics, Luxembourg and Andorra, the syndicate established a fifty-year concession to conduct sweepstakes on famous horse races. The project was not short on ambition; it shot at the moon. Among its several targets were the English Derby, the Melbourne Cup and the English Grand National Hurdle Race.

The idea was to sell a million sweep tickets per race, and to offer big payouts. It would be a gambler's feast, putting common lotteries in the shade. The syndicate was invited to anticipate one hundred per cent net profits as a consequence. Investors were told that the 'Broom' in the syndicate's title represented a 'clean sweep'. Who would be swept and sent to the cleaners? Tallis remarked, 'I may be doing my money in cold blood as I have sometimes done before. But the scheme could work'.

After his retirement, George missed all the business challenges. Where was the fun? To heighten his interest, he attacked the international stock markets. He had mixed success, and his London broker was unsympathetic:

The heavy fall in the American shares has made all the banks and finance houses call for a 30 per cent margin. I must ask you to increase your deposit ...

Tallis was getting some action now; he was gearing his stock market purchases.

He visited London in 1936 and 1938, and involved himself with his share dealings. At night George would return to his flat either euphoric or depressed. 'Let's eat dinner at the Ritz tonight. I'm starving,' signalled that the day had been good, while, 'I'm not very hungry tonight; let's eat at Lyons [the McDonalds of 1930s London],' warned George's dinner guests that his day had been bad.

When he returned to Australia his broker had more to say:

I received your cable yesterday. It drifted from the financial to the psychological aspects of share investing. I emphasise the impossibility of putting money in the scales on one side, anxiety on the other, and making the two balance.

Once you had the 'wind up' with your American shares. I told you then as I do now; it is bad to hold shares speculatively on loan in times of international stress. That advice holds good for eternity. If you give that to your son as a legacy, you will give him an asset that is not taxable by Succession Duties.

George's gearing strategy, once a powerful tool of his early business life, hit turbulence on the sliding world markets. By 1939 he was seventy, and his thirst for risks was quenched. Clouds were forming over Europe, and he cabled his London broker for advice in the face of international turmoil. The broker responded:

I have got your cable today: 'What would you advise?' You do put it up to one. Now I wish to God I could advise you. I do not know how you see the situation in Europe. I do not think that affairs there will lead to war. Equally, I do not think one will ever get nearer to war without having it.

Convinced by the reply that sharebrokers are also mortals, George closed his international account.

'Those who indulge in theatre management play a dangerous game.' This old cliche was reiterated by JC Williamson himself many times. Ted Tait satisfied himself that the chances of success for Williamson-produced theatrical pieces were no more than a third. Naturally, some theatre managers did better than others, but it was hard to tell if a run of flops was due to bad choice, bad production, changed circumstances or just a string of bad luck.

It was the duty of all managers to increase their, at best, meagre success rate as much as possible. A careful weeding out of doubtful shows helped, as did high production standards. The winds of change were more difficult to monitor. It was a wise entrepreneur who was one step ahead in the right direction; he was the survivor.

George followed these principles in all his business dealings, but he added one more – diversity. During his life he held significant portfolios in live theatre, films, radio, real estate and the equity markets. Had he overlooked the newspapers?

In a letter to Lord Northcliffe of the *London Times* on 13 March 1922, Keith Murdoch of the Melbourne *Herald* – later Sir Keith – introduced Tallis as 'king of the theatres and picture shows of Australia and New Zealand', and as one of Murdoch's partners. Tallis and Murdoch held a joint interest in the London *Evening News*, a newspaper with which Lord Northcliffe was evidently also associated. The pairing of Murdoch and Tallis was another loose partnership, like the Tallis–Thring combination, which yielded prime results. It featured in the 3LO story of the 1920s.

So George had the newspaper business covered as well, it seems.

Occupation: retired grazier. This was how George filled out official forms in his later years. There was no hint of a life spent at the top of Australian entertainment. Some cows, sheep and an orchard made him a mixed farmer, and he enjoyed his rural ties. They went back to his father and grandfather, who supported their families in Ireland by turning a sod.

The 1940s put an end to overseas trips, and George became more involved in the management of his two farms. His sons Pat and Mick were in the armed forces, leaving him the job of growing food and wool for the 'boys'. During these years he got to know his grandchildren, and the protective streak he had shown his own children spilled over to the next generation. One of his granddaughters observed that she and her brother had been so shielded from the ugly realities of the world as youngsters, largely due to George's influence, that for them the Second World War passed by almost unnoticed.

George may have had trouble adjusting to this retirement of semi-seclusion. His inherent restlessness, promoted by the demands of his job, must have been hard to curb. Because he kept most of his thoughts to himself, we don't know how fully his family understood his problems. He became quiet and pensive, and perhaps the adage of 'the bigger they are the harder they fall' applied as well to him as it did to his Firm.

The causes of withdrawal are not hard to find. In the 1920s he was at the pinnacle of the entertainment business in Australia, and on his many overseas journeys he represented the Firm, and often his country. This put him in demand socially and professionally; it was life at the top.

However, Tallis had one main problem; he was tied to the Firm's hostile board. In the end, he was unable to have his ideas implemented. Even the suggestion of a staff share-buy scheme was continually refused by the Tait managing directors.[2] What was the use? His sense of redundancy must have been strong. Only when he was out of the country did he get the illusion of independence that comes with distance from trouble.

In 1928 George had moved most of his family to England. Why? Perhaps if there had been no bad luck dogging his assault on London, and the financial losses had been big profits, and the depression had not arrived, then he might have stayed in England permanently as the Firm's managing director in charge of an expanding London business, far away from head office. An idle speculation, but George had more than a year's experience in producing plays in London. That theatre world certainly took him seriously, and gave him every chance of success. But luck had taken a holiday.

Moving abruptly from world heights into the oblivion of retirement was like engaging reverse gear in a car that is moving rapidly forward. There was much for George to be pensive about.

Tallis spent summers at Mornington, where he supervised his Ayrshire stud, shearing, hay-making and apple-picking. This was mixed farming, and George spread the risks here as he had with his theatre business.

The summers seemed hotter then. The New South Wales property at Wagga Wagga was at risk, for with the warm weather came fires. Fires were even a problem at Mornington, although not all of them were unavoidable. As George's health deteriorated, it interfered with his main diversion of 'burning-off'. Around his old house, *Beleura,* were large pines, gums and plenty of tinder. When he felt the urge for a fire, he wandered into the shady reserves full of twigs, cones and stumps. Armed with a rake and a box of matches, in no time he got a good blaze going.

He prodded the embers, and wandered off in search of more fuel. When he returned the fire was often out, or out of control. Gardeners with hoses, and even the fire brigade, came to douse the flames. The ashes were then combed for the trusty rake. There it was, with a charred handle only a few inches long.

Perhaps it occurred to George on such occasions that these regular conflagrations mimicked his last decade as chairman of the giant theatrical company. In those exhilarating days he built it up, and then was away searching for prime theatrical fare to import from America and Europe, or busy with negotiations involving massive corporate deals in films and radio. When he returned to his routine management duties, there was usually trouble in one or another of the Williamson departments. Always, it seemed, there were new rows in the boardroom, and then it was George who attended the flames.

Over the years the old mansion *Sunnyside*, which George had once owned, was transformed into a Roman Catholic boys' remand centre. When the boys tired of losing fights with the priests, they invented an excellent game. With the assistance of a stiff north wind, they torched George's grassland, which was adjacent to their quarters. Then, in the following confusion of fire brigades and smoke, half the residents of *Sunnyside* escaped. News of their progress around the district trickled in to police stations, and it was months before the last escapee was rounded up.

George was always grateful for the swift and efficient services of the local fire brigade, and he ordered kegs of beer to the site of the holocaust. Weary battlers of the flames refreshed themselves with a light brown ale, and the party was on. Year after year a 'spontaneous' blaze started on the grassland and, during the celebration of a job well done, the cause of the fire was discussed but never quite identified.

Fires on the Wagga property, *Braehour*, were a more serious proposition. Close by was the air force's Forest Hill camp, full of young airmen and WAAAFs who found it convenient to party on George's property. These affairs did not have a strict protocol, and fires erupted with a devastating effect on local farms. George wrote a long letter to the commanding officer in 1944:

The last fire occurred a week ago – the usual bottle party. The glow of the fire was seen from the house, a half a mile away . . . Last year we lost four bullocks, shot in the legs. Your people were welcome at all times to roam all over the property shooting rabbits, hares and ducks, and to bathe and fish, so long as they refrained from lighting fires and shooting down our livestock . . .

The strain was starting to tell, and George felt frail. He had migrated to Australia, as much as anything, to evade the Irish winters. Now he noticed the cold and rainy weather that slashed his home at Mornington, where winter seemed to last for ever. For his dose of sunshine he escaped more frequently, and for longer spells, to the banks of the Murrumbidgee River.

George's old friends dropped off one by one. Fred Smith appeared from time to time, but each visit led to trouble. In 1946, Fred wrote to George:

I have looked at the spectacles I brought back, but they are both mine. I think you will find that whatever spectacles are remaining at Beleura *belong to yourself. I appreciate your habit of leaving your glasses round about. I have three pairs for long sight and three for reading but I rarely know where more than one pair is. The rest are hidden; a bit like the dog and his bone . . . I am following your diet to the letter – weak tea, whole-meal bread etc. I feel rotten, but may survive in spite of the treatment.*

Two years later George was peering out of the window of his study. He couldn't count the number of times he had done that already, and the morning was still young. He saw the trees leaning under the force of strong winds, as rain came in bursts and pounded the garden and paths. Australia had better weather on offer. He noticed with annoyance a large bough that had been stripped from its moorings, and which lay in the middle of the bowling green. Well, there would be no game today!

He sat down. In truth, there had been no bowling now for a number of years. The 'club' membership had vanished as the once ardent competitors succumbed to illness. Some had checked out permanently. As for golf, he could hardly remember the last time he had played. He had given up his membership at Riversdale Golf Club, where he had fought those competitive tussles with Jo Wasley and a handful of other old friends. He had been president of the club in 1916, and more recently he had lent his support to local clubs. In 1924 he had been on the formation committee of the Peninsula Country Golf Club as a foundation member, and much later he had leased some of his prime grazing land to the Mornington Country Golf Club, later facilitating the club's ownership of it.

George was no longer a fire hazard to himself or his neighbours. The flames from the hearth that were now warming his hands would have to serve as a reminder of better times.

He heard the rumbling of a tea-trolley, and somewhere in the depths of the house a clock chimed eleven. There followed a perfunctory knock and the door was pushed open as his housekeeper, Christina McKeller, trundled in the morning spread: buttered scones, orange cake and biscuits. Standing in the middle of all this over-catering were two enormous silver pots, one for tea and the other for hot water.

George looked at the woman who had created the diversion. She was neatly dressed in black, with trimmings of white at the collar and a big white apron tied around her waist. Christina dated back to a time when *Beleura* and its inhabitants were young. Hers was the uniform of an era that might have supported this absurd morning tea. The two were good friends, with a common bond: they were both migrants – George from Ireland and Christina from Scotland.

'You really must find something to do, sir', said Christina as she poured out the tea.

George smiled. 'You're right, of course. But what?'

'Well, why not write your memoirs?'

There is nothing like the Scots, thought George, they shoot straight from the shoulder every time. 'Anything else?'

'Isn't it time for you to be thinking of heading to Wagga again? The winter has set in here; just look at it.'

His memoirs! These he had already started some years before. He went to his desk and rummaged. There they were, a few pages of handwriting. He started to read:

George Tallis at the age of 17 arrived in Australia in November 1886, having already had two years experience as a junior reporter on a newspaper in Ireland. Within a week joined Williamson, Garner and Musgrove as secretary to James Cassius Williamson and was shortly afterwards appointed treasurer at the Theatre Royal and Princess and then Business Manager in charge of companies touring Australia.

That was his autobiography; it needed trimming. The rest of the writing was about partnerships, shows and personalities of the golden era of the Australian theatre between 1880 and 1910, with no mention of himself. He felt comfortably tired and settled back in the chair. The fire was crackling. He was remembering.

The names of shows flashed through his mind: *The Sign of the Cross, The Belle of New York, San Toy, Lightnin', Mr Cinders* and countless others. They all meant something to him. They marked off his life better than any calendar. But they were all details, and they had to be pushed aside to reveal the core.

The journalists had it wrong, of course. They knew nothing of his Irish background, and therefore had over-emphasised his good luck in joining JC Williamson all those years ago. Of course, that had been at once fortunate, hard work and marvellous. But the real turning point in his life had come at the expense of his two brothers, John and Henry. They were the first to test Australia for his generation of Tallises, and they were in serious trouble shortly after their arrival. Soon John had died, and Henry was drifting. It was the Irish family's push to save Henry that gave him, George, his opportunity of making a start in a new country at the tender age of seventeen. Moreover, it was his brothers' demise that convinced him of the need to have a plan.

The mercy trip that he and his sister Charlotte had made to Australia to save Henry was an abject failure; Henry died less than two years later. For George, it was his making. He remembered clearly his own enthusiasm and energy in those days, and he would settle for one-tenth of it now. Charlotte returned to Ireland, married and had a family. She died in 1927 but, long before, sporadic communication had dwindled to zero. Even Charlotte's sisters in Ireland complained that she had dropped out of sight.

Only recently, his last surviving sister, Susan, had died. The pair had written to each other regularly over sixty years. They were good letters; fond letters. They kept the vestiges of the Irish connection intact. Now, with Susan gone, he was the last of the Tallises from Callan. Here it was, halfway through 1948. In a few months he'd be celebrating his seventy-ninth birthday. Seventeen years had passed since he had written that 'forty-five years makes a canvas crowded with memories of men, women and events.' Where had it all gone?

Son Mick entered George's study and saw him asleep by the dying fire. Mick teased the fire to life and turned to inspect his father. But he was too late; the old man was already awake.

'What's the time, Mick?'

'About twelve; how are you feeling, Dad?'

'Bloody awful!'

Mick thought that his father looked older and frailer that morning than he had ever seen him.

'The doctor came again this morning and said that I need another transfusion. Do you think that the silly devils know what they're doing?'

'Of course they do, Dad. They have all the latest equipment down at the hospital these days.' Mick hoped that he sounded more confident than he felt. He, too, mistrusted the medical profession.

George continued: 'The trouble is that I get so bored sitting here and sleeping all day. My mind is perfectly all right, you know.'

Mick did know. His father still had incisive perceptions and a prodigious memory. 'Well Dad, how are your memoirs going? Christina tells me you are going to make a start on them.'

George picked up the pages he had been reading and handed them to his son.

'Not bad for an hour's work,' said Mick with a smile as he leafed through the pages. 'Now, how about the rest?'

George laughed, and was silent. Mick knew the silences only too well, and he changed tack.

'It's about time for Wagga again, don't you think? I'm free to drive you there any time you like.'

George nodded. He fell to reverie again after Mick had left.

He thought of size, and how the giant theatrical concern of JC Williamson had become the leader in providing entertainment for the masses. Its very size had proved its downfall; swept away by the depression. He recalled how the problems of the troubled board of that period were so dwarfed by those brought on by the new technological, economic and social forces that they were of minor influence in determining the destiny of the company.

Perhaps the two elements of the 1920 Amalgamation – JCW Ltd and J&N Tait – would have withstood the depression years better had there been no coming together. Each would have been administratively nimbler; each would have made its own decisions and each, therefore, could have had better prospects of survival.

What negative thinking! The 1920s were positive years, filled with optimism that had not been seen since. They were years crying out for experimentation, courage and big achievement.

The Firm made many mistakes, but no one claimed that it lacked courage in its investment in the future of Australian entertainment. Nor was there courage lacking among its managing directors, who backed boardroom decisions with their own money. In the process, the company was successful beyond the wildest dreams. If its demise was as spectacular as its rise to fame, then history was the richer, leaving important lessons for all who followed.

George thought about these issues. He had been there: he had participated, and there was no need for writing. He also decided that the early years of his awakening to the stage and its business were his most enjoyable and rewarding years. Since his notes covered this period well enough, his job was done. He stood up, and put the memoirs back in the desk drawer.

When Christina came in with his lunch at one sharp, she found George looking out of the window as usual. Somehow he did not appear to be as restless. He turned and said, 'You'll be pleased to know that I have finished my memoirs, and that I'll be leaving for Wagga at the end of the week.'

George Tallis died on 15 August 1948 at Wagga Wagga, New South Wales. Perhaps his most poignant memorial was from the little town he had made part of his life for more than thirty years. George may have been surprised at the rare honour the Shire of Mornington bestowed upon him; he would surely have been touched by the warm message of friendship and appreciation that the council expressed on behalf of the community. The letter, dated 22 September 1948, was addressed to George's son Mick:

At the last meeting of the above Shire Council, a resolution was passed that a letter of condolence, under seal, be forwarded to you and the members of the family in your recent bereavement.

It was also resolved that a minute of appreciation of the public service rendered to the community by the late Sir George Tallis, be placed on record. In passing this resolution, reference was made to his high sense of citizenship, his many generous gifts to public institutions and charities and particularly to his warm-hearted and kindly disposition towards his fellowmen. These qualities, with which he was so richly endowed, served as an example and an inspiration to all who knew him.

As a further mark of respect to the memory of your late father, the meeting observed two minutes silence.

Running order of shows in Melbourne theatres under the Firm's management 1886–1931

This 'running order' of Williamson shows in Melbourne has been compiled largely from the amusement columns of the Melbourne *Argus* newspaper. The time span is that of George Tallis's direct involvement with JC Williamson managements, and Melbourne theatres were used because that city was his home base.

We have listed shows under the name of the managing company, or the names of the principal actors, where possible. We use the letters M, P and O for Musical, Play and Opera; Pa, B and R for Pantomime, Ballet and Review, and Bu for Burlesque; WG & M for Williamson, Garner and Musgrove; JCW for JC Williamson.

Melbourne theatres under the Firm's control 1886–1931

Date	Royal	Princess	HMT	Kings	Comedy	Partnership/ Company
1886–1891	✯	✯				Williamson, Garner and Musgrove
1892–1899		✯				Williamson, Musgrove
1900–1903			✯			Williamson
1904–1910		✯	✯			Williamson, Tallis, Ramaciotti
1910–1912		✯	✯			JC Williamson Ltd
1912–1919	✯		✯			JC Williamson Ltd
1920–1927	✯		✯	✯		JC Williamson Ltd
1928–1929	✯		✯	✯	✯	JC Williamson Ltd
1930–1931	✯			✯	✯	JC Williamson Ltd

Theatre Royal

			weeks
1886			
George Titheradge			**5**
Oct	30	*Human Nature* (P)	
Carrie Swain			**3**
Dec	4	*The Tomboy* (P)	
WG & M production			**6**
	27	*Robinson Crusoe* (Pa)	
1887			
George Rignold & Kate Bishop			**9**
Feb	5	*Siberia* (P)	3
	26	*The Tempest* (P)	4
Mar	26	*Called Back* (P)	2
Bland Holt			**11**
Apr	9	*A Run of Luck* (P)	5
May	14	*Alone in London* (P)	4
Jun	11	*The World* (P)	2
JC Williamson & Maggie Moore			**8**
	25	*Struck Oil* (P) 10th Revival	3
Jul	16	*Shadows of a Great City* (P) and *The Chinese Question* (P)	1
	23	*Streets of London* (P)	2
Aug	6	*Rip Van Winkle* (P)	1
	13	*Eureka* (P)	1
George Darrell & Royal Dramatic Co.			**5**
Nov	19	*Sunny South* (P)	2
Dec	3	*First Class* (P)	3
WG & M production			**6**
	26	*Jack the Giant Killer & Little Bo Peep* (Pa)	
1888			
Capt De Burgh & Isabel Morris with Royal Dramatic Co.			**1**
Feb	11	*Sentenced to Death* (P)	
Charles Warner			**6**
	18	*Drink* (P)	4
Mar	17	*The Road to Ruin* (P)	2
Bland Holt			**9**
	31	*New Babylon* (P)	4
Apr	28	*Mankind or Beggar Your Neighbour* (P)	2
May	12	*Alone in London* (P)	2
	26	*Taken from Life* (P)	1
Carrie Swain			**13**
Jun	2	*The Tomboy* (P)	3
	23	*The Miner's Daughter* (P)	2
Jul	7	*Uncle Tom's Cabin* (P)	3
	28	*Jack and I* (P)	2
Aug	11	*Little Nell & the Marchioness* (P)	2
	25	*The Tomboy* (P)	1
Signor & Signora Majeroni & George Darrell			**4**
Sep	1	*Mr Barnes of New York* (P)	3
	22	*The Old Corporal* (P)	1
Charles Warner			**10**
	29	*Hands across the Sea* (P)	8
Dec	8	*It's Never Too Late to Mend* (P)	2
WG & M production			**10**
	26	*Sinbad the Sailor* (Pa)	
1889			
Bland Holt			**10**
Mar	16	*Union Jack* (P)	2
	30	*The World* (P)	2
Apr	13	*A Run of Luck* (P)	1
	20	*The Ruling Passion* (P)	3
May	11	*New Babylon* (P)	2
The New London Dramatic Co.			**18**
	25	*The Pointsman* (P) Matinee – Testimonial to Brough & Boucicault	4
Jun	29	*The Bells of Haslemere* (P)	5

Theatre Royal

			weeks
Jul	6	Matinee – Testimonial to William Marshall	
Aug	3	*The Silver King* (P)	4
	31	*Harbour Lights* (P)	2
Sep	14	*The Silver Falls* (P)	3
WG & M production			**2**
Oct	5	*Human Nature* (P)	
Royal Dramatic Co.			**1**
	19	*The Merchant of Venice* (P)	
Dion Boucicault & Janet Achurch			**1**
	26	*Led Astray* (P)	
Janet Achurch,Charles Charrington & The New London Dramatic Co.			**1**
Nov	4	*The Pointsman* (P)	
Grattan Riggs			**6**
	9	*The Shaughraun* (P)	2
	23	*The Irish Detective* (P)	1
	30	*The Octoroon* (P)	1
Dec	7	*Shin Fane* (P)	1
	14	*The Colleen Bawn* (P)	1
	21	Farewell Benefit – Grattan Riggs	
Royal Comic Opera Co.			**8**
	26	*Cinderella* (Pa)	

1890

			weeks
Charles Warner & Royal Dramatic Co.			**17**
Feb	22	*Hands across the Sea* (P)	2
Mar	8	*The Streets of London* (P)	2
	22	*A Man's Shadow* (P)	2
Apr	5	*Drink* (P)	2
	19	*It's Never Too Late to Mend* (P)	1
	26	*The Noble Vagabond* (P)	2
May	10	*After Dark* (P)	3
	31	*The Silver King* (P)	2
Jun	14	*Dora* (P) and *The Barrister* (P)	1
George & Christine Darrell & Royal Dramatic Co.			**19**
	21	*The Flying Scud* (P)	3
Jul	12	*The Black Country* (P)	2
	26	*Formosa or Road to Ruin* (P)	2
Aug	9	*The Lucky Lot* (P)	3
	30	*Potter of Texas* (P)	1
Sep	9	*The Mystery of a Hansom Cab* (P)	1
	13	*The Famine* (P)	3
Oct	4	Theatre sub-leased to Simonsen Opera Co.	
Nov	1	*The English Rose* (P)	4
Grattan Riggs			**3**
	29	*Arrah-na-Pogue* (P)	1
		Maggie Moore	
Dec	6	*The Irish Detective* (P)	1
	13	*Shin Fane* (P)	1
	20	*The Colleen Bawn* (P)	
WG & M production			**8**
	26	*Aladdin* (Pa)	

1891

			weeks
Charles Cartright & Olga Nethersole			**7**
Feb	21	*The Middleman* (P)	2
Mar	7	*The Fortune of War* (P)	3
	28	*Moths* (P)	2
George & Christine Darrell			**3**
Apr	18	*Transported for Life* (P)	1
	25	*The Sunny North* (P)	1
May	2	*The New Rush* (P)	1
	9	*Back from the Grave* (P)	
	13	Matinee benefit for Capt. De Burgh	
John H Sheridan			**6**
	13	*Bridget O'Brien Esq.* (M)	5
Jun	20	*Fun on the Bristol* (M)	1

Theatre Royal

			weeks
Jun	29	Matinee Testimonial to John H Sheridan	
		After nine years at the Theatre Royal, JC Williamson and Arthur Garner relinquish the lease.	

1911

JCW Comic Opera Co.			**3**
Sep	30	*The Chocolate Soldier* (M)	
Oct	28	HB Irving Farewell – *The Lyons Mail* (P)	
Ethel Irving			**5**
Nov	4	*Lady Frederick* (P)	2
	18	*Dame Nature* (P)	3
Hilda Spong			**8**
Dec	16	*Every Woman* (P)	5

1912

Jan	27	*Passers-By* (P)	3
JCW Comic Opera Co.			**1**
Feb	17	*The Chocolate Soldier* (M)	
William Desmond & Dorothy Dix			**2**
	24	*Alias Jimmy Valentine* (P)	
Cyril Mackay, Harcourt Beatty & Dorothy Dix			**3**
Mar	9	*The House of Temperley* (P)	
Oscar Asche & Lily Brayton			**10**
Apr	6	*Kismet* (P)	7
Jun	1	*Othello* (P)	2
	15	*The Virgin Goddess* (P)	1
Frederick Harrison's Haymarket Theatre Co.			**7**
	22	*The Blue Bird* (P)	5
Jul	27	*You Never Can Tell* (P)	2
Aug	31	Reopening of the Theatre after alterations.	
Gen Lew Wallace's Religious Romance			**6**
Aug	31	*Ben Hur* (P)	
Dorothy Dix & Drury Lane Theatre Co.			**2**
Oct	19	*The Whip* (P)	2
Nov	1	*Raffles* (P) Amateur Performance in aid of the poor	
Fred Niblo & JCW Co. of Comedians			**4**
	20	*Get-Rich-Quick Wallingford* (P)	
Oscar Asche & Lily Brayton			**11**
Dec	26	*Anthony and Cleopatra* (P)	5

1913

Feb	1	*The Taming of the Shrew* (P)	1
	8	*A Midsummer Night's Dream* (P)	4
Mar	11	*Merchant of Venice* (P)	
	14	*Othello* (P)	
	17	*The Taming of the Shrew* (P)	
Julius Knight, Irene Brown & New English Comedy Co.			**11**
	22	*Milestones* (P)	9
	28	Matinee in aid of the Captain Scott Memorial Fund by the Puss in Boots Co. and the Oscar Asche and Lily Brayton Co.	
May	3	*Man and Superman* (P)	2
Muriel Starr, EW Morrison, Mary Worth & Lincoln Plumer			**12**
	17	*Within the Law* (P)	
Jul	21	Farewell Matinee Benefit to Frances Ross prior to her departure for America	

Theatre Royal

			weeks
Fred Niblo & JCW Co. of Comedians			**10**
Aug	16	*The Fortune Hunter* (P)	8
Oct	11	*Excuse Me* (P)	2
Lewis Waller & Madge Titheradge			**10**
	25	*A Marriage of Convenience* (P)	2
Nov	8	*A Butterfly on the Wheel* (P)	4
Dec	13	*Miss Elizabeth's Prisoner* (P)	2
	27	*Monsieur Beaucaire* (P)	2

1914

Julius Knight & Irene Brown			**3**
Jan	10	*Diplomacy* (P)	2
	29	*Man and Superman* (P)	
	31	*Milestones* (P)	
Feb	7	*The Lion and the Mouse* (P)	1
Louis N Parke's Pageant Play – Ethel Warwick & JCW Dramatic Co.			**6**
	14	*Joseph and His Brethren* (P)	
Muriel Starr & Lincoln Plumer			**5**
Mar	28	*Madame X* (P)	
JCW's New Comic Opera Co.			**1**
May	9	*Dorothy* (M)	
Fred Niblo & Josephine Cohan			**10**
	16	*Never Say Die* (P)	6
Jun	29	*Officer 666* (P)	4
Julius Knight, Irene Browne & JCW Dramatic Co.			**11**
Aug	1	*A Royal Divorce* (P)	5

WAR DECLARED BETWEEN ENGLAND AND GERMANY

			weeks
Sep	5	*The Scarlet Pimpernel* (P)	1
	12	*Monsieur Beaucaire* (P)	1
	19	*The Sign of the Cross* (P)	2
Oct	3	*The Silver King* (P)	2
Charles A Millward & William Harrigan			**2**
	17	*The Argyle Case* (P)	
Muriel Starr			**3**
	31	*Within the Law* (P)	
Muriel Starr & Charles A Millward			**15**
Nov	21	*The Yellow Ticket* (P)	3
Dec	12	*The Chorus Lady* (P)	2
	26	*Bought and Paid For* (P)	10

1915

Mar	11	Bridge afternoon and Café Chantant in aid of the Belgium Relief Fund. 'Stars who will entertain include those from Theatre Royal, Her Majesty's Theatre, Tivoli and Fuller and Brennan Co.'	
Fred Niblo & Josephine Cohan			**12**
Mar	13	*Seven Keys to Baldpate* (P)	6
Apr	24	*Broadway Jones* (P)	6
May	16	Matinee in aid of British and Australian Red Cross Funds	
	28	Matinee in aid of the Benevolent Fund for the Actors Association	
Jun	4	*The Importance of Being Earnest* (P) in aid of St John Ambulance Service	
Frank Harvey & JCW Dramatic Co.			**4**
	5	*The Man Who Stayed at Home* (P)	
Paul Burns & Sam Howard & Artists from New York			**6**
Jul	10	*Potash and Perlmutter* (P)	

Theatre Royal

			weeks
Muriel Starr & Charles A Millward			**11**
Aug	28	*Under Cover* (P)	6
Oct	9	*Nobody's Widow* (P)	2
	22	*Within the Law* (P)	1
	30	*Bought and Paid For* (P)	1
Nov	6	*Madame X* (P)	1
	11	Farewell performance for Muriel Starr	
JCW Farce Co.			**4**
	13	*A Pair of Sixes* (P)	3
Dec	4	*Stop Thief* (P)	1
Frank Harvey & JCW Dramatic Co.			**3**
	11	*Kick In* (P)	2
	25	Festival of Sacred Songs	
	26	*The Man Who Stayed at Home* (P)	1

1916

Frank Harvey & L Kimball			**4**
Jan	1	*Under Fire* (P)	
Hale Hamilton & Myrtle Tannerhill			**15**
Comedians with George M Cohan at Astor Theatre, New York			
	29	*It Pays to Advertise* (P)	7
Mar	25	*Twin Beds* (P)	4
Apr	22	*The Boomerang* (P)	2
May	6	*Get-Rich-Quick Wallingford* (P)	2
DW Griffiths Motion Picture			**2**
	20	*The Birth of a Nation*	
Madge Fabian & Frank Harvey			**14**
Jun	3	*On Trial* (P)	4
Jul	5	*Madame X* (P)	
	8	*Romance* (P)	4
Aug	5	*The Story of the Rosary* (P)	3
	26	*The Land of Promise* (P)	3
Hale Hamilton & Myrtle Tannerhill			**4**
Sep	16	*Too Many Cooks* (P)	1
	23	*It Pays to Advertise* (P)	1
	30	*A Full House* (P)	1
Oct	14	*Get-Rich-Quick Wallingford* (P)	1
Julius Knight			**13**
	21	*Under Fire* (P)	1
	28	*A Royal Divorce* (P)	2
Nov	11	*The Silver King* (P)	2
	25	*The Sign of the Cross* (P)	1
Dec	2	*Damaged Goods* (P)	5

1917

Jan	6	*The Woman* (P)	2
Florence Rockwell & Frank Harvey			**5**
	20	*The House of Glass* (P)	3
Feb	10	*The Misleading Lady* (P)	2
DW Griffiths Motion Picture			**2**
	24	*Intolerance*	
JCW New English Comedy Co.			**3**
Mar	17	*Fair and Warmer* (P)	
Apr	6	Good Friday Night Concert of Sacred Songs	
Marie Tempest & Graham Browne			**6**
	7	*The Marriage of Kitty* (P)	4
May	7	*Penelope* (P)	2
JCW Dramatic Co.			**2**
	19	*London Pride* (P)	
	22	Matinee Benefit in aid of the widow of Tom Dawson, comedian killed in the Battle of Pozieres	
JCW New English Comedy Co.			**2**
Jun	2	*A Little Bit of Fluff* (P)	
Cyril Maude			**6**
	16	*Grumpy* (P)	

Theatre Royal

weeks

Kathlene MacDonell & Charles Waldron **12**

Jul 28 *Daddy Long Legs* (P) 5
Sep 8 *Outcast* (P) 4
Oct 6 *L'Aiglon* (P) 3

Marie Tempest & Graham Browne **7**

27 *Good Gracious Annabelle* (P) 2
Nov 10 *Mary Goes First* (P) 1
17 *A Pair of Silk Stockings* (P) 1
Dec 1 *Mrs Dot* (P) 3

Muriel Starr, Frank Harvey & Louis Kimball **14**

22 *The Bird of Paradise* (P) 6

1918

Feb 2 *The Easiest Way* (P) 5
Mar 9 *Within the Law* (P) 3
12 Matinee in aid of the State War Councils Appeal Theatrical Café Chantant and Card Afternoon
29 Good Friday Night – Concert of Sacred Music

Kathlene MacDonell & Charles Waldron **9**

30 *The Cinderella Man* (P) 2
Apr 13 *The Rainbow* (P) 2
27 *The Willow Tree* (P) 2
May 11 *Outcasts* (P) 1
18 *Daddy Long Legs* (P) 2

Graham Browne **4**

Jun 1 *General Post* (P)

Muriel Starr, Frank Harvey & Louis Kimball **6**

29 *The Man Who Came Back* (P) 5
Aug 10 *Bought and Paid For* (P) 1

weeks

Margaret Wycherly & Brimsley Shaw **4**

17 *The 13th Chair* (P)

JCW New Musical Comedy Co. **3**

Sep 14 *Oh, Boy* (M)

Nick Adam, James E. Waters & JCW Comedy Co. **8**

Oct 5 *Business before Pleasure* (P) 5
Nov 9 *The High Cost of Loving* (P) 2

11 END OF WAR

23 *Potash and Perlmutter* (P) 1

DW Griffiths Motion Picture **3**

30 *Hearts of the World*

MB Figman & Lolita Robertson **5**

Dec 26 *Nothing But the Truth* (P)

1919

All Theatres closed 29 January to 8 March 1919 due to influenza epidemic.

Muriel Starr, Frank Harvey & Louis Kimball **17**

Mar 8 *The Great Divide* (P) 4
Apr 7 *Madame X* (P) 1
13 *Three Faces East* (P) preceded by *The Monkey's Paw* (P) 4
18 Good Friday Night Annual Festival of Sacred Music
May 10 *Common Clay* (P) 3
31 *The Silent Witness* (P) 4
Jun 28 *Bought and Paid For* (P) 1

MB Figman & Lolita Robertson **6**

Jul 5 *A Tailor-Made Man* (P) 5
Aug 9 *Nothing but the Truth* (P) 1

Theatre Royal

			weeks
John D O'Hara			**15**
	15	*Lightnin'* (P)	
Royal Comic Opera Co. with Theodore Leonard & Florence Young			**14**
Nov	29	*Theodore and Co.* (M)	8

1920

Jan	31	*Kissing Time* (M) (Maude Fane and Gladys Moncrieff)	6
Muriel Starr			**1**
Mar	13	*The Silent Witness* (P)	
JCW Comedy Co.			**10**
	20	*Tilly of Bloomsbury* (P)	
Apr	2	Good Friday *The Truant Soul* (film)	
JCW Musical Comedy Co.			**14**
May	28	*Going Up* (M)	2
Jun	12	*Yes, Uncle* (M)	10
Aug	21	*The Girl in the Taxi* (M)	2
Marie Tempest & Graham Browne			**5**
Sep	4	*Outcast* (P)	1
		Duke of Killiecrankie (P)	1
		Penelope (P)	1
		The Marriage of Kitty (P)	1
		Mrs Dot (P)	1
Royal Comic Opera Co.			**40**
Oct	9	*Kissing Time* (M)	2
	23	*The Boy* (M)	12

1921

			weeks
Jan	22	*The Maid of the Mountains* (M) (Gladys Moncrieff)	24
Jul	2	*Katinka* (M)	2
Jamieson Dodds & Rene Maxwell			**2**
	16	*The Lilac Domino* (M) transferred to HMT	
Joseph Coyne			**13**
	30	*Nightie Night* (P)	6
Sep	10	*His Lady Friends* (P) (Blanche Browne)	5
Oct	15	*Wedding Bells* (P)	2
JCW Royal Comic Opera Co.			**3**
	29	*Firefly* (M)	
Maude Hannaford & Frank Harvey			**4**
Nov	19	*The Sign on the Door* (P)	
	22	Matinee in aid of the Funds for the Victorian Civil Ambulance – Café Chantant and Card Afternoon	
Royal Comic Opera Co.			**2**
Dec	22	*Merrie England* (M)	

1922

Jan	5	*Yeomen of the Guard* (M)	
John D O'Hara			**2**
Jan	7	*The Laughter of Fools* (P)	
Maude Fane & JCW New English Comedy Co.			**5**
	21	*A Night Out* (M)	
Isobel Brosnan & JCW New English Comedy Co.			**16**
Feb	25	*Paddy the Next Best Thing* (P)	10
May	6	*The Bat* (P)	6
	13	Gala Performance for Boat Race Night, Moving Pictures of the Race	
	19	Matinee in Aid of Distressed Diggers and their families. Every theatre represented by principal artists	
Maire O'Neil & Original Abbey Theatre Co. (Ireland)			**3**
Jun	17	*The White Headed Boy* (P)	

Theatre Royal

weeks

JCW Gilbert & Sullivan Opera Co. **4**

Jul 8 *The Chocolate Solider* (M)
Dorothy (M)
The Mikado (M)
The Gondoliers (M)
The Pirates of Penzance (M)
The Yeomen of the Guard (M)
Iolanthe (M)
Pinafore (M) and
Trial by Jury (M)

Maire O'Neil & Abbey Theatre Co.

Jul 24 *In the Shadow of the Glen* (P)
The Building Fund (P)
The Workhouse Ward (P)

JCW Comedy Co. **4**

Aug 12 *Parlour, Bedroom, Bath* (P)

Louis Bennison **4**

Sep 9 *The Great Lover* (P)

Maude Fane, Madge Elliot, Cyril Ritchard & JCW Musical Comedy Co. **10**

Oct 7 *Mary* (M) 2
21 *The Peep Show* (Revue) 8

Royal Comic Opera Co. **6**

Dec 16 *The Maid of the Mountains* (M)

1923

Produced by Oscar Asche for JCW with Gladys Moncrieff **3**

Jan 27 *A Southern Maid* (M)

Gertrude Elliott (Lady Forbes Robertson) & her English Dramatic Co. **13**

Mar 24 *Woman to Woman* (P) 6
May 3 *Smilin' Through* (P) 5
Jun 9 *Enter Madame* (P) 2

weeks

Garry Marsh, Muriel Martin-Harvey & JCW New English Dramatic Co. **7**

23 *If Winter Comes* (P) 3
Jul 14 *The Cat and the Canary* (P) 4

Bert Bailey & Julius Grant **3**

Aug 13 *The Sentimental Bloke* (P)
Theatre Royal closed September 1–15 for extensive alterations.

Josie Melville & JCW Musical Comedy Co. **25**

Sep 5 *Sally* (M)
This JCW Co. also took *Sally* into the wards of the Repatriation Hospitals.

1924

Gertrude Elliott **2**

Mar 8 *Bluebeard's Eighth Wife* (P)

Alfred Frith, Madge Elliott, Cyril Ritchard & JCW Musical Comedy Co. **13**

25 *The Cabaret Girl* (M) 9
May 24 *Kissing Time* (M) 3
Jun 14 *Whirled into Happiness* (M) 1

Muriel Starr & Frank Harvey **1**

21 *The Garden of Allah* (P)
Jun 28 Theatre Royal closed until July 5 for alterations to make it suitable for vaudeville.

Bransby Williams & JCW (Vaudeville) Ltd **15**

Jul 5 *Vaudeville Deluxe*

Muriel Starr & Frank Harvey **1**

Oct 27 *The Silent Witness* (P)

John D O'Hara **5**

Nov 8 *Kempy* (P) 3
29 *Lightnin'* (P) 2

Theatre Royal

			weeks
Maurice Moscovitch			**7**
Dec	13	*The Merchant of Venice* (P)	2
	27	*The Outsider* (P)	5

1925

Josie Melville, George Gee & JCW Musical Comedy Co.			**2**
Feb	7	*Sally* (M) 632 performances in Australia	
Thurston Hall			**7**
	21	*So This Is London* (P)	
Pauline Frederick			**11**
Apr	11	*Spring Cleaning* (P)	8
Jun	6	*The Lady* (P)	3
	14	Grand Instrumental and Vocal Concert in aid of the unemployed	
Muriel Starr & Frank Harvey			**4**
	27	*Secrets* (P)	
Thurston Hall			**1**
Jul	25	*So This Is London* (P)	
Marie Burke & Gus Bluett			**4**
Aug	1	*Wildflower* (M)	
Muriel Starr & Frank Harvey			**8**
	29	*Within the Law* (P)	2
Sep	12	*The Silver King* (P)	3
Oct	3	*A Royal Divorce* (P)	3
Royal Comic Opera Co. & Gladys Moncrieff			**4**
	24	*The Street Singer* (M)	
Townsend Whitling & Doris Johnstone			**4**
Nov	21	*The Farmer's Wife* (P)	
Royal Comic Opera Co., Gladys Moncrieff & Claude Fleming			**3**
Dec	19	*The Street Singer* (M)	1
	26	*The Maid of the Mountains* (M)	1

1926

			weeks
Jan	3	*The Merry Widow* (M)	1
Royal Comic Opera Co. & Harriet Bennett			**15**
	9	*Lilac Time* (M)	
Guy Bates Post			**6**
Apr	24	*The Bad Man* (P)	
Margery Hicklin & JCW New Musical Co.			**8**
Jun	5	*Leave It to Jane* (M)	6
Jul	17	*Tell Me More* (M)	2
Harry Greer & Roy Rene			**2**
	31	*Give and Take* (P)	
Leon Gordon			**5**
Aug	14	*White Cargo* (P)	
Marie Burke, Claude Fleming & Cecil Kellaway			**4**
Sep	18	*Katja* (M)	
Richard Taber & Hale Norcross			**2**
Oct	16	*Is Zat So* (P)	
Renee Kelly			**4**
	30	*Brown Sugar* (P)	
Marie Burke & R Barrett-Lennard			**4**
Nov	27	*Wildflower* (M)	
Motion Picture			
Dec	16	Dempsey v Tunney heavy weight bout	
Ada Reeve & Jack Morrison			**8**
Dec	27	*Pins and Needles* (R)	

1927

Repertory Theatre Society			**1**
Feb	26	*Androcles and the Lion* (P)	
Nellie Stewart			**3**
Mar	5	*Sweet Nell of Old Drury* (P)	
Judith Anderson & Leon Gordon			**2**
Apr	2	*Tea for Three* (P)	

Theatre Royal

			weeks
Maurice Moscovitch			**11**
	20	*The Fare* (P)	1
	30	*The Ringer* (P)	10
Marie Burke			**4**
Jul	9	*Frasquita* (M)	
Victorian Opera Co.			
Aug	8	*Florodora* (M)	
Thurza Rogers & JCW Musical Comedy Co.			**4**
	13	*Tip Toes* (M)	
Peter Gawthorne			**1**
Sep	1	Matinees: *Hamlet* (P)	
Marie Burke & R Barrett-Lennard			**6**
Oct	13	*The Whole Town's Talking* (P)	5
Nov	19	*Outward Bound* (P)	1
Margaret Lawrence & Louis Bennison			**3**
	26	*Our Wife* (P)	
R Barrett-Lennard, Cecil Kellaway, Irene North & The New Musical Comedy Co.			**5**
Dec	23	*Queen High* (M)	

1928

Maurice Moscovitch			**8**
Jan	28	*The Terror* (P)	
Leon Gordon			**4**
Mar	31	*The Trial of Mary Dugan* (P)	
Annie Croft, Richard Sharland & JCW New Musical Comedy Co.			**11**
Apr	28	*The Girl Friend* (M)	
Jun	14	Gala Performance for Kingsford Smith and his Comrades in their epoch making Flight from America	
Irene Homer			**9**
Jul	14	*The Patsy* (P)	
Maurice Moscovitch			**7**
Sep	22	*The Ringer* (P)	
Leon Gordon			**4**
Nov	24	*Interference* (P)	
Margaret Bannerman & Anthony Prinsep's London Co.			**13**
Dec	22	*Other Men's Wives* (P)	4

1929

Jan	26	*Victory* (P)	4
Feb	23	*The Marionettes* (P)	5
Maisie Gay			**7**
Mar	30	*This Year of Grace* (P)	
Alfred Frith & Helen Patterson			**6**
May	18	*The Five O'Clock Girl* (M) Transferred to HMT June 25	
Jun	29	Sir Harry Lauder	2
Nat Madison			**3**
Jul	20	*Dracula* (P) (Trained nurse in attendance at theatre)	
RC Sheriff & Maurice Brown producers			**10**
Aug	10	*Journey's End* (P)	
Leon Gordon			**1**
Oct	26	*Brewster's Millions* (P) to Comedy Theatre Nov 2	
Alfred Frith & Cecil Kellaway			**3**
Nov	2	*Hold Everything* (M)	
Gus Bluett, Leo Franklyn & Cecil Kellaway			**11**
Dec	26	*Turned Up* (M)	6

1930

Feb	8	*Follow Through* (M)	5
Gladys Moncrieff			**9**
Mar	15	*The Maid of the Mountains* (M)	6
Apr	26	*The Merry Widow* (M)	2

Theatre Royal

			weeks
May	17	*Katinka* (M)	1
Marie Bremner & Leo Franklyn			**15**
	31	*The Belle of New York* (M)	5
Jun	16	Gala Performance for Amy Johnson British flyer	
Jul	6	*A Country Girl* (M)	1
	19	*New Moon* (M)	6
Sep	4	*Lilac Time* (M)	3
Josie Melville & Hindle Edgar			**8**
Oct	11	*Mr Cinders* (M)	4
Nov	15	*The Cingalee* (M)	4
Arthur Stigant & Roy Rene			**5**
Dec	20	*The House That Jack Built* (Pa)	

1931

			weeks
Elsie Prince, Gus Bluett, Cecil Kellaway, Leo Franklyn & Bertha Riccardo			**9**
Jan	31	*Sons O'Guns* (M)	
Ivan Menzies, Marie Bremner, Gregory Stroud & JCW Gilbert & Sullivan Opera Co.			**13**
Apr	11	*Gondoliers* (M)	3
May	2	*The Pirates of Penzance* (M) and *Trial by Jury* (M)	1
	16	*Iolanthe* (M)	2
	30	*The Mikado* (M)	3
Jun	27	*The Yeomen of the Guard* (M)	2
Jul	11	*Pinafore* (M) and *Cox and Box* (M)	2
	25	*Patience* (M)	
Grand Opera Season with Bernard Heinze, Alice Orff-Solscher, Joseph Hislop			**1**
Aug	1	*Carmen* (O)	
		Faust (O)	
		La Tosca (O)	
Dorothy Brunton & JCW Comic Opera Co.			**14**
	22	*The Duchess of Dantzic* (M)	3
Sep	12	*Dearest Enemy* (M)	4
Oct	10	*Florodora* (M)	4
Nov	7	*The Merry Widow* (M)	2
	10	Gala Performance for South African Cricketers	
	21	*Oh Lady Lady* (M)	1
Gladys Moncrieff			**2**
Dec	5	*Maid of the Mountains* (M)	
JCW Production			**5**
	26	*Sinbad the Sailor* (Pa)	

Princess Theatre

1886

Refurbished by William Pitt for Williamson, Garner and Musgrove, the theatre reopened on Dec 18 1886.

			weeks
Nellie Stewart & Royal Comic Opera Co.			**7**
Dec	18	*The Mikado* (M)	2

1887

			weeks
Jan	8	*The Pirates of Penzance* (M)	2
	22	*Iolanthe* (M)	1
	29	*Patience* (M)	1
Feb	4	*Mikado* (M) – Benefit for Nellie Stewart	
	5	*Billee Taylor* (M) and *Charity Begins at Home* (M)	1
	14	Farewell Performances of Royal Comic Opera Co.	
William Elton & Royal Comedy Co.			**10**
	26	*Harbour Lights* (P)	8
Apr	2	Matinee Benefit for family of actor–manager William Hoskins	
	30	*The Magistrate* (P)	2
GW Anson, Alfred Maltby & George Titherage			**8**
May	14	*Hazel Kirke* (P)	1
	14	Matinee – *The Palace of Truth* (P) with Kate Bishop (Hospital Benefit)	
	21	*A Night Off* (P)	3
	28	Matinee Performance Benefit for Mr S Genese	
Jubilee Performances for Queen Victoria's reign 1837–1887			**4**
Jun	18	*Betsy* (P)	
	21	*A Night Off* (P)	
	23	*The Professor* (P)	
	25	*The Silver King* (P)	
Royal Comic Opera Co.			**30**
Jul	16	*Princess Ida* (M)	4
Aug	20	*Dorothy* (M)	4
Sep	24	*The Mikado* (M)	1
Oct	1	*Les Cloches de Corneville* (M)	1
	8	*La Mascotte* (M)	1
	15	*La Fille Du Tambour Major* (M)	2
	29	*La Mascotte* (M)	2
Nov	12	*The Mikado* (M)	1
	19	*Iolanthe* (M)	1
	26	*Patience* (M)	1
Dec	3	*Pinafore* (M)	2
	17	*The Pirates of Penzance* (M)	1
	26	*Erminie* (M)	4

1888

			weeks
	28	*Dorothy* (M) (Nellie Stewart)	5
Royal Opera Co.			**2**
Mar	3	*Faust* (O) In English with Federici as Mephistopheles	
Mar	17	*Faust* – Benefit for Federici, who died while performing	
Charles Warner			**11**
	31	*School for Scandal* (P)	1
Apr	7	*London Assurance* (P)	1
	14	*The Fools Revenge* (P)	1
	21	*Old Heads and Young Hearts* (P)	1
	28	*The Lady of Lyons* (P)	1
May	5	*The Barrister* (P)	2
	19	*Dora* (P)	1
	26	*Hamlet* (P)	1
Jun	2	*School for Scandal* (P)	
	5	*The Fool's Revenge* (P)	

Princess Theatre

			weeks
	7	*Old Heads & Young Hearts* (P)	
	9	*The Lady of Lyons* (P)	
	12	*London Assurance* (P)	
	14	Farewell Benefit for Charles Warner	
Nellie Farren, Fred Leslie and London Gaiety Burlesque Co.			**9**
	16	*Monte Cristo* (Bu)	5
Jul	21	*Miss Esmerelda* (Bu)	4
Essie Jenyns & WJ Holloway's Shakespearean Co.			**9**
Aug	18	*Merchant of Venice* (P)	1
	25	*As You Like It* (P)	1
Sep	1	*Much Ado about Nothing* (P)	2
	15	*Pygmalion and Galatea* (P)	2
	29	*Romeo and Juliet* (P)	1
Oct	6	*Twelfth Night* (P)	2
	13	Matinee in aid of sick children *Cymbelink, King of Britain* (P)	
	16	Matinee Benefit for Essie Jenyns	
Royal Comic Opera Co.			**36**
	20	*Olivette* (M)	2
Nov	3	*The Mikado* (M)	2
	17	*La Mascotte* (M)	2
Dec	1	*Iolanthe* (M)	1
	8	*Princess Ida* (M)	2
	26	*Dorothy* (M)	5

1889

			weeks
Feb	2	*The Mikado* (M)	1
	9	*Pepita* (M)	5
Mar	16	*Erminie* (M) and *Charity Begins at Home* (Musical Proverb)	2
Mar	30	*Pirates of Penzance* (M) and *Charity Begins at Home* (M)	2
Apr	13	*Dorothy* (M)	1
	20	*The Yeomen of the Guard* (M)	7
Jun	8	*Patience* (M)	2
	22	*HMS Pinafore* (M)	1
	29	*Dorothy* (M)	1
Jennie Lee			**9**
Jul	6	*Jo* (P)	3
	27	*The Grasshopper* (P)	3
Aug	17	*Jack in the Box* (P)	3
Sep	7	Matinee – Testimonial Benefit to Signor & Signora Majeroni	
Janet Achurch & Charles Charrington			**5**
	14	*A Doll's House* (P)	2
	28	*The New Magdalen* (P)	2
Oct	12	*Pygmalion and Galatea* (P)	1
Henry Edwards & Olive Berkley			**8**
	19	*Little Lord Fauntleroy* (P)	
Royal Comic Opera Co.			**1**
Dec	14	*Yeomen of the Guard* (M)	
William Elton & Janet Achurch			**7**
	26	*That Dr Cupid* (P)	4

1890

			weeks
Jan	25	*The Guv'nor* (P)	2
Feb	8	*Our Boys* (P)	1
Janet Achurch			**2**
	15	*Two Nights in Rome* (P)	
Mrs Brown-Potter & Kyrle Bellew			**4**
Mar	1	*Camille* (P)	1
	8	*The Lady of Lyons* (P)	1
	15	*La Tosca* (P)	2
JL Toole			**8**
Apr	5	*A Fool and His Money* (P)	1
	12	*Artful Cards* (P) and *The Steeplechase* (P)	1
	19	*Dot or the Cricket on the Hearth* (P)	1

Princess Theatre

			weeks
	26	*The Don* (P)	1
May	3	*Paul Pry* (P) and *Off the Line* (P)	1
	10	*Uncle Dick's Darling* (P)	1
	17	*The Serious Family* (P)	1
	24	*The Don* (P) and Burlesque Scientific Lectures	
	29	*Artful Cards* (P) The Trial Scene from Pickwick (P)	
Jun	2	*The Serious Family* (P) and *The Birthplace of Podgers* (P)	
	4	*Off the Line* (P) and *The Steeplechase* (P)	
	5	Benefit for JL Toole – Various scenes and acts from his plays	
Henry Edwards & Olive Berkley			**2**
	7	*Little Lord Fauntleroy* (P)	
Mrs Brown-Potter & Kyrle Bellew			**11**
	21	*Our Bitterest Foe* (P)	2
Jul	7	*Romeo and Juliet* (P)	3
Aug	2	*La Tosca* (P)	1
	9	*Frou Frou* (P)	1
	16	*Mademoiselle de Bressier* (P)	1
	23	*Hero and Leander* (P) (first production on any stage in the world)	2
Sep	6	*Camille* (P)	1
Royal Comic Opera Co.			**37**
	13	*Dorothy* (M)	2
	27	*The Mikado* (M)	2
Oct	11	*La Mascotte* (M)	2
	25	*The Gondoliers* (M)	8
Dec	20	*Marjorie* (M)	5

1891

			weeks
Jan	17	*The Pirates of Penzance* (M)	1
	24	*Iolanthe* (M)	2
Feb	7	*Princess Ida* (M)	1
	14	*Yeomen of the Guard* (M)	1
	21	*The Gondoliers* (M)	2
Mar	14	*Pepita* (M)	4
Apr	11	*The Old Guard* (M)	7
Sarah Bernhardt			**4**
May	30	Season of 24 nights and 4 matinees includes: *La Tosca* (P) *Fedora* (P) *La Dame aux camelias* (P) *Cleopatra* (P) *Adrienne Lecouvreur* (P) *Theodora* (P) *Frou Frou* (P) *Jeanne D'Arc* (P) *Camille* (P)	
Nellie Farren, Fred Leslie & London Gaiety Burlesque Co.			**10**
Jun	27	*Ruy Blas and Blasé Roué* (Bu)	7
Aug	22	*Cinder Ellen up Too Late* (Bu)	3
Maggie Moore & GH Snazelle			**5**
Sep	12	*The Late Lamented* (P)	2
	26	*Kindred Souls* (P)	1
Oct	5	*Our Flat* (P)	2
JC Williamson			**1**
	24	*Kerry* (P) (1 act) *Rip Van Winkle* (P) (3 acts)	
Royal Comic Opera Co.			**27**
	31	*The Old Guard* (M)	3
Nov	21	*The Gondoliers* (M)	2
Dec	5	*Marjorie* (M)	1
	12	*Iolanthe* (M)	1
	19	*Yeomen of the Guard* (M)	1
	26	*The Merry Monach* (M)	4

Princess Theatre

1892

			weeks
		Australia is gripped by financial crisis. End of land boom.	
Jan	9	Matinee Benefit for Aust Drama & Music Assoc.	
	23	*The Old Guard* (M)	2
Feb	6	*Iolanthe* (M)	1
		Charity Begins at Home (M)	
	13	*La Cigale* (M)	5
Mar	26	*Dorothy* (M)	2
Apr	9	*The Gondoliers* (M)	1
	14	Matinee – Testimonial to William Elton	
	16	*Carmen* (M)	2
	30	*The Mikado* (M)	1
May	7	*La Cigale* (M)	1
Grand Italian Opera Season			**6**
	14	*Lucia di Lammermoor* (O)	
		La Traviata (O)	
		The Barber of Seville (O)	
		Faust (O)	
		Rigoletto (O)	
Jun	8	Grand Festival Concert with Italian Artists	
	11	*Rigoletto* (O)	
	15	*Maritana* (O) – English Opera	
	16	*Lucia di Lammermoor* (O)	
	21	*La Sonnambula* (O)	
	22	Foli Combination Concerts –	
	25	Italian & English Opera Singers	
	25	Matinee – Testimonial to Alfred Dampier	
		Theatre sub-leased to George Rignold Jul 2–Aug 17. JCW resumes direction Aug 20	
Walter Bentley			**5**
Aug	20	*The Silver King* (P)	4
Sep	17	*Hamlet* (P)	
	20	*The Bells* (P)	
	23	Farewell Benefit to Walter Bentley	
George Carey & E Sass & Co.			**2**
	24	*The Lost Paradise* (P)	
Henrietta Watson, E Sass, Maud Williamson & Albert Lucas			**1**
Oct	8	*The Pointsman* (P)	
		The Theatre leased 15–28 to Tom Pollard for the first appearance of his Juvenile Opera Co.	
London Gaiety Burlesque Co. (managed by George Musgrove)			**6**
	29	*Faust up to Date* (Bu)	1
Nov	5	*Carmen up to Date* (Bu)	1
	12	*Joan of Arc* (Bu)	1
	19	*Miss Esmeralda* (Bu)	3
Dec	12	Closed until Boxing Day	
Williamson & Musgrove production			**7**
	26	*Ali Baba and the Forty Thieves* (Pa)	

1893

			weeks
Royal Comic Opera Co.			**16**
Feb	18	*Dorothy* (M)	1
	22	Matinee Benefit for Brisbane flood victims	
	25	*Pepita* (M)	1
Mar	4	*The Gondoliers* (M)	1
	11	*The Old Guard* (M)	2
		Iolanthe (M)	1
		Yeomen of the Guard (M)	
		The Mikado (M)	
Apr	1	*The Mountebanks* (M)	5
May	6	*La Cigale* (M)	2
	20	*The Vicar of Bray* (M)	2

Princess Theatre

			weeks
Jun	3	*Trial by Jury* (M) and *The Vicar of Bray* (M)	1
London Gaiety Burlesque Co.			**2**
	17	*Faust up to Date* (Bu) *Joan of Arc* (Bu) *Carmen up to Date* (Bu) *Miss Esmeralda* (Bu)	
Jul	7	Grand Farewell Performance	
Bland Holt			**2**
	8	*A Million of Money* (P)	
	20	Matinee Benefit for Aust Drama and Music Association	
Ed Terry			**5**
	29	*Sweet Lavender* (P)	1
Aug	7	*In Chancery* (P)	1
	12	*Liberty Hall* (P)	1
	19	*The Churchwarden* (P)	1
	26	*The Rocket* (P)	1
	31	Farewell Performance of Ed Terry	
Robert Courtneidge & Ethel Haydon			**1**
Sep	2	*On Change* (P)	
Italian Opera & Grand Ballet			**6**
	9	*I Pagliacci* (O) *Turquoisette* (B)	2
	25	*Cavalleria Rusticana* (O)	
Oct	14	*I Pagliacci* (O)	
	19	*L'Amico Fritz* (O)	
Brough Boucicault Co.			**6**
Oct	21	*The Amazons* (P)	2
Nov	4	*The Magistrate* (P) *The Idler* (P) *Niobe* (P)	1
	11	*A Village Priest* (P)	1
	18	*The Guardsman* (P) and *Open Gate* (P)	
	22	*Lady Bountiful* (P)	
	25	*Joseph's Sweetheart* (P) *Diplomacy* (P) *The Times* (P) *Dandy Dick* (P)	
Dec	8	Grand Farewell Performance	
Italian Opera Co.			**2**
	9	*I Pagliacci* (O) *Cavalleria Rusticana* (O) *Faust* (O) *L'Amico Fritz* (O)	
Williamson & Musgrove production			**6**
	26	*Little Red Riding Hood* (Pa) or *Harlequin Boy Blue*	

1894

			weeks
Nellie Stewart with Williamson & Musgrove's Royal Comic Opera Co.			**9**
Feb	10	*The Gondoliers* (M)	1
	17	*Dorothy* (M)	1
	24	*The Mountebanks* (M)	1
Mar	3	*The Mikado* (M)	1
	7	*The Pirates of Penzance* (M)	
	10	*La Mascotte* (M)	2
	24	*Paul Jones* (M)	2
Apr	7	*La Cigale* (M)	
	10	*Princess Ida* (M)	
Bland Holt			**8**
	14	*A Woman's Revenge* (P)	2
	28	*The Prodigal Daughter* (P)	3
May	19	*A Life of Pleasure* (P)	3
Royal Comic Opera Co.			**7**
Jun	9	*The Vicar of Bray* (M)	1
	16	*Ma Mie Rosette* (M)	6
	22	Matinee Performance for Charles Ryley of Royal Comic Opera	
Jul	28	Theatre sub-leased to Brough–Boucicault – Oct 5	
William Elton			**4**
Oct	6	*Morocco Bound* (P)	3
	27	*Charley's Aunt* (P)	1

Princess Theatre

weeks

Royal Comic Opera Co. **6**

Nov 3 *Ma Mie Rosette* (M)
Paul Jones (M)
La Mascotte (M)
M'zelle Nitouche (M)
Predatoros (M)
La Cigale (M)

Dec 19 Mr Ernest Hosking performs two public seances

Williamson & Musgrove production **5**

22 *Beauty and the Beast* (Pa)

1895

Winter & Wheatley **4**

Feb 2 *Cinderella* (Bu)

Mar 8 Matinee Benefit to Horace Wheatley

Company of English Actors **4**

9 *The New Boy* (P) and *New Tableaux* – a series of 18 'Living Pictures'

Apr 9 Marie Elster's Farewell

George Edwardes Co. **7**

10 *HMS. Pinafore* (M) Benefit for Jewish Philanthropic Society

13 *A Gaiety Girl* (M) 3

May 4 *In Town* (M) 3

25 *The Shop Girl* (M) 1

Jun 1 Theatre sub-leased to Brough–Boucicault, Jun 1–Aug 23.

Royal Comic Opera Co. **4**

24 *La Fille de Madame Angot* (M) 1

31 *Ma Mie Rosette* (M) 1

Sep 7 *An Arcadian Eve* (M) 1

14 *Paul Jones* (M)

17 *Dorothy* (M)

19 *The Mikado* (M)

weeks

George Edwardes Co. **5**

21 *Gentleman Joe* (M) 1

28 *The Shop Girl* (M) 2

Oct 12 *A Gaiety Girl* (M) 1

19 *In Town* (M) 1

Royal Comic Opera Co. **8**

26 *The Old Guard* (M) 1

Nov 1 Matinee Benefit for George Lauri

2 *Ma Mie Rosette* (M)

4 *La Fille de Madame Angot* (M)

5 *The Old Guard* (M)

6 *La Mascotte* (M)

8 *An Arcadian Eve* (M) and *The Vicar of Bray* (M)

9 *The Gondoliers* (M) 2

23 *The Yeomen of the Guard* (M) 1

30 *The Mikado* and *Charity Begins at Home* (M) 1

Dec 4 Matinee Benefit for Signora Majeroni

7 *La Belle Therese* (M) 2

25 Festival of sacred songs

Williamson & Musgrove production **7**

26 *Djin-Djin (The Japanese Bogie Man)* (Pa)

1896

Theatre sub-leased to Brough and Boucicault from Feb 15. Last season of their partnership formed in 1886.

Mar 28 Matinee – Testimonial to Boucicault – *The Amazons* (P)

Palmer's & Brady's New York Co. **5**

Apr 6 *Trilby* (P)

Royal Comic Opera Co. **3**

May 16 *Miss Decima* (M) 1

23 *In Town* (M) 2

Princess Theatre

			weeks
Mrs Brown-Potter & Kyrle Bellew			**6**
Jun	6	*As You Like It* (P)	2
	20	*Charlotte Corday* (P)	1
	27	*Camille* (P)	1
Jul	4	*La Tosca* (P)	1
	11	*David Garrick* (P) and *Cavalleria Rusticana* (P)	1
	18	Special Farewell Performance	
	21	*Trilby* (P)	
Nat Goodwin's Co.			**5**
	25	*A Gilded Fool* (P)	1
Aug	1	*In Mizzoura* (P)	1
	8	*The Rivals* (P)	1
	15	*The Ballad Monger* (P) and *The Rivals* (P)	1
	22	*The Nominee* (P)	1
Hoyt's Comedians			**9**
	29	*A Trip to Chinatown* (M)	6
Oct	10	*A Milk White Flag* (M)	3
Royal Comic Opera Co.			**9**
	31	*Djin-Djin* (Pa) and First Exhibition in Melbourne of Lumière Cinématographe	3
Nov	11	Matinee of the above showing Flemington on Cup Day	
		Theatre leased to Phil Goatcher for 4 weeks from Nov 21.	
Dec	26	*Matsa: The Queen of Fire* (Pa) (by Bert Royle and JC Williamson)	6

1897

Julius Knight with English & Australian Actors			**7**
Feb	13	*Prisoner of Zenda* (P)	4
Mar	13	*The Two Little Vagabonds* (P)	2
Apr	3	Matinee Benefit for Distressed Actors	
	3	*Prisoner of Zenda* (P)	1
	10	Farewell program of the two above plays	
Mrs Brown-Potter & Kyrle Bellew			**3**
	17	*Romeo and Juliet* (P)	
	22	*The School for Scandal* (P)	
	24	*Francillon* (P)	
	28	*The Ironmaster* (P)	
May	1	*The Merchant of Venice* (P)	
	5	*The Lady of Lyons* (P)	
	6	*David Garrick* (P) and *Cavalleria Rusticana* (P)	
Royal Comic Opera Co.			**2**
	8	*Lelamine* (M) Benefit for distressed actors	1
	15	*Matsa: The Queen of Fire* (Pa)	1
Paulton & Stanley Comedy Co.			**5**
	22	*A Night Out* (P)	2
Jun	10	Matinee: Concert in aid of Queen's Memorial Hospital and Melbourne Poor	
	12	*My Friend from India* (P)	2
	26	*My Friend from India* (P) and *Charity Begins at Home* (P)	
	29	Farewell to George Lauri of Royal Comic Opera	
	30	*Lelamine* (M) Benefit for abused children and distressed actors	
Jul	1	Matinee – Testimonial Concert to Alfred Moulton, composer of *Lelamine*	
Julius Knight			**9**
	3	*Sign of the Cross* (P)	
	5	Invitation to clergymen to attend free matinee	
	14	Matinee Benefit for infants in distress	

Princess Theatre

			weeks
Paulton & Stanley with Williamson & Musgrove Comedy Co.			**3**
Sep	4	*Too Much Johnson* (P)	1
	11	*Niobe* (P)	
	18	*In a Locket* (P)	1
	25	*My Friend from India* (P)	
Julius Knight & Ada Farrar			**4**
Oct	2	*A Royal Divorce* (P)	
Musical Comedy Co.			**6**
	30	*The Gay Parisienne* (M)	3
Nov	27	*The French Maid* (M)	3
Wilson Barrett & London Co.			**8**
Dec	18	*Claudian* (P)	2

1898

			weeks
Jan	8	*The Manxman* (P)	2
	26	*Virginius* (P)	
	29	*Ben-My-Chree* (P)	
Feb	12	*The Silver King* (P)	2
	25	Matinee – concert in aid of theatrical charities	
	26	*Hamlet* (P)	
Mar	1	*Othello* (P)	
	2	*Virginius* (P)	
Williamson & Musgrove Musical Comedy Co.			**9**
Mar	5	*The French Maid* (M)	2
	19	*The Gay Parisienne* (M)	2
Apr	2	*Babes in the Wood* (M)	5
Julius Knight			**2**
May	7	*The Royal Divorce*	
Wilson Barrett			**2**
	21	*The Manxman* (P)	
	24	*Claudian* (P)	
	26	*Ben-My-Chree* (P)	
	27	*Virginius* (P)	
	28	*Hamlet* (P)	
May	31	*The Silver King* (P)	
Jun	2	*Othello* (P)	
Pattie Browne			**5**
	4	*The Little Minister* (P)	4
Jul	2	*Sweet Nancy* (P)	1
		Theatre leased to Temple & Moulton on Jul 9.	
Julius Knight & Ada Farrar			**11**
	19	*Prisoner of Zenda* (P)	
	23	*The Sign of the Cross* (P)	2
Aug	9	250th performance of *Sign of the Cross*	
	13	*The Harbour Lights* (P)	4
Sep	17	*The Prisoner of Zenda* (P)	1
	24	*Under the Bed Robe* (P)	4
Royal Comic Opera Co.			**11**
Oct	26	*La Poupée* (M)	4
Nov	24	Matinee Benefit for family of John Hennings	
	26	*The Mikado* (M)	1
Dec	3	*The Gondoliers* (M)	1
	10	*Yeomen of the Guard* (M)	
	17	*The Geisha* (M)	5

1899

			weeks
Jan	24	Concert in aid of Funds for Theatrical Charities	
		Theatre sub-leased to Robert Brough on Feb 4.	
Company of Comedians from Casino Theatre, New York			**5**
Apr	1	*The Belle of New York* (M)	
Julius Knight & Ada Farrar			**2**
May	6	*Pygmalion and Galatea* (P) and *A White Stocking* (P)	
	9	*The Prisoner of Zenda* (P)	
	11	*The Harbour Lights* (P)	
	15	*A Royal Divorce* (P)	
	17	*The Sign of the Cross* (P)	

Princess Theatre

			weeks
	18	Farewell Matinee for Julius Knight – *The Sign of the Cross*	
Williamson & Musgrove production			**6**
Jun	17	*The King's Musketeer* (P)	
The Harry Conor Comedy Season			**5**
Jul	29	*A Trip to China Town* (P)	2
Aug	12	*A Stranger in New York* (P)	2
Sep	2	*A Trip to China Town* (P)	1
Royal Comic Opera Co.			**7**
	8	*The Geisha* (M)	3
	30	*Iolanthe* (M)	2
Oct	14	*La Poupée* (M)	1
	21	*Ma Mie Rosette* (M)	1
	28	*The Gondoliers* (M)	
Nov	1	*The Mikado* (M)	
		Theatre sub-leased to Robert Brough for 6 weeks from Nov 4.	
Dec	16	Giant Benefit in aid of the Old Actors' Homes and theatrical charities for which Williamson & Musgrove were responsible	

1900

Feb	24	*Little Red Riding Hood* (Pa)	6
Mar	17	Anglo-American Bio-Tableau featuring 'first time ever Genuine War Pictures, including capture of Boer's stronghold'	
Apr	4	Grand Combination Matinee by entire entertainment industry in Melbourne, in aid of Melbourne Hospital Bazaar	

1904

Proprietor and lessee George Musgrove.

			weeks
JCW New Comedy Co.			**2**
Apr	30	*The Marriage of Kitty* (P)	
George Edwardes London Gaiety Co.			**7**
May	21	*Three Little Maids* (M)	1
Jun	4	*The Girl from Kay's* (M)	3
	25	*Kitty Grey* (M)	3
Minnie Tittell Brune & JCW Dramatic Co.			**5**
Dec	24	*L'Aiglon* (P)	2

1905

Jan	11	*Camille* (P)	1
	21	*Romeo and Juliet* (P)	2
JCW Comedy Co.			**2**
Mar	11	*The Duke of Killiecrankie* (P)	
Minnie Tittell Brune & JCW Dramatic Co.			**4**
Apr	22	*Theodora* (P)	2
May	10	*Camille* (P)	
	13	*Sunday* (P)	
	20	*L'Aiglon* (P)	
	24	*Romeo and Juliet* (P)	
	27	*The Second Mrs Tanqueray* (P)	1
JJ Dallas & Florence Lloyd with Strand Comedy Co.			**2**
Sep	9	*The JP* (P)	
Maud Jeffries & Julius Knight			**4**
	23	*His Majesty's Servant* (P)	1
Oct	4	*Monsieur Beaucaire* (P)	
	7	*The Darling of the Gods* (P)	1
	14	*Davy Garrick* (P) and *Comedy and Tragedy* (P)	1
	21	*The Silver King* (P)	
	25	*A Royal Divorce* (P)	
	27	*The Lady of Lyons* (P)	

Princess Theatre

			weeks
JCW's Gilbert & Sullivan Opera Co.			**6**
Dec	23	*HMS. Pinafore* (M)	
	25	Concert by Principal Ladies of Gilbert & Sullivan Opera Co.	

1906

Jan	3	*The Gondoliers* (M)	
	6	*Princess Ida* (M)	
	13	*The Sorcerer* (M) and *Trial by Jury* (M)	
	17	*The Yeomen of the Guard* (M)	
	20	*Utopia Ltd* (M)	2
Feb	10	*Patience* (M)	
	15	*The Mikado* (M)	

1907

Jun	12	*Mother Goose* (Pa)	1
JCW New Musical Comedy Co.			**9**
	22	*The Blue Moon* (M)	7
Aug	3	*Lady Madcap* (M)	2
Ernest Leicester			**2**
	17	*Human Hearts* (P)	
Julius Knight			**6**
	31	*Robin Hood* (P)	2
Sep	14	*Raffles* (P)	2
Oct	5	*Monsieur Beaucaire* (P)	1
	12	*Brigadier Gerard* (P)	1
Andrew Mack			**1**
Nov	23	*Tom Moore* (P)	

1908

			weeks
JCW's New Comedy Co.			**2**
Mar	7	*Brewsters Millions* (P) moved Mar 21 to HMT	
Minnie Tittell Brune			**10**
Apr	18	*Peter Pan* (P)	4
May	9	Matinee – seats reserved for children from all the charitable organisations in Melbourne	
Jun	27	*Mrs Wiggs of the Cabbage Patch* (P)	6
JCW's Musical Co.			**11**
Aug	29	*The Red Mill* (M)	5
Sep	26	Matinee *The Vicissitudes of Vivienne* (P) Benefit for the City Newsboys Building Fund	
Oct	31	*The Prince of Pilsen* (M)	4
Nov	21	Matinee *The Liars* (P) Benefit for the Foundling Hospital and Infants Home, East Melbourne	
	28	*The Red Mill* (M)	1
Dec	5	*The Belle of New York* (M)	1
		Matinee *The Liars* (P) in aid of the Distressed Actors Fund	

1909

Nellie Stewart			**7**
Apr	10	*Sweet Kitty Bellairs* (P)	
Julius Knight & JCW Dramatic Co.			**4**
Jun	26	*A Royal Divorce* (P)	3
Aug	28	*The Flag Lieutenant* (P)	1
GS Titheradge			**1**
Sep	4	*The Village Priest* (P)	
Thomas Kingston			**1**
	11	*Sherlock Holmes* (P)	
GS Titheradge & Wilfred Denver			**1**
	18	*The Silver King* (P)	
Nellie Stewart			**8**
Oct	30	*Sweet Kitty Bellairs* (P)	1
Nov	3	*Sweet Nell of Old Drury* (P)	
	6	*Za Za* (P)	2

Princess Theatre

weeks

1910

Mar 26 *What Every Woman Knows* (P) 3

Apr 23 *When Knighthood Was in Flower* (P) 2

Royal Comic Opera Co. 1

Jul 30 *The Girls of Gottenberg* (M)

Julius Knight 6

Aug 20 *The Third Degree* (P) with Katherine Grey 2

Sep 10 *Henry of Navarre* (P) with Ethel Warwick 2

24 *Sign of the Cross* (P) 2

Oct 6 Farewell Matinee for Julius Knight. Special performance of *Pygmalion and Galatea* (P) with Maud Jeffries. 'Souvenir photograph of Knight (produced by Syd Day) given to every lady in the audience.'

weeks

New English Farce Co. 2

10 *The Brass Bottle* (P)

New Comic Opera Co. 6

29 *A Knight for a Day* (M) 4

Nov 26 *The Dollar Princess* (M) 2

1911

Apr 12 *Olivetta* (P) Benefit for Old Colonists Home Fund

Katherine Grey & William Desmond 6

15 *Paid in Full* (P) 2

29 *The Dawn of Tomorrow* (P) 2

May 13 *Arms and the Man* (P) 1

20 *The Third Degree* (P) and *The Lion and the Mouse* (P) 1

Jul 29 *Veronique* (P) Benefit for the Austin Hospital

William Desmond 6

5 *Silver King* (P) 1

12 *Via Wireless* (P) 2

Sep 2 *The Speckled Band* (P) 3

Her Majesty's Theatre

			weeks
1900			
		The former Alexandra Theatre commences its new career.	
Williamson Opera Co.			**2**
May	19	Grand Opening Performance *HMS Pinafore* (M)	1
	26	*The Pirates of Penzance* (M) plus Bio-Tableau – new war films	1
Nance O'Neill			**12**
Jun	2	*Magda* (P)	2
	16	*Queen Elizabeth* (P)	2
	30	*School for Scandal* (P)	1
Jul	1	*Camille* (P)	2
	20	Matinee in aid of Melbourne Hospital – *Hedda Gabler* (P)	
	21	*Peg Woffington* (P)	1
	28	*Fedora* (P)	2
Aug	11	*Tess of the T'Urbervilles* (P)	1
	23	*Magda* (P)	
	24	*Hedda Gabler* (P)	
	25	*Ingomar* (P)	
	29	Combined program for last night of season	
JCW Dramatic Co. & Crane-Power Co.			**5**
Sep	1	*Trilby* (P)	1
	8	*The Christian* (P)	2
	26	*Tess of the D'Urbervilles* (P)	
	29	*The Only Way* (P)	2
Oct	13	*Trilby* (P)	
		Her Majesty's Theatre Closed for Alterations until Oct 27	
JCW Opera Co.			**17**
	27	*The Rose of Persia* (M)	4
Nov	24	*The Old Guard* (M)	2
Dec	8	*HMS. Pinafore* (M)	1
	15	*Florodora* (M) with Grace Palotta	10
1901			
Feb	2	Theatre closed. Day of national mourning for Queen Victoria who died Jan 24	
	8	Complimentary Send-off to George Darrell	
Nance O'Neill			**6**
Apr	6	*La Tosca* (P)	
	13	*Magda* (P)	
	16	*Fedora* (P)	
	18	*Peg Woffington* (P)	
	20	*Lady Inger of Ostrat* (P)	
	27	*Queen Elizabeth* (P)	
May	1	*Camille* (P)	
	2	*School for Scandal* (P)	
	4	*Macbeth* (P)	
JCW Dramatic Co.			**2**
	17	*A Royal Divorce* (P)	
JCW Italian Opera Co.			**8**
Jun	1	*Aida* (O) (250 persons in production)	
	6	*Lucia Di Lammermoor* (O)	
	8	*Aida* (O)	
	10	*Lucia Di Lammermoor* (O)	
	12	*Aida* (O)	
	13	*Lucia Di Lammermoor* (O)	
	15	*Ernani* (O)	
	19	*Lucia Di Lammermoor* (O)	
	20	*Ernani* (O)	
	22	*Lucia Di Lammermoor* (O)	
	24	*Ernani* (O)	
	25	*Aida* (O)	
	29	*I Pagliacci* and *Cavalleria Rusticana* (O)	

Her Majesty's Theatre

			weeks
Jul	6	*I Pagliacci* and *Cavalleria Rusticana* (O)	
	13	*La Bohème* (O)	
	20	*Un Ballo in Maschera* (O)	
	24	*La Bohème* (O)	
	27	*Rigoletto* (O)	
	31	Last night of season. Artists in Favourite Roles	
Wilson Barrett & his London Co.			**8**
Aug	3	*Man and His Makers* (P)	
	10	*The Manxman* (P)	
	17	*The Sign of the Cross* (P)	
	31	*The Silver King* (P)	
Sept	10	*Quo Vadis* (P)	
	14	*The Christian King* (P)	
	27	*The Christian King* (P) matinee in aid of The World's Fair	
	28	*Virginius* (P)	
	30	*Hamlet* (P)	
Oct	1	*Othello* (P)	
	2	*Claudian* (P)	
JCW Comic Opera Co.			**5**
	5	*The Casino Girl* (M)	3
	26	*The Gondoliers* (M)	1
Nov	2	*Florodora* (M)	
	9	*The Old Guard* (M)	
	14	Matinee concert in aid of Theatrical Charities for 1901	
Italian Opera Co.			**5**
	16	*Faust* (O)	
	19	*Il Trovatore* (O)	
	23	*Otello* (O)	
	26	*La Bohème* (O)	
	27	*Lucia* (O)	
	28	*Otello* (O)	
	29	*La Bohème* (O)	
Dec	2	*La Giocondo* (O)	
	3	*Rigoletto* (O)	
	4	Matinee: *La Bohème* (O) Evening: La Gioconda (O)	
	5	*Faust* (O)	
	6	*La Gioconda* (O)	
	7	*La Traviata* (O)	
	10	*Otello* (O)	
	11	*Rigoletto* (O)	
	12	*Otello* (O)	
	13	*La Traviata* (O)	
	14	*Fedora* (O)	
	17	*La Gioconda* (O)	
	18	*I Pagliacci* and *Cavalleria Rusticana* (O)	
	19	*Fedora* and *I Promessi Sposi*(O)	
	20	Farewell Program	
Royal Comic Opera Co.			**18**
	21	*San Toy* or *Emperors Own* (M) 'Florence Young appears on the Australian stage after an absence of 5 years'	8

1902

Feb	15	*A Runaway Girl* (M)	8
Apr	19	*Dorothy* (M)	2
	30	Complimentary concert to George Lauri	
Janet Waldorf & JCW Dramatic Co.			**4**
May	3	*As You Like It* (P)	1
	10	*Romeo and Juliet* (P)	1
	17	*Twelfth Night* (P)	
	22	*Camille* (P)	
	24	*A Royal Divorce* (P)	1
Jun	4	*Much Ado about Nothing* (P)	
	9	*Ingomar the Barbarian* (P)	
	10	*The Lady of Lyons* (P)	
	11	*Twelfth Night* (P)	

Her Majesty's Theatre

			weeks
	12	Complimentary benefit for Janet Waldorf featuring scenes from 5 of the above plays	
Royal Comic Opera Co.			**11**
	14	*Dorothy* (M)	1
	21	*Florodora* (M)	2
Jul	5	*Iolanthe* (M) and *Trial by Jury* (M)	2
	19	*A Circus Girl* (M)	2
Aug	9	*A Runaway Girl* (M)	1
	16	*Robin Hood* (M)	3
JCW Dramatic Co.			**3**
Sep	13	*Sherlock Holmes* (P)	
Royal Comic Opera Co.			**22**
Oct	11	*The Toreador* (M)	5
Nov	22	*The Mikado* (M)	2
Dec	6	*Paul Jones* (M)	2
JCW & George Musgrove production			
	26	*Dick Whittington & His Cat* (Pa)	5

1903

			weeks
Feb	28	*The Geisha* (M)	2
Mar	17	*The Emerald Isle* (M)	2
Apr	11	*Ma Mie Rosette* (M)	2
	25	*Paul Jones* (M)	1
May	2	*The Toreador* (M)	1
JCW Comedy Opera Co.			**3**
	9	*My Lady Molly* (M)	
	27	Farewell Matinee for Carrie Moore on her departure from Australia to work in London with George Edwardes	
Daniel Frawley & his American Co.			**5**
	30	*Secret Service* (P)	
Jun	13	*Madame Sans Gene* (P)	
	20	*Arizona* (P)	
Jul	7	Send-off to Hugh Ward on his departure for England	
JCW Musical Comedy Co.			**5**
	11	*The Belle of New York* (M)	
	25	*The Messenger Boy* (M)	
Aug	8	*A Runaway Girl* (M)	
	12	*San Toy* (250th performance in Australia) (M)	
JCW Dramatic Co.			**3**
	22	*If I Were King* (P)	
Julius Knight, Maud Jeffries & Beerbohm Tree's Co.			**11**
Sep	12	*Resurrection* (P)	4
Oct	10	*Monsieur Beaucaire* (P)	3
Nov	2	Matinee in aid of theatrical charities	
	7	*The Eternal City* (P)	3
	30	*Monsieur Beaucaire* (P)	1
Dec	12	*The Eternal City* (P)	
Royal Comic Opera Co.			**12**
Dec	26	*A Country Girl* (M)	11

1904

			weeks
Mar	21	*Ma Mie Rosette* (M)	1
	26	Matinee farewell to Peter Hughes	
Beerbohm Tree's Co.			**7**
Apr	2	*The Darling of the Gods* (P)	4
May	7	*The Sign of the Cross* (P) Played 500 times under JCW management.	2
	23	*The Silver King* (P)	1
	27	Farewell matinee to Johnny Wallace, veteran actor, producer and stage manager	
Jun		Theatre closed for extensive renovations 4–18	

Her Majesty's Theatre

			weeks
JCW Dramatic Co.			**7**
	18	*Sherlock Holmes* (P)	1
	25	*Admiral Crichton* (P)	2
Jul	13	*The Christian* (P)	
	16	*The Light That Failed* (P)	2
Aug	6	*Sunday* (P)	2
Royal Comic Opera Co.			**20**
	20	*Tapu* (M)	1
Sep	3	*My Lady Molly* (M)	1
	14	*The Mikado* (M)	
	17	*Patience* (M) and *Charity Begins at Home* (M)	2
Oct	5	*Dorothy* (M)	
	8	*Yeomen of the Guard* (M)	1
	15	*A Country Girl* (M)	1
	29	*The Orchid* (M)	10

1905

			weeks
Jan	7	*Florodora* (M)	2
	20	Complimentary night to George Lauri to celebrate his 14 years with the Royal Comic Opera Co.	
	21	*The Geisha* (M)	2
Feb	4	*Paul Jones* (M)	
	10	Send-Off to Florence Young *Paul Jones* (M)	
New English Comedy Co.			**2**
	11	*Cousin Kate* (P) and *The Rough Diamond* (P)	1
	18	*The Marriage of Kitty* (P)	1
Julius Knight & Maud Jeffries			**6**
	25	*A Royal Divorce* (P)	
Mar	18	*If I Were King* (P)	
	25	*Monsieur Beaucaire* (P)	
	29	*The Eternal City* (P)	
Apr	1	*The Sign of the Cross* (P)	
	5	*The Silver King* (P)	
	8	*Pygmalion and Galatea* (P)	
	12	*The Lady of Lyons* (P)	
Andrew Mack & his Co.			**8**
	15	*Tom Moore* (P)	3
May	6	*The Way to Kenmare* (P)	2
	20	*Arrah-na-Pogue* (P)	3
Jun	8	Matinee benefit to veteran manager and showman, GBW Lewis	
	10	*Tom Moore* (P)	
	14	*The Way to Kenmare* (P)	
Nance O'Neill & her Co.			**6**
	17	*Magda* (P)	1
	24	*The Fires of St John* (P)	1
Jul	1	*Queen Elizabeth* (P)	1
	8	*The School for Scandal* (P)	1
	15	*Ingomar* (P)	1
	22	*Trilby* (P)	1
Gilbert & Sullivan Repertoire Co.			**3**
Aug	5	*The Gondoliers* (M)	1
	12	*The Pirates of Penzance* (M)	
	16	*The Mikado* (M)	
	19	*Iolanthe* (M)	
	23	*HMS Pinafore* (M)	
Royal Comic Opera Co.			**16**
	26	*The Cingalee* (M)	9
Oct	21	*The Orchid* (M)	2
Nov	4	*A Country Girl* (M)	
	7	*Paul Jones* (M)	
	11	*Veronique* (M)	4
Dec	9	*The Girl from Kay's* (M)	1
	21	Theatrical Carnival at Prince's Court for theatrical charities	
Minnie Tittell Brune			**19**
Dec	26	*Merely Mary Ann* (P)	4

1906

Jan	27	*L'Aiglon* (P)	1
Feb	3	*Sunday* (P)	2

Her Majesty's Theatre

			weeks
	17	*La Tosca* (P)	1
Mar	3	*Leah Kleschna* (P)	3
	28	*L'Aiglon* (P)	1
Apr	7	*Camille* (P)	1
	14	*Dorothy Vernon* (P)	5
May	19	*Sunday* (P)	1
William Collier Co. with John Barrymore			**11**
	26	*The Dictator* (P)	3
Jun	16	*On the Quiet* (P)	3
Jul	7	*The Squaw Man* (P)	5
Aug	10	*The Christian* (P)	
Royal Comic Opera Co.			**17**
	11	*The Little Michus* (M)	4
Sep	8	Matinee in aid of the Foundling Hospital and Infants Home *La Poupée* (M)	
	15	*La Mascotte* (M)	2
Oct	1	*Paul Jones* (M)	
	6	*The Belle of New York* (M)	3
	27	*The Shop Girl* (M)	1
Nov	3	*The Spring Chicken* (M)	5
Dec	8	*The Girl from Kay's* (M)	2
JCW production			**12**
	22	*Mother Goose* (Pa)	

1907

Minnie Tittell Brune & JCW Dramatic Co.			**8**
Mar	23	*Parsifal* (P)	5
Apr	27	*Dorothy Vernon* (P)	1
May	4	*Sunday* (P)	1
	11	*Leah Kleshna* (P)	
	15	*Merely Mary Ann* (P)	
	18	*Romeo and Juliet* (P)	
	22	*Camille* (P)	
	25	*La Tosca* (P)	
	30	Farewell Program	
Charles Waldron & Ola Humphrey			**5**
Jun	1	*The Virginian* (P)	2
	15	*The Squaw Man* (P)	2
	29	*The Christian* (P)	1
Andrew Mack & his Co.			**8**
Jul	6	Grand Irish Welcome to Andrew Mack during *Tom Moore* (P)	
	13	*The Way to Kenmare* (P)	
	16	Matinee in aid of the Distressed Actors Fund	
	20	*Arrah-na-Pogue* (P)	
	27	*The Ragged Earl* (P) and *Jack Shannon* (P)	
Aug	17	*Tom Moore* (P)	
	27	*The Way to Kenmare* (P)	
	28	*Arrah-na-Pogue* (P)	
	29	Final Appearance of Andrew Mack	
Royal Comic Opera Co.			**14**
	31	*The Spring Chicken* (M)	1
Sep	7	*The Dairymaids* (M)	6
Oct	19	*Dorothy* (M)	
	26	*The Girls of Gottenberg* (M)	7
JCW production			**12**
Dec	21	*Humpty-Dumpty* (Pa)	10

1908

Mar	7	*Mother Goose* (Pa)	2
JCW New Comedy Co.			**5**
	21	*Brewsters Millions* (P)	
	30	Benefit for Jenny Lee (Jo) on her departure for Europe	
Thomas Kingston, Mrs Robert Brough & JCW Dramatic Co.			**3**
Apr	25	*John Glayde's Honour* (P)	2
May	9	*Sherlock Holmes* (P)	1

Her Majesty's Theatre

			weeks
George Edwardes & Royal Comic Opera Co. present Carrie Moore			**12**
	16	*Merry Widow* (M)	
		Merry Widow trips from country centres arranged with the Victorian Railways	
	30	*Pygmalion and Galatea* (P)	
		Matinee to equip new operating theatre at the Alfred Hospital	
Jul	30	Matinee by musical and dramatic profession for Actors Benevolent Fund	
Aug	1	*The Dairymaids* (M)	1
Minnie Tittell Brune & Special Co.			**2**
	8	*Peter Pan* (P)	
Margaret Anglin & George Titheradge			**9**
	22	*The Thief* (P)	2
Sep	12	*The Truth* (P)	2
	26	*The Taming of the Shrew* (P)	2
Oct	10	*Camille* (P)	1
	17	*Zira* (P)	1
	24	Farewell Performance – *Twelfth Night* (P)	1
Julius Knight & JCW Dramatic Co.			**5**
	31	*The Scarlet Pimpernel* (P)	5
Dec	2	*The Lady of Lyons* (P)	
	5	*Prisoner of Zenda* (P)	
JCW production			**14**
	19	*Jack and Jill* (Pa) featuring an ensemble of 350 people	

1909

			weeks
Minnie Tittell Brune & JCW Dramatic Co.			**6**
Mar	27	*The Girl of the Golden West* (P)	3
Apr	24	*Diana of Dobson's* (P)	2
May	5	*Sunday* (P)	1
JCW Presents			**3**
	15	*An Englishman's Home* (P)	
Ola Humphrey & Henry Kolker			**1**
Jun	5	*The Silver King* (P)	
JCW Presents			**5**
	12	*The King of Cadonia* (M)	
JCW New Comic Opera Co.			**2**
Jul	24	*Havana* (M)	
George Titherage, Ethel Warwick, Dorothy Grimston & Thomas Kingston			**2**
Aug	14	*The Flag Lieutenant* (P)	
Royal Comic Opera Co.			**14**
	28	*The Duchess of Dantzic* (M)	4
Sep	25	*The Girls of Gottenberg* (M)	1
Oct	2	*The Catch of the Season* (M)	3
	30	*The Merry Widow* (M)	3
Nov	20	*The Lady Dandies* (M)	3
JCW production			**10**
Dec	18	*Aladdin* (Pa)	

1910

			weeks
Julius Knight & JCW Dramatic Co.			**3**
Mar	5	*The Lion and the Mouse* (P)	
JCW New Comic Opera Co.			**6**
	26	*A Country Girl* (M)	2
Apr	9	*The Dollar Princess* (M)	4
May	9	Women's Hospital Bazaar Building Fund Matinee given by JCW Comic Opera Co.	
Farewell Appearance of Nellie Stewart			**1**
	14	*Sweet Nell of Old Drury* (P)	
Royal Comic Opera Co.			**10**
	21	*A Waltz Dream* (M)	6
Jun	10	Performance for Royal Comic Opera Co. Benefit's Fund	
Jul	2	*The Orchid* (M)	3

Her Majesty's Theatre

			weeks
	23	*The Girls of Gottenberg* (M)	1
Grand Opera in English with Bel Sorel & Amy Castles			**4**
	30	*Madame Butterfly* (O)	
Aug	27	*Carmen* (O)	
	29	*La Bohème* (O)	
	30	*Madame Butterfly* (O)	
	31	*Carmen* (O)	
Sep	1	*La Bohème* (O)	
	2	*Carmen* (O)	
	3	*La Bohème* (O)	
	5	*Carmen* (O)	
	6	*La Bohème* (O)	
	10	*Madame Butterfly* (O) Farewell Performance	
London Co. from Drury Lane			**12**
	17	*The Whip*	10
Nov	26	Harbour Lights (P)	2
JCW production			**14**
Dec	17	*Jack and the Beanstalk* (Pa)	

1911

			weeks
JCW Juvenile Opera Co.			
Apr	3	*The Geisha* (M)	
The New Comic Opera Co.			**14**
	8	*A Waltz Dream* (M)	2
	22	*The Merry Widow* (M)	2
May	1	Florence Young and the Opera Co. give an At Home in the lounge of Her Majesty's Theatre in aid of Funds for the Alfred Hospital	
	13	*Our Miss Gibbs* (M)	10
	16	A Testimonial matinee for Gerard Coventry	
Aug	5	Theatre closed for alterations 5–12	
HB Irving & Dorothea Baird			**8**
	26	*Hamlet* (P)	3
Sep	23	*The Lyons Mail* (P)	1
	30	*The Bells* (P)	2
Oct	14	*Louis XI* (P)	1
	21	*Dr Jekyll and Mr Hyde* (P)	1
The Melba–Williamson Grand Opera Season			**6**
	30	*Samson and Delilah* (O)	
	31	*Madame Butterfly* (O)	
Nov	1	Matinee – *Samson and Delilah* (O)	
		Evening – *La Traviata* (O)	
	2	*Madame Butterfly* (O)	
	3	*La Bohème* (O)	
	4	*Samson and Delilah* (O)	
	6	*Faust* (O)	
	7	*Carmen* (O)	
	8	*La Tosca* (O)	
	9	*Samson and Delilah* (O)	
	10	*La Tosca* (O)	
	11	*Faust* (O)	
	13	*Samson and Delilah* (O)	
	14	*La Bohème* (O)	
	18	*Carmen* (O)	
	20	*Romeo and Juliet* (O)	
	21	*Samson and Delilah* (O)	
	22	*La Bohème* (O)	
	23	*La Tosca* (O)	
	24	*Romeo and Juliet* (O)	
	25	*Lohengrin* (O)	
	27	*Faust* (O)	
	28	*Lohengrin* (O)	
	29	*Rigoletto* (O)	
	30	*Carmen* (O)	
Dec	1	*La Tosca* (O)	
	2	*Othello* (O)	
	4	*La Tosca* (O)	

Her Majesty's Theatre

			weeks
	5	*Rigoletto* (O)	
	6	*Aida* (O)	
	7	*Faust* (O)	
	8	*Samson and Delilah* (O)	
	9	Farewell Mixed Program (O)	
Royal Comic Opera Co.			**1**
	9	*Our Miss Gibbs* (M)	
JCW production			**14**
	23	*Sinbad the Sailor* (Pa)	

1912

			weeks
Mar	1	Melba's Matinee. A program of selected acts from various plays and operas in aid of the Building Fund for the New Concert Hall of the University Conservatorium of Music	
	22	At East Melbourne Cricket Ground Monster Theatrical Carnival in aid of the JCW Comic Opera Co. Sick Fund and the Musical and Dramatic Benevolent Fund. 'One Pound's Worth of Amusement For One Shilling'	
	23	Matinee by members of the Sinbad the Sailor Pantomime Co. and the New Comic Opera Co. for ET Steyne, producer of *The Girl in the Train* and *Sinbad the Sailor*	
JCW New Opera Co.			**9**
Apr	6	*The Girl in the Train* (M)	7
May	25	*The Cingalee* (M)	2
Quinlan Grand Opera Co.			**5**
Jun	8	Grand Opera in English	
		The Tales of Hoffman (O)	
		Tannhauser (O)	
		The Girl of the Golden West (O)	
		Rigoletto (O)	
		Tristan and Isolde (O)	
		The Prodigal Son (O)	
		Hansel and Gretel (O)	
		Valkyrie (O)	
		Aida (O)	
		La Bohème (O)	
		Carmen (O)	
		Lohengrin (O)	
		Madame Butterfly (O)	
		Faust (O)	
JCW Opera Co.			**12**
Jul	13	*The Quaker Girl* (M)	
Royal Comic Opera Co.			**9**
Oct	12	*Florodora* (M)	3
Nov	2	*Night Buds* (M)	6
JCW production			**11**
Dec	21	*Puss in Boots* (Pa) (350 in cast)	

1913

JCW New Comic Opera Co.			**9**
Mar	15	*The Chocolate Soldier* (M)	2
	29	*The Count of Luxembourg* (M)	7
May	12	*The Cingalee* (M)	
Royal Comic Opera Co.			**4**
	17	*The Sunshine Girl* (M)	3
Jun	14	*Miss Hook of Holland* (M)	1
Adeline Genée & Alexander Volinine & the Imperial Russian Ballet			**5**
	21	Repertoire includes	
		The Secret of Susanna (B)	
		Coppelia (B) *(from the Tales of Hoffman)*	
		Divertissements (B)	

			weeks
		JC Williamson dies in Paris on Jul 6. As a token of respect no performances were given at Her Majesty's Theatre and the Theatre Royal in Melbourne on Jul 7. All the theatres under the Firm's management in Sydney, Adelaide and New Zealand close for the day.	
Julius Knight & Irene Brown			**2**
Aug	2	*Bella Donna* (P)	
Quinlan Opera Co.			**8**
	16	*The Meistersingers* (O)	
		Rigoletto (O)	
		Rhinegold (O)	
		The Valkyrie (O)	
		Siegfried (O)	
		Twilight of the Gods (O)	
		Tales of Hoffman (O)	
		La Tosca (O)	
		Samson and Delilah (O)	
		Faust (O)	
		The Barber of Seville (O)	
		Aida (O)	
		Tannhauser (O)	
		Louise (O)	
		Lohengrin (O)	
		Marriage of Figaro (O)	
		La Bohème (O)	
Lewis Waller & Madge Titheradge			**2**
Oct	11	*Henry V* (P)	
New Comic Opera Co.			**8**
	25	*The Arcadians* (M)	3
Nov	15	*Autumn Manoeuvres* (M)	2
	29	*The Balkan Princess* (M)	3
JCW production			**14**
Dec	20	*The Forty Thieves* (Pa)	

1914

			weeks
First Revue Season			**8**
Mar	28	*Come over Here* (R)	
JCW Dramatic Co.			**4**
May	30	*Sealed Orders* (P)	
Gilbert & Sullivan Opera Co.			**7**
Jun	29	*The Gondoliers* (M)	
Jul	2	*The Mikado* (M)	
	11	*Iolanthe* (M)	
	18	*Yeomen of the Guard* (M)	
	25	*The Pirates of Penzance* (M) and *Trial by Jury* (M)	
Aug	1	**WAR DECLARED BETWEEN ENGLAND AND GERMANY**	
Aug	15	*Patience* (M)	
	22	*HMS Pinafore* (M) and *Trial by Jury* (M)	
	28	Matinee in aid of the Australian Patriotic Fund by Combined Theatrical Managements	
JCW production			**1**
	29	*Forty Thieves* (Pa)	
Royal Comic Opera Co.			**15**
Sep	5	*Gipsy Love* (M)	7
Oct	17	*Princess Caprice* (M)	1
	24	*The Girl in the Taxi* (M)	7
Dec	5	Matinee of opera in aid of the British Red Cross Society	
JCW production			**8**
	29	*Cinderella* (Pa)	

Her Majesty's Theatre

1915

			weeks
Gilbert & Sullivan Opera Co.			**3**
Mar	6	*The Yeomen of the Guard* (M)	
	13	*The Gondoliers* (M)	
		The Pirates of Penzance (M) and *Trial by Jury* (M)	
	20	*HMS Pinafore* (M)	
		Trial by Jury (M)	
		Mikado (M)	
JCW's New English Musical Comedy Co.			**8**
	27	*High Jinks* (M)	
JCW's Royal Comic Opera Co.			**6**
May	22	*The Marriage Market* (M)	4
Jun	26	*The Arcadians* (M)	2
JCW's New English Musical Co.			**2**
Jul	10	*The Girl on the Film* (M)	1
	21	*The Chocolate Soldier* (M)	1
	30	Australia Day – Theatrical matinee for Australian sick and wounded soldiers	
Muriel Starr			**3**
Aug	7	*The Law of the Land* (P)	
Royal Comic Opera Co.			**12**
	28	*After the Girl* (M)	1
Sep	4	*Our Miss Gibbs* (M)	2
	18	*Ma Mie Rosette* (M)	1
	25	*The Quaker Girl* (M)	1
Oct	2	*Paul Jones* (M)	2
	16	*The Dancing Mistress* (M)	2
	30	*The Old Guard* (M)	2
Nov	11	Monster Carnival Matinee in Aid of Comic Opera Benevolent Fund	
	13	*Our Miss Gibbs* (M)	
	17	*Ma Mie Rosette* (M)	
New English Comic Opera Co.			**3**
	20	*High Jinks* (M)	2
Dec	4	*The Girl in the Taxi* (M)	1
JCW production			**11**
	18	*Mother Goose* (Pa)	

1916

			weeks
Royal Comic Opera Co.			**7**
Mar	4	*Gipsy Love* (M)	1
	11	*The Belle of New York* (M)	2
	25	*The Merry Widow* (M)	2
Apr	8	*The Arcadians* (M)	1
	15	*The Quaker Girl* (M)	
	17	*Paul Jones* (M)	
	18	*Ma Mie Rosette* (M)	
	19	*Our Miss Gibbs* (M)	
	20	*Gipsy Love* (M)	
JCW New English Musical Comedy Co.			**21**
	22	*So Long Letty* (M)	9
Jun	24	*High Jinks* (M)	2
Jul	8	*Tonight's the Night* (M)	5
Aug	19	*The Girl in the Train* (M)	2
	28	Madame Melba's Matinee in aid of the Actor's Benevolent Fund and the Royal Comic Opera Co., Sick Fund	
Sep	1	*The Girl on the Film* (M)	1
	8	*The Girl in the Taxi* (M)	1
	16	*High Jinks* (M)	1
JCW Royal Comic Opera Co. with Florence Young			**12**
	23	*The Geisha* (M)	2
Oct	7	*The Cinema Star* (M)	6
Nov	26	*The Orchid* (M)	2
Dec	9	*Florodora* (M)	2
JCW production			**10**
	23	*The House That Jack Built* (Pa)	

Her Majesty's Theatre

			weeks
1917			
Mar	2	Matinee – Children's performance of pantomime in aid of the Children's Hospital and the Comic Opera Benevolent Fund	
JCW New English Musical Comedy Co.			**11**
	10	*A Waltz Dream* (M)	2
	24	*Canary Cottage* (M)	7
Apr	6	Good Friday Night Concert of Sacred Music	
May	12	*So Long Letty* (M)	1
	19	*High Jinks* (M)	1
Royal Comic Opera Co.			**16**
	26	*Three Twins* (M)	2
Jun	9	*The Pink Lady* (M)	5
Jul	14	*The Mikado* (M)	2
	24	Matinee in aid of the 'State War Council's Amelioraton Fund For Wounded Soldiers and their Families in Want or Distress, Organised by Madame Melba and Cyril Maude'	
	28	*The Arcadians* (M)	1
Aug	4	*The Red Widow* (M)	3
	25	*The Belle of New York* (M)	1
Sep	1	*The Merry Widow* (M)	1
	8	*The Cinema Star* (M)	1
JCW Musical Comedy Co.			**4**
	15	*Mr Manhattan* (M)	
Cyril Maude			**3**
Oct	13	*Grumpy* (P)	
	17	*General John Regan* (P)	
		Caste (P)	
JCW New English Musical Comedy Co.			**6**
Nov	3	*You're in Love* (M)	
JCW production			**11**
Dec	22	*Dick Whittington* (Pa)	
1918			
JCW New English Musical Comedy Co.			**5**
Mar	7	*You're in Love* (M)	3
	30	*Canary Cottage* (M)	1
Apr	6	*So Long Letty* (M)	1
JCW Revue Co.			**8**
	13	*The Bing Boys are Here* (R)	
	15	Red Cross Day Matinee – address about the Red Cross at the Front Line and a Variety Program by the Bing Boys Co.	
May	16	Matinee – 'Gala Performance by 300 artists from every Co. with every penny made going to the Red Cross'	
Royal Comic Opera Co. with Florence Young			**17**
Jun	8	*Katinka* (M)	13
Aug	1	Matinee in aid of the Actors Association of Australia and the JCW Employees Sick Fund	
Sep	7	*Oh! Oh! Delphine* (M)	4
JCW New Musical Comedy Co.			**3**
Oct	4	*Oh Boy* (M) Transferred from Theatre Royal	2
	19	*High Jinks* (M)	1
Nov	11	**END OF WAR**	
JCW Revue Co.			**7**
	26	*Hello Everybody* (R)	

Her Majesty's Theatre

			weeks
JCW production			**7**
Dec	21	*Goody Two Shoes* (Pa)	

1919

		Theatre closed from Jan 1 to Mar 8 influenza epidemic.	
Mar	8	Re-opening Gala Performance of Pantomime	
Apr	18	Good Friday Night Sacred Concert	
Ethel Erskine with New Musical Comedy Co.			**18**
	19	*Going Up* (M)	15
Jul	19	PEACE DAY CELEBRATIONS *Going Up* (M) Grand Victory Prelude – Australia in Peacetime, The Call to Arms, The Trenches, Peace	
Aug	2	*You're In Love* (M)	1
	9	*Oh Boy* (M)	1
	16	*High Jinks* (M)	1
Royal Comic Opera Co. with Florence Young			**10**
	23	*Maytime* (M)	7
Oct	11	*Katinka* (M)	3
JCW Grand Opera Co. with Amy Castles			**6**
Nov	1	*Madame Butterfly* (O)	
		Cavalleria Rusticana (O)	
		I Pagliacci (O)	
		Faust (O)	
		Il Trovatore (O)	
		Tales of Hoffman (O)	
		La Bohème (O)	
		Rigoletto (O)	
		Carmen (O)	

			weeks
JCW production			**12**
	20	*The Sleeping Beauty* (Pa)	

1920

Feb	5	Gala Performance of *Sleeping Beauty* 'in honour of General Sir William Birdwood' (British Field Marshall)	
	25	'Official Performance to honour Captain Sir Ross Smith, Lieutenant Sir Keith Smith, Sergeant J Bennett and Sergeant WH Shiers whose flight from England to Australia thrilled the world'	
	26	Professional Matinee – for artists appearing in other theatres, the opportunity to see *Sleeping Beauty*	
Mar	5	Matinee In Aid of the Children's Hospital and JCW Sick Fund. Children's Day at *Sleeping Beauty*	
Royal Comic Opera Co.			**10**
	13	*Kissing Time* (M)	
Apr	2	Good Friday Sacred Concert including Gladys Moncrieff, Maude Fane and Walter Kirby	
JCW Revue Co.			**11**
May	22	*The Bing Boys on Broadway* (R)	5
	31	Matinee HMS Renown (Prince of Wales's ship). Variety Concert – vocal, instrumental, comedy and acrobatic feats – in aid of the YMCA	

Her Majesty's Theatre

			weeks
Jun	5	In Honour of the Prince of Wales, gala performance – The Bing Boys on Broadway; a Pageant of Princes with historic tableaux and Amy Castles appears with the band of HMS Renown	
	26	*The Passing Show of 1920* (R)	6

Charles R Walenn, James Hay & Eileen Castles with JCW Gilbert & Sullivan Co. — 15

Aug	7	*The Mikado* (M)	2
	21	*The Yeomen of the Guard* (M)	2
Sep	4	*Iolanthe* (M)	2
	18	*The Gondoliers* (M)	3
Oct	9	*Patience* (M)	1
	16	*Pinafore* (M)	2
Nov	1	*The Mikado* (M)	
	2	*Iolanthe* (M)	1
	5	*Yeomen of the Guard* (M)	
	6	*The Pirates of Penzance* (M)	
	11	Matinee Benefit for Howard Vernon *The Mikado* (M)	2
	20	Travel Talk and Motion Picture by Lowell Thomas, traveller and explorer. Also the Anzacs in Palestine and Lawrence in Arabia	

JCW production — 10

Dec	18	*Humpty Dumpty* (Pa)	

1921

Dorothy Brunton & JCW New English Musical Comedy Co. — 22

Feb	26	*Baby Bunting* (M)	5
Apr	2	*So Long Letty* (M)	1
	9	*Irene* (M)	7
May	28	Farewell Season to Dorothy Brunton *Going Up* (M)	2
Jun	2	Benefit Matinee in aid of The Blind Apeal	
	11	*Oh Lady, Lady* (M)	7

Jamieson Dodds & Rene Maxwell — 7

Jul	30	*The Lilac Domino* (M)	

JCW Extravaganza — 2

Sep	17	*Chu Chin Chow* (M)	

Rene Maxwell, Ralph Errolle & Claude Fleming — 4

Oct	1	*Firefly* (M)	

JCW Gilbert & Sullivan Opera Co. — 7

	29	*The Gondoliers* (M)	3
		The Yeomen of the Guard (M)	
		The Mikado (M)	
		Princess Ida (M)	
		Iolanthe (M)	
		HMS Pinafore (M)	
		Patience (M)	
		The Pirates of Penzance (M)	
Nov	19	*Merrie England* (M)	4

JCW production — 9

Dec	24	*Babes in the Wood* (Pa)	

1922

Maude Fane — 14

Feb	25	*A Night Out* (M)	12
Apr	6	Matinee Benefit in aid of Old Actors Fund and JCW Employees Fund – Shakespeare, Grand Opera, Farce and Comedy and Vaudeville	
May	19	Matinee for Distressed Diggers and their Families	
	20	*You're in Love* (M)	1
	27	*Going Up* (M) (Alfred Frith)	1

Her Majesty's Theatre

weeks

JCW New Comic Opera Co. **28**

Jun 3 *A Little Dutch Girl* (M) 7
On Jun 6 members of *The Little Dutch Girl, The Bat,* and The Humphrey Bishop Co. from the Kings, together with the orchestras and staff from the three theatres under JCW Ltd Management in Melbourne, gather in the foyer of Her Majesty's Theatre to mark the knighthood of Sir George Tallis, the Chairman of Directors of the Firm

Jul 22 *The Naughty Princess* (M) (Gladys Moncrieff and Jack Cannot) 6

Sep 2 Melba Matinee Benefit for the Soldiers War Memorial Fund

2 *The Merry Widow* (M) (Gladys Moncrieff) 7

Oct 21 *Mary* (M) from the Theatre Royal 8

Nov 5 HMT lent by JCW for an afternoon of music, song and recitation in aid of the Adam Lindsay Gordon Memorial Fund

Oscar Asche & his Complete London Production **8**

Dec 23 *Cairo* (P)

1923

JCW & Oscar Asche present **5**

Feb 17 *Julius Caesar* (P) 2

Mar 7 *Chu Chin Chow* (M) 3

Royal Comic Opera Co. **9**

24 *A Southern Maid* (M) 6

weeks

May 6 *The Arcadians* (M) 3

Maude Fane **1**

26 *A Night Out* (P)

Kathlyn Hilliard & New English Musical Comedy Co. **2**

Jun 5 *Mary* (M)

Royal Comic Opera Co. with Gladys Moncrieff **16**

23 *Sybil* (M) 10

Jul 9 Monster Matinee organised by Mrs Stanley Bruce, wife of the Prime Minister, in aid of the Renown Free Kindergarten Building Fund

Sep 8 *Ma Mie Rosette* (M) 3

29 *Katinka* (M) 2

Oct 13 *The Merry Widow* (M) 1

A Howett-Worster, Pauline Bindley & Jack Cannot **3**

20 *The Beggars Opera* (M)

The Hon Mrs Pitt Rivers & the Sydney Repertory Theatre Society

Nov 13 *Pygmalion* (P)Benefit for the Queen Victoria Hospital Appeal and Actors Benevolent Fund and JCW Sick Fund

Emelie Polini & Frank Harvey **4**

17 *De Luxe Annie* (P) 2

Dec 1 *Eyes of Youth* (P) 2

Ada Reeve & JCW production **9**

22 *Aladdin* (Pa)

1924

Lawrence Grossmith **2**

Feb 23 *Ambrose Applejohn's Adventure* (P) 1

30 *The Silver Fox* (P) 1

His Majesty's Theatre

weeks

Alfred Frith, Madge Elliott & JCW New English Musical Comedy Co. 2

Mar 8 *The Cabaret Girl* (M)
Her Majesty's Theatre renamed His Majesty's Theatre
Official Commonwealth Government Gala Performance of *Cabaret Girl,* tendered by JCW Ltd in honour of Vice-Admiral Sir Frederick L Field and the Officers of the British Special Service Squadron

Dame Nellie Melba – A Season of Grand Opera 12

Mar 20 Gala Performance in the presence of Goveror General & Lady Forster, Prime Minister & Mrs Bruce, State Premier Mr Lawson. Theatre redecorated for this season, new seating and a new drop curtain.
Repertoire for the season:
La Bohème (O)
Barber of Seville (O)
Lucia (O)
Tales of Hoffman (O)
Madame Butterfly (O)
Carmen (O)
La Tosca (O)
Samson and Delilah (O)
Faust (O)
Cavalleria and *I Pagliacci* (O)
Romeo and Juliet (O)
Don Pasquale (O)
Othello (O)
Il Trovatore (O)
Aida (O)
Andrew Chenier (O)
Rigoletto (O)

Apr 18 Good Friday Night Concert by artists from the Grand Opera Co.

JCW New English Musical Comedy Co. 9

Jun 21 *Whirled into Happiness* (M)

Winnie Collins, Alfred Frith with JCW Musical Comedy Co. 4

Aug 23 *A Night Out* (M) 2

Sep 6 Farewell to the Operatic Stage in Australia of Nellie Melba and the last appearance in Australia of Toti Dal Monte 2

Howett Worster 3

20 *The Lady of the Rose* (M)

Oct 13 Final Grand Opera Performance *La Bohème* in aid of the Appeal for the Limbless and Tubercular Soldiers
Dame Nellie Melba's Farewell.
Opening broadcast of radio station 3LO from HMT

Royal Comic Opera Co. with Gladys Moncrieff 5

Nov 15 *The Maid of the Mountains* (M)

Dec 20 *Sybil* (M)
The Merry Widow (M)
A Southern Maid (M)

25 Grand Opera at His Majesty's concert

Josie Melville & George Gee 6

26 *Good Morning Dearie* (M)

1925

Maude Fane, Alfred Frith with JCW New Musical Comedy Co. 21

Feb 7 *Betty* (M) 9

His Majesty's Theatre

weeks

Apr 11 *Primrose* (M) 11

May 21 Matinee Benefit for the Old Actors Fund and the JCW Ltd Employees Fund

Jun 19 Gala Performance of *Primrose* in honour of and in the presence of Commandante De Pinedo and Chief Warrant-Officer Ernesto Campanelli to celebrate their epoch making flight from Rome to Melbourne

27 *Whirled into Happiness* (M) 1

Josie Melville & George Gee 7

Jul 4 *Kid Boots* (M)

Jul 25 Official Fleet Gala Performance of *Kid Boots* tendered by JCW Ltd for Commonwealth and State Governments. 'In the presence of the Admiral and Officers of the US Fleet. Gala Decorations and Pageant will be retained for the entire visit of the Fleet.' All officers and men of the Fleet invited as guests to any JCW theatre during their visit

Marie Burke & Gus Bluett 13

Aug 29 *Wild Flower* (M)

Oct 13 Testimonial matinee to Maggie Moore prior to her departure for America

22 Matinee Follies for St Vincent's Hospital Appeal

Royal Comic Opera Co. & Gladys Moncrieff 14

Nov 21 *The Street Singer* (M) transferred from Theatre Royal 4

weeks

JCW Production

Dec 26 *Aladdin* (Pa) 10

1926

Anna Pavlova with Laurent Novikoff & Entire London & Paris Organisation 5

Mar 13 Repertoire includes:
The Fairy Doll (B)
Chopiniana (B)
Divertissements (B)
Other ballets performed during the season:
Amarilla (B)
Autumn Leaves (B)
Don Quixote (B)
The Magic Flute (B)
Snow Flakes (B)
The Swan (B)
Russian Dance (B)
Bolero (B)

Gilbert & Sullivan & JCW Specially Organised Co. 15

Apr 17 *The Gondoliers* (M) 2

May 1 *The Yeomen of the Guard* (M) 2

15 *The Pirates of Penzance* (M) 2

29 *The Mikado* (M) 3

Jun 21 *Pinafore* (M) and *Trial by Jury* (M) 2

Jul 3 *Iolanthe* (M) 2

17 *Princess Ida* (M) 2

23 Matinee farewell to Pavlova

JCW New English Musical Comedy Co. 7

31 *Tell Me More* (M) from Theatre Royal

His Majesty's Theatre

weeks

Aug 17 Gala Night for Alan Cobham and the 'Intrepid Airmen, whose flight from England to Australia has made new history'

Sep 30 Matinee in aid of the Free Kindergarten Union of Victoria

Marie Burke **10**

Sep 18 *Katja* (M) from Theatre Royal

Maude Fane, George Gee & Gus Bluett & JCW New English Musical Co. **11**

Nov 27 *A Night Out* (M) 2

Dec 11 *Primrose* (M) 1

Dec 18 *The Cousin from Nowhere* (M) 8

1927

Margery Hicklin & Leo Franklyn **1**

Feb 12 *Kissing Time* (M)

Harriet Bennet & Frederic Bentley **27**

19 *Rose Marie* (M)

Aug 23 Patchwork Revue organised by Lady Tallis presented by Members of 'Melbourne's Younger Set' in aid of the Victorian Civil Ambulance. After the performance on opening night, a supper dance was held on the stage

Royal Comic Opera Co. & Beppie DeVries & Frank Webster **28**

27 *Madame Pompadour* (M) 10

Nov 5 *The Student Prince* (M) (Beppie DeVries & James Liddy) 18

weeks

1928

Charles Walenn, Strella Wilson & Gilbert & Sullivan Opera Co. **6**

Mar 10 *Ruddigore* (M)
The Gondoliers (M)
The Pirates of Penzance (M)
The Mikado (M)
Yeomen of the Guard (M)
Iolanthe (M)
Pinafore (M)
Princess Ida (M)
Patience (M)

Mar 19 Bert Hinkler's Gala Night – 'Various Stages of Hinkler's Flight from London to Melbourne will be depicted by an electrical device. Moving pictures of Hinkler's landing at Flemington Racecourse will be shown'

Williamson–Melba Grand Opera Season repertoire **8**

May 12 *The Barber of Seville* (O)
Manon Lescaut (O)
Aida (O)
Lohengrin (O)
La Bohème (O)
Lucia di Lammermoor (O)
Suor Angelica (O)
Rigoletto (O)
La Tosca (O)
La Traviata (O)
Madame Butterfly (O)
The Daughter of the Regiment (O)
Don Pasquale (O)

His Majesty's Theatre

			weeks
		Tannhauser (O)	
		Andrea Chenier (O)	
		The Valkyrie (O)	
		Carmen (O)	
		The Tales of Hoffman (O)	
		Cavalleria Rusticana (O)	
		L'amore dei tre re (The Love of Three Kings) (O)	
		Il Trovatore (O)	
		Turandot (O)	
		Il Tabaro (O)	
		Faust (O)	
		I Pagliacci (O)	
The Victorian Opera Co.			**1**
Jul	7	*The Quaker Girl* (O)	
Annie Croft & JCW New Musical Comedy Co.			**9**
	14	*The Girl Friend* (M)	2
	28	*Hit the Deck* (M)	7
Virginia Perry & Herbert Mundin			**28**
Sep	15	*The Desert Song* (M)	
Oct	27	Gala Performance of *The Desert Song* for the English Cricket Team	

1929

			weeks
James Liddy & Strella Wilson			**4**
Mar	30	*The Vagabond King* (M)	
James Liddy & Arthur Stigant			**3**
May	4	*The Student Prince* (M)	
Anna Pavlova, Pierre Vladimiroff, Ruth French & Nina Kirsanova & the complete European Company			**4**
	25	Repertoire includes:	
		The Sleeping Beauty	
		The Swan	
		Amarilla	
		Oriental Impressions	
		Giselle (B)	
		Divertissements (B)	
		including *Gavotte Pavlova* (B)	
		The Dance of the Hours (B)	
		Pastorale (B)	
		La Fille Mal Gardée (B)	
		Autumn Leaves (B)	
		Don Quixote (B)	
		The Californian Poppy (B)	
		The Fairy Doll (B)	
		Invitation to Dance (B)	
Alfred Frith, Gus Bluett & Helen Patterson			**5**
Jun	25	*The Five O'Clock Girl* transferred from Theatre Royal	2
Jul	13	*A Night Out* (M)	3
Madge Aubrey, Nydia d'Arnell & Frederic Bentley			**9**
Aug	3	*Show Boat* (M)	
	13	Charity Matinee for Women's Hospital Appeal and Lord Mayor's Unemployed Fund	
Frederic Bentley, Marie Bremner & Glen Dale			**1**
Oct	12	*Rose Marie* (M)	
	24	Fire occurred after workmen preparing for *Brewster's Millions* had left the theatre. Due to the Depression, the fire-damaged shell of HMT was not renovated until June 1931, when it was reopened by Efftee Films as a film studio.	

King's Theatre

			weeks
1920			
John D O'Hara			**13**
Aug	14	*Three Wise Fools* (P)	*7*
		Theatre lent by JCW to students of the Conservatorium to stage 'Scenes From Opera' in aid of the appeal for Queen Victoria Memorial Hospital.	
Oct	30	*Lightnin'* (P)	2
Nov	13	*Shore Acres* (P)	3
Dec	4	*Three Wise Fools* (P)	1
J & N Tait production			**9**
	18	*Sinbad the Sailor* (Pa)	
1921			
Fred Collier & A Howett-Worster			**2**
Feb	26	*The Marriage of Figaro* (O)	
J & N Tait's All Diggers Co.			**2**
Mar	12	*Mademoiselle Mimi* (M)	
John D O'Hara & Jules Jordan			**6**
	26	*Welcome Stranger* (P)	
Marie Tempest & Graham Browne			**3**
Jul	11	*The Great Adventure* (P)	
	16	*Cousin Kate* (P)	2
	30	*Mr Pim Passes By* (P)	1
Maude Hannaford & Frank Harvey			**6**
Aug	6	*Scandal* (P)	
Bert Bailey & Julius Grant			**5**
Sep	17	*Jefferson Wins Through* (P)	3
Oct	15	*On Our Selection* (P)	2
Joseph Coyne (from Theatre Royal)			**1**
	29	*Wedding Bells* (P)	
Maude Hannaford			**2**
Nov	5	*The Sign on the Door* (P)	
(to Theatre Royal)			
Marie Tempest & Graham Browne			**9**
	19	*Mr Pim Passes By* (P)	4
Dec	17	*Penelope* (P)	1

			weeks
	24	*Tea for Three* (P)	*4*
1922			
John D O'Hara			**5**
Jan	21	*The Laughter of Fools* (P)	
Isobel Brosnan & the New English Comedy Co.			**2**
Mar	4	*Paddy the Next Best Thing* (P)	
Nicola			**4**
	18	*Nicola – Magician*	
Phillip Tead, Marjorie Bennett &			**4**
J & N Tait's New Comedy Co.			**6**
Apr	15	*The First Year* (P)	
Humphrey Bishop Comedy & Operatic Co.			**5**
May	27	18 Star Acts including Burlesque and Variety	
Emelie Polini & Frank Harvey			**14**
Jul	1	*My Lady's Dress* (P)	9
Sep	2	*The Lie* (P)	5
JCW production			**6**
Dec	23	*The Forty Thieves* (Pa)	
1923			
Lawrence Grossmith			**21**
Feb	10	*Ambrose Applejohn's Adventure* (P)	9
Apr	14	*The Silver Fox* (P)	6
May	26	*Quarantine* (P)	6
Jul	7	**Harry Lauder**	**4**
Irene Vanbrugh & Dion Boucicault & their London Co.			**19**
Aug	4	*His House in Order* (P)	5
Sep	8	*The Twelve Pound Look* (P) and *Mr Pim Passes By* (P)	3
	29	*Mis' Nell O' New Orleans* (P)	4
Oct	27	*Belinda* (P) and *The Will* (P)	3

King's Theatre

			weeks
Nov	17	*The Second Mrs Tanqueray* (P)	4
Emelie Polini & Frank Harvey			**7**
Dec	22	*French Leave* (P)	4

1924

Jan	19	*My Lady's Dress* (P)	3
Oscar Asche			**6**
Feb	9	*Othello* (P)	4
Mar	8	*Iris* (P)	1
	15	*The Taming of the Shrew* (P)	1
Gertrude Elliott			**6**
	25	*Blue Beard's Eighth Wife* (P)	2
Apr	12	*Enter Madame* (P)	1
	19	*Woman to Woman* (P)	1
	26	*Smilin' Through* (P)	2
Oscar Asche			**7**
May	10	*The Skin Game* (P)	
Muriel Starr & Frank Harvey			**17**
Jun	28	*The Garden of Allah* (P)	4
Jul	26	*Madame X* (P)	3
Aug	16	*East of Suez* (P)	8
Oct	11	*Bought and Paid For* (P)	2
Irene Vanbrugh & Dion Boucicault			**17**
	25	*Aren't We All* (P)	7
Dec	26	Grand Matinee for Travellers Aid Society	
	20	*The Truth about Blayds* (P)	4

1925

			weeks
Jan	17	*Trelawney of the Wells* (P)	4
Feb	14	*Mr Pim Passes By* (P)	1
	19	*His House in Order* (P)	1
Guy Bates Post			**13**
	28	*The Green Goddess* (P)	7
Apr	18	*The Masquerader* (P)	4
May	16	*The Nigger* (P)	2
Bert Bailey & Julius Grant			**6**
	30	*On Our Selection* (P)	
Thurston Hall			**2**
Jul	11	*The Broken Wing* (P)	
Muriel Starr & Frank Harvey			**5**
	25	*The Pelican* (P)	4
Aug	22	*Within the Law* (P)	1
Maurice Moscovitch			**5**
	29	*The Great Lover* (P)	2
Sep	12	*The Merchant of Venice* (P)	1
	19	*The Outsider* (P)	2
Bailey & Grant			
Oct	3	*Rip Van Winkle* (P) (transferred from Playhouse)	1
Nellie Bromley Co.			**7**
	17	*Fair and Warmer* (P)	3
Nov	7	*Peg O' My Heart* (P)	1
	14	*Madame X* (P)	1
	21	*Paddy the Next Best Thing* (P)	1
	28	*It Pays to Advertise* (P)	1
William Russell			**2**
Dec	5	*Fair and Warmer* (P)	
Renee Kelly			**13**
	19	*Polly with a Past* (P)	9

1926

Feb	20	*Daddy Long Legs* (P)	4
Dion Boucicault's London Co. in a Series of JM Barrie Plays			**14**
Mar	20	*Quality Street* (P)	5
Apr	24	*The Admirable Crichton* (P)	5
May	29	*What Every Woman Knows* (P)	4
Leon Gordon			**7**
Jun	26	*White Cargo* (P)	
Bert Bailey			**5**
Aug	14	*The Sentimental Bloke* (P)	
Richard Taber & Hale Norcross			**4**
Sep	18	*Is Zat So* (P)	
Gregan McMahon & Lily Titheradge			**1**
Oct	16	*Old English* (P)	

King's Theatre

			weeks
Dion Boucicault & his London Co.			**5**
	23	*Aren't We All* (P)	2
Nov	7	*Mary Rose* (P)	3
Renee Kelly			**15**
	27	*Brown Sugar* (P) from Theatre Royal	3
Dec	18	*The Naughty Wife* (P)	4

1927

Jan	29	*The Last of Mrs Cheyney* (P)	7
Mar	19	*Daddy Long Legs* (P)	1
Maurice Moscovitch			**4**
	26	*They Knew What They Wanted* (P)	2
Apr	9	*The Fare* (P)	2
Judith Anderson & Leon Gordon			**5**
	18	*Tea for Three* (P)	1
	30	*The Green Hat* (P)	4
Richard Taber & Hale Norcross			**4**
May	28	*Six-Cylinder Love* (P)	
Melbourne Repertory Theatre			**1**
Jun	25	*Little Mary* (P)	
Jul	5	*Six Characters in Search of an Author* (P)	
Maurice Moscovitch			**4**
	9	*Trilby* (P)	
Olive Stone			**9**
Aug	6	*Cradle Snatchers* (P)	
Melbourne Repertory Theatre			**2**
Oct	13	*Liliom* (P)	1
	22	*The Old Adam* (P)	1
Irene Vanbrugh & Dion Boucicault			**11**
Nov	5	*Caroline* (P)	4
Dec	3	*The Letter* (P)	4
	31	*All the King's Horses* (P)	3

1928

			weeks
New English Comedy Co.			**4**
Jan	28	*A Cuckoo in the Nest* (P)	
New London Comedy Co.			**4**
Feb	25	*Thark* (P)	
Bailey & Grant			**4**
Mar	31	*On Our Selection* (P)	
Leon Gordon			**2**
Apr	28	*The Trial of Mary Dugan* (P)	
The Gregan McMahon Play Co.			**6**
May	12	*Getting Married* (P)	2
	26	*Dear Brutus* (P)	2
Jun	9	*Anna Christie* (P)	2
Irene Homer			**6**
	23	*The Patsy* (P)	3
Jul	14	*The Rudd Family* (P)	3
William Anderson's Dramatic Co.			**1**
Aug	11	*When London Sleeps* (P)	
Muriel Starr			**16**
Sep	1	*The Donovan Affair* (P)	5
Oct	6	*Declassee* (P)	2
	20	*Whispering Wires* (P)	3
Nov	10	*Cheating Cheaters* (P)	2
	24	*Within the Law* (P)	4
Nicola			
Dec	22	*World's Greatest Wizard*	4

1929

Leon Gordon			**15**
Jan	19	*White Cargo* (P)	4
Feb	16	*The Flying Squad* (P)	7
Apr	6	*The Ghost Upstairs* (P)	4
Nellie Stewart			**3**
May	11	*Trilby* (P)	
Irene Homer & AS Byron			**4**
Jun	1	*The Patsy* (P)	

King's Theatre

			weeks
Josephine Wilson & Clayton Greene			**1**
	29	*The Wrecker* (P)	
William Anderson Dramatic Plays			**4**
Jul	20	*The Squatter's Daughter* (P)	1
	27	*The Face at the Window* (P)	1
Aug	3	*The Prince and the Beggar Maid* (P)	1
	10	*Dracula* (P)	1
Nat Madison			**2**
	17	*No. 17* (P)	
Ziegfield's Musical Romance with Charley Sylber, Genevieve McCormack & Forrest Yarnall			**12**
	31	*Whoopee* (M)	
Ann Penn, Roy Rene & Hector St Clair			**8**
Nov	30	*Clowns in Clover* (M)	4
Dec	26	*Mother Goose* (Pa) (Matinee)	4
		Clowns in Clover (M) (Evenings)	

1930

			weeks
Frank Neil's Comedians			**1**
Jan	25	*Nightie Night* (P)	
Allan Wilkie			**5**
Feb	22	*The School for Scandal* (P)	
		The Merchant of Venice (P)	
		Twelfth Night (P)	
		The Rivals (P)	
		She Stoops to Conquer (P)	
		The Jealous Wife (P)	
		A Midsummer Night's Dream (P)	
		Macbeth (P)	
		Julius Caesar (P)	
		Much Ado About Nothing (P)	
Clem Dawe			**6**
Apr	5	*Love Lies* (M)	4
May	10	*So This Is Love* (M)	1
	28	*Journey's End* (P)	
Leon Gordon			**5**
Jun	7	*This Thing Called Love* (P)	4
Jul	19	*Scandal* (P)	1
	29	*White Cargo* (P)	
Jim Gerald, Mary MacGregor & Ethel Morrison			**3**
Aug	30	*Little Accident* (P)	
Edith Taliaferro & Ethel Morrison			**5**
Sep	23	*Let Us Be Gay* (P)	
Gregan McMahon			**1**
Dec	26	*Uncle Tom's Cabin* (M)	

1931

			weeks
George Marlow, Nat Phillips & Syd Beck			**2**
Jul	25	*Revue* (R)	
Ethel Morrison & Iris Darbyshire			**7**
Dec	26	*As Husbands Go* (P)	

Comedy Theatre

weeks

1928

Margaret Bannerman & Anthony Prinsep's London Co. **6**

Apr 28 *Our Betters* (P) 3

May 19 *Diplomacy* (P) 3

New English Co. **4**

Jun 16 *Rookery Nook* (P)

Victorian Opera Co. **1**

Jul 14 *Quaker Girl* (O) (from HMT)

Vanbrugh–Boucicault Co. **17**

21 *The High Road* (P) 4

Aug 18 *The Notorious Mrs Ebbsmith* (P) 2

Sep 1 *Belinda* (P) 2

15 *All the King's Horses* (P) 3

Oct 6 *Mis' Nell O' New Orleans* (P) 2

20 *On Approval* (P) 4

Leon Gordon **3**

Dec 22 *Scandal* (P)

1929

JCW New Comedy Co. with Allan Bruce & Ruth Nugent **12**

Jan 18 *Pigs* (P) 7

Mar 16 *Applesauce* (P) 4

Apr 13 *Kempy* (P) 1

Nellie Stewart **3**

20 *Sweet Nell of Old Drury* (P)

Natalie Moya, Lewis Shaw & New English Co. **4**

May 11 *Young Woodley* (P)

Aug 3 Farewell Performance of *A Night Out* (from HMT.)

Leon Gordon **16**

Nov 2 *Brewster's Millions* (P) from Theatre Royal 7

weeks

Dec 21 *The Murder on the Second Floor* (P) 4

1930

Jan 18 *The Land of Promise* (P) 2

Feb 8 *White Cargo* (P) 1

15 *The Poppy God* (P) 2

Leo Carrillo **6**

Mar 1 *Lombardi Ltd* (P)

Nellie Stewart **3**

Apr 17 *Romance* (P)

William Faversham **6**

May 10 *The Hawk* (P) 2

24 *The Prince and the Pauper* (P) 2

Jun 7 *Lord and Lady Algy* (P) 2

14 Charity Matinee in aid of the Alfred Hospital

Leon Gordon & Ann Davis **2**

Jul 4 *Tea for Three* (P)

Edith Taliaferro **3**

Nov 1 *The Road to Romance* (P) 2

22 *Peg O' My Heart* (P) 1

Ethel Morrison, JB Rowe & Mary Macgregor **11**

Dec 1 *The First Mrs Fraser* (P) 8

1931

Feb 21 *Mary Rose* (P) 3

Frank Harvey **9**

Apr 4 *On the Spot* (P) 4

May 2 *Loyalties* (P) 3

23 *The Calendar* (P) 2

Ethel Morrison, Cecil Kellaway & JCW Comedy Co. **1**

Aug 29 *A Warm Corner* (P)

Comedy Theatre

			weeks
Frank Harvey & Iris Darbyshire			**1**
Sep	26	*Cape Forlorn* (P)	
New English Co.			**5**
Jun	16	*Rookery Nook* (P)	4
Jul	14	*Quaker Girl* (O) from HMT	1

			weeks
Vanbrugh–Boucicault Co.			**11**
	21	*The High Road* (P)	4
Aug	18	*Notorious Mrs Ebbsmith* (P)	2
Sep	1	*Belinda* (P)	2
	15	*All the King's Horses* (P)	3

Notes

1 With a Little Bit of Luck

[1] The theatre was known as the Princess's Theatre until replaced in 1886 by a new theatre designed by William Pitt, to emerge as the Princess Theatre on the new letterheads. We note that the amusement columns in the newspapers continued to refer to this theatre as the Princess's.

2 The Irish Connection

[1] Melbourne *Punch*, 2 April 1908

[2] Melbourne *Herald*, 14 March 1923

[3] G Mauresceaux, *Old Kilkenny Review*

[4] Melbourne *Herald*, 'Sir George Tallis Looks Back', 13 November 1931

3 The Firm

[1] Ronald J Walker, Foreword, *Melbourne's Yesterdays*

[2] *Encyclopaedia Britannica*, Eleventh Edition, Vol 18, p 90

[3] Katharine Brisbane, *Entertaining Australia*, p 12

[4] JC Williamson, *Life-Story Told in His Own Words with Valedictory Messages*, p 18

[5] cited in Ian Dicker, *JCW: A Short Biography of James Cassius Williamson*, pp 80, 81

[6] Nellie Stewart, *My Life's Story*, p 45

[7] *JC Williamson's Life Story*, p 21

[8] *Theatre Magazine*, 1 March 1913

[9] cited in Dicker, p 103

[10] Melbourne *Punch*, 22 May 1913

[11] *Theatre Magazine*, 1913

[12] *Punch*, 1913

[13] cited in Dicker, p 107

4 Preparation of an Irish Immigrant

[1] *Punch,* 1908

[2] *The Stage,* 8 April 1920

[3] *The Stage,* 1920

[4] *Punch,* 1913

[5] greenroom: a backstage room in a theatre where performers revitalise.

[6] Melbourne *Herald,* 'Sir George Tallis Looks Back', 13 Nov 1931

[7] *New York Times,* 9 February 1891

[8] Melbourne *Herald,* 13 November 1931

[9] *Punch,* 1908

[10] *Punch,* 1913

[11] Williamson, p 36

[12] Melbourne *Herald,* 5 December 1931

[13] Melbourne *Herald,* 13 November 1931

5 Tour Manager

[1] Ian Bevan, *The Story of the Theatre Royal,* p 115

[2] Stewart, p 161

[3] *Theatre Magazine,* March 1914

[4] *Theatre Magazine,* 1914

[5] *Punch,* 1913

[6] Peter Downes, *Shadows on the Stage.* This book gives a detailed treatment of New Zealand's early theatre history, including a description of JC Williamson companies in New Zealand and their influence on an isolated colony.

[7] *Theatre Magazine,* August 1914

6 Partnerships

[1] cited in Viola Tait, *A Family of Brothers,* p 66

[2] Dicker, p 137

[3] Tait, p 70

[4] Dicker, p 138

[5] *Sydney Morning Herald,* 8 May 1899

[6] Melbourne *Midnight Sun,* 'In the Limelight', c June 1922

[7] Melbourne *Argus,* 29 October 1900

[8] *Punch,* 1913

[9] Melbourne *Herald,* 5 December 1931

[10] Melbourne *Herald,* 1931

[11] Williamson, p 22

[12] We are unable to throw any light on the claim made in a letter by a four-year junior in the Firm, Ted Tait, that he helped George raise the 'entrance fee' into the partnership. A loan from The Bank of New South Wales was allegedly involved. The bank's archives should have a record of such a transaction, but we have found no trace of it. Moreover, no trace has been found in the records of George's estate of any need for such a loan. Interestingly, Ted Tait went on to assert that he managed Tallis's affairs during 1900–1904. This also seems unlikely; Tallis used his cousin, Fred Nicholson, as his personal accountant and manager during those years.

7 Very Firm

[1] *Otago Witness,* 9 July 1913

[2] Melbourne *Argus,* 25 September 1906

[3] *Lyttelton Times,* 9 February 1907

[4] Melbourne *Argus,* 1906

[5] *The Theatre Magazine,* February 1913

[6] Melbourne *New Idea,* 6 February 1907

[7] *Otago Witness,* 9 July 1913

[8] *Theatre Magazine,* March 1913

[9] Josephine V Fantasia, PhD Thesis 'Entrepreneurs, Empires and Pantomimes', University of Sydney, 1996, p 339

[10] Claude Kingston, *It Don't Seem a Day Too Much,* p 168

[11] *Punch,* 1908

8 Santoi George

[1] *Punch,* 1908

[2] Undated article in *The Australian Home Builder* entitled 'To Have and to Hold', reproduced in Tallis J, Knight S & Tallis M, *In Search of the Sun,* p 72;

[3] Some information supplied by Bruce Horsley, a grandson of JC Williamson

[4] Melbourne *Punch,* 4 July 1912

[5] *Australian,* 30 July 1974

[6] Melbourne *Age,* 10 August 1911

[7] *Table Talk,* 24 December 1925

[8] *Punch,* 1913

9 The Passing of Williamson

[1] *Otago Witness,* 18 January 1905

[2] *Punch,* 1913

[3] *JC Williamson's Life-Story,* p 39

[4] cited in Dicker, p 199

[5] Melbourne *Argus,* 8 July 1913

10 Faith, Hope and Charity

[1] *Theatre Magazine,* December 1915

[2] *The South African Dictionary of Biography,* pp 884–885

[3] FCL Bosman (ed.), *Drama en toneel in Suid-Afrika*

[4] *Theatre Magazine,* 1915

[5] Melbourne *Argus,* 8 November 1918

11 Amalgamation

[1] John West, *Theatre in Australia,* p 116

[2] Theodore Fink trained as a solicitor. With Robert Best he formed a respected legal firm in Melbourne from where he practised his profession, and maintained very wide business interests. Fink was well connected at every level of academics, politics and the newspaper world. Known as a lawyer, a man of the arts, a theatre buff and a popular public speaker, Theodore Fink was a

bon vivant who made his audiences laugh. One might suppose that he was a significant addition to the Firm's board, although interestingly this appointment is not mentioned in his recently published biography *Theodore Fink: A Talent for Ubiquity* by Don Garden.

[3] This chapter is compiled from the George Tallis Theatre Collection. Use is also made of Viola Tait's *A Family of Brothers,* and Katharine Brisbane's (ed.) *Entertaining Australia.* Details of the major share-holdings in JCW Ltd were gleaned from business letters, while the story of the Lambs Club affair comes mainly from letters written to Tallis around 1918.

12 What's This I Hear?

[1] *Australian Home Beautiful,* 7 May 1926

[2] *Table Talk,* 24 December 1925

[3] Melbourne *Age,* 18 February 1989

[4] *Theatre Magazine,* 1 November 1912

[5] Melbourne *Herald,* 28 February 1956

[6] *New Zealand Herald,* Auckland Supplement, 22 July 1922

[7] Melbourne *Herald,* 18 December 1922

13 Celluloid and Ether

[1] *Theatre Magazine,* August 1921

[2] *Sydney Mail,* September 1926

[3] *Theatre Magazine,* April 1920

[4] Frank Van Straten, *Regent Theatre, Melbourne: Palace of Dreams*

[5] Colin MacKinnon, unpublished article 'The History of Australasian Wireless Company'

[6] Philip Geeves, *The Dawn of Australian Radio Broadcasting,* p 29

[7] Peter Game, *The Music Sellers,* p 238

[8] *Smith's Weekly,* 5 May 1928

[9] Melbourne *Wireless Weekly,* 12 April 1929

[10] Melbourne *Wireless Weekly,* 17 May 1929

[11] The Diaries of Arthur Wigram Allen, 3 October 1925

14 Old Lightnin'

[1] *Theatre Magazine,* March 1922

[2] Kingston, p 168

[3] Tait, p 98

[4] *Daily Sketch,* 16 January 1925

[5] *London Times,* 28 January 1925

[6] Melbourne *Argus,* 19 December 1927

[7] This information is gathered from legal documents concerning the sale kindly supplied by the legal firm of Allen, Allen and Hemsley.

15 London Calling

[1] Unidentified newspaper article entitled 'New Melbourne Theatre', reproduced in Tallis *et al,* p 38

[2] Brisbane, p 114

[3] Melbourne *Argus,* 30 April 1928

[4] Melbourne *Herald,* 14 March 1923

[5] Melbourne *Herald,* 17 April 1926

[6] Unidentified newspaper article entitled 'Tallis Play Succeeds in London', 20 December 1928, reproduced in Tallis *et al,* p 44

[7] London *Times,* 21 December 1928

[8] W MacQueen-Pope, *The Footlights Flickered,* p 223

16 Not So Firm

[1] Adelaide *Advertiser,* 31 July 1929, Melbourne *Age,* 6 August 1929

[2] *Smith's Weekly,* 26 September 1931

[3] The Diaries of Arthur Wigram Allen, 28 November 1930

[4] Melbourne *Age,* 13 November 1931

[5] *Washington Evening News,* 4 August 1925

[6] Alan Thomas, *Broadcast and Be Damned,* p 9

[7] Melbourne *Argus,* 23 May 1932

[8] Ken Inglis, *This Is the ABC,* p 11

[9] Game, p 241

[10] Melbourne *Herald*, 17 April 1926

17 Too Many Cooks

[1] *Smith's Weekly*, 26 September 1931

[2] Melbourne *Herald*, 5 December 1931

18 Rangatira

[1] The Diaries of Arthur Wigram Allen are on microfilm at the Mitchell Library, Sydney, and give a daily coverage of the events surrounding the sale of the Tallis–Allen shares to Rangatira. Since Allen was one of the main players, and because, as the Firm's solicitor, he was meticulous with his records, his impeccable diaries are a main source of facts surrounding this transaction. We have used a copy of two agreements between George Tallis and Rangatira, a detailed memo, dated 1 December 1937, written by Allen to Robert Hill (one of the Firm's accountants) concerning the events leading up to the sale of the shares, and other old legal documents to provide background information. We have also used personal communications from Sir Roy MacKenzie, many years a managing director of Rangatira, and standard sources such as *A Family of Brothers* and *It Don't Seem a Day Too Much* to throw additional light on the share transaction.

[2] Some of the details in this chronology have been generously supplied, or confirmed, by JC Williamson's grandson Bruce Horsley.

The Allen Diaries, in general, provide significant details of important managerial and financial difficulties besetting the Firm in the 1930s.

19 Rien ne va Plus

[1] *Smith's Weekly*, 23 August 1930

[2] Kingston, p 169

Bibliography

Books

Atkinson, B (1970) *Broadway*, Macmillan, New York

Australian Dictionary of Biography, Melbourne University Press

Bagot, A (1965) *Coppin the Great*, Melbourne University Press

Bennetts, D (1976) *Melbourne's Yesterdays*, Souvenir Press, Adelaide

Bevan, I (1993) *The Story of the Theatre Royal*, Currency Press, Sydney

Beyers, CJ (ed.) (1987) *Dictionary of South African Biography*, Volume V, Human Sciences Research Council, Pretoria

Bosman, FCL *Drama en toneel in Suid-Afrika*, Deel 2 1856–1912

Brisbane, K (ed.) (1991) *Entertaining Australia*, Currency Press, Sydney

Dicker, IG (1974) *A Short Biography of James Cassius Williamson*, The Elizabeth Tudor Press, Sydney

Downes, P (1975) *Shadows of the Stage*, John McIndoe, Dunedin

Dreyfus, K (ed.) (1985) *The Farthest North of Humanness* (letters of Percy Grainger 1901–1914), Macmillan, Melbourne

Encyclopaedia Britannica (1910) Eleventh Edition, Volume 18, New York

Fantasia, JV (1996) *Entrepreneurs, empires and pantomimes*, PhD Thesis, University of Sydney

Game, P (1976) *The Music Sellers*, Hawthorn Press, Melbourne

Garden, Don (1998) Theodore Fink, *A Talent for Ubiquity*, Melbourne University Press

Geeves, P (1993) *The Dawn of Australian Broadcasting*, Federal Publishing, Alexandria NSW

Hetherington, J (1967) *A Biography of Melba*, Faber and Cheshire, Victoria

Inglis, K (1983) *This Is the ABC*, Melbourne University Press

Irvin, E (1985) *Dictionary of the Australian Theatre 1788–1914*, Hale and Iremonger, Sydney

Kingston, C (1971) *It Don't Seem a Day Too Much*, Rigby Ltd, Adelaide

Lawson, Valerie (1995) *The Allens Affair,* Macmillan, Sydney

Legrand, J (1993) *Chronicle of Australia,* Griffin Press, Adelaide

Long, J (1982) *The Pictures That Moved: a picture history of the Australian cinema,* Hutchinson, Melbourne

MacQueen-Pope, W (1959) *The Footlights Flickered,* Herbert Jenkins, London

McGuire, P (1948) *The Australian Theatre,* Oxford University Press, Melbourne

Mauresceaux, G (1974) *Old Kilkenny Review*

Parsons, P & Chance, V (eds.) (1995) *Companion to Theatre in Australia,* Currency Press, Sydney

Pask, Edward H (1979) *Enter the Colonies Dancing: A History of Dance in Australia 1835–1940,* Oxford University Press, Melbourne

Porter, Hal (1965) *Stars of Australian Stage and Screen,* Rigby Ltd, Adelaide

Reid, A (1986) *Those Were the Days,* Hesperian Press, W. Aust

Sands & McDougall's Directory (1886) Melbourne

Sierp, A (1972) *Colonial Life in Victoria,* Rigby Ltd, Adelaide

Stewart, N (1923) *My Life's Story,* John Sands, Sydney

Tait, V (1971) *A Family of Brothers,* Heinemann, Melbourne

Tallis, J, Knight, S & Tallis, M (1988) *In Search of the Sun,* Lutheran Publishing House, Adelaide

Tallis, J & M (1992) *The Family of John & Sarah Tallis,* Investigator Press, Adelaide

Thomas, A (1980) *Broadcast and Be Damned,* Melbourne University Press

Van Straten, F (1996) *The Regent Theatre: Melbourne's Palace of Dreams,* ELM Publishing, Melbourne

Vestey, P (1996) *Melba a Family Memoir,* Phoebe Publishing, Melbourne

West, J (1978) *Theatre in Australia,* Cassell, Sydney

Williamson, JC (1913) *Life-Story Told in His Own Words with Valedictory Messages,* Bookstall Co., Sydney

Unpublished

Arthur Wigram Allen Diaries 1914–1941, Mitchell Library, Sydney

Diaries of George Tallis, Victoria

MacKinnon, C *The Sydney Sealed Set Stations 2FC, 2BL,* NSW

MacKinnon, C 'The History of the Australasian Wireless Company', NSW

Sir George Tallis Memoirs, 1948, Victoria

Newspapers

Advertiser, Adelaide

Age, Melbourne

Argus, Melbourne

Australian

Daily News, London

Daily Sketch, London

Daily Telegraph, London

Evening Standard, London

Herald, Melbourne

Lyttelton Times, New Zealand

Midnight Sun, 1920–1923, Melbourne

Morning Telegraph, New York

New York Times

New Zealand Herald

New Zealand Mail

Otago Witness, New Zealand

Register, Adelaide

Smith's Weekly, Melbourne

Sun News Pictorial, Melbourne

Sydney Mail

Sydney Morning Herald

Times, London

Washington Evening News

Periodicals

The Australian Home Builder

The Australian Home Beautiful

New Idea Magazine

Nation

Punch, Melbourne

Table Talk

J.C. Williamson Ltd Magazine

The Stage

Wireless Weekly, South Australia, Victoria

The Theatre Magazine

Archives

Allen, Allen & Hemsley

Australian Securities Commission microfiche

Barr Smith Library, Special Collections, University of Adelaide, South Australia

Dennis Wolanski Performing Arts Library, The Opera House, Sydney

La Trobe Library, Melbourne

Lillydale Museum, Victoria

Mitchell Library, Sydney

Mortlock Library, Adelaide

National Library, Canberra

Performing Arts Museum, Victoria

Royal Historical Society of Victoria, Melbourne

Sir George Tallis Theatre Collection, National Library of Australia, Canberra

State Library of South Australia

State Library of Victoria

Photograph Acknowledgments

We gratefully acknowledge photographs other than those from the Sir George Tallis collection, National Library of Australia, Canberra.

Pictorial Sources and Abbreviations

Barr Smith Library, Special Collections, The Allan Wilkie-Frediswyde Hunter-Watts Theatre Collection, University of Adelaide, South Australia; BSLSA

Lillydale Museum, Lilydale, Victoria; LMV

National Library of Australia, Canberra; NLA

Royal Historical Society of Victoria, Melbourne; RHSV

Mortlock Library of South Australia, Adelaide; SLSA:MLSA

State Library of Victoria; SLV

La Trobe Picture Collection, State Library of Victoria, Melbourne; LTPC:SLV

The Harold Paynting Collection; State Library of Victoria, HPC: SLV

David Allen, DA; Sue Bowler, SB; Ann Heath, AH; The Horsley Family, HF; Sir Roy McKenzie, RMcK; Mark Tapping, MT

Chapter 1	Spring Street, Melbourne, RHSV; Theatre Royal, Melbourne, LTPC:SLV
Chapter 2	Bourke St, Melbourne, RHSV; Bland Holt, NLA
Chapter 3	Bert Levy, BSLSA; Nellie Stewart, BSLSA; Sarah Bernhardt, NLA
Chapter 5	Julius Knight, BSLSA; Theatre Royal, Adelaide, SLSA: MLSA B8347
	Royal Comic Opera program, SB; *Mikado* program, SB; *Dorothy* program, SB
Chapter 6	Julius Knight, BSLSA; Nellie Stewart, BSLSA; *Belle of New York*, NLA
Chapter 7	Florence Young, BSLSA; *Aladdin*, BSLSA; *Mother Goose*, NLA
	Mary Weir, HF
	Jennie Brenan, AH
	Parsifal, NLA; Percy Grainger, NLA
Chapter 9	JC Williamson, HF
Chapter 10	HMT, Johannesburg, MT; Florence Young, NLA
Chapter 11	Gladys Moncrieff, BSLSA
Chapter 12	Pavlova, *Herald* 7 April 1926, SLV

Chapter 13 Regent Theatre, Melbourne, HPC:SLV; Regent Theatre, Adelaide, SLSA:MLSA B8347; Dame Nellie Melba, LMV

Chapter 14 Melba Program, LMV; Melba in *La Bohème*, LMV

Chapter 18 Arthur Allen, DA; Sir John McKenzie, portrait by Edward Halliday, R McK

Index

Illustrations are indicated by *italic* page numbers

N

O

P

Q

R

S

T